Nanobiotechnology and Artificial Intelligence in Gastrointestinal Diseases

Online at: https://doi.org/10.1088/978-0-7503-6134-7

IOP Series in Artificial Intelligence in the Biomedical Sciences

Series Editor

**Ge Wang, Clark and Crossan Endowed Chair Professor,
Rensselaer Polytechnic Institute, Troy New York, USA**

About the Series

The *IOP Series in Artificial Intelligence in the Biomedical Sciences* aims to develop a library of key texts and reference works encompassing the broad range of artificial intelligence, machine learning, deep learning and neural networks within all applicable fields of biomedicine. There is now significant focus in using advancements in the field of AI to improve diagnosis, management, and better therapeutic options of various diseases. Some examples and applications incorporated would be AI in cancer diagnosis/prognosis, implementing artificial intelligence, data mining of electronic health records data, ambient intelligence in hospitals, AI in virus detection, AI in infectious diseases, biomarkers and genomics utilizing machine learning and clinical decision support with AR. These are just a few of the many applications that AI and related technologies can bring to the biomedical sciences. The series contains two broad types of approach. Those addressing a particular field of application and reviewing the numerous relevant artificial intelligence methods applicable to the field, and those that focus on a specific AI method which will permit a greater in-depth review of the theory and appropriate technology.

A full list of titles published in this series can be found here:
https://iopscience.iop.org/bookListInfo/iop-series-in-artificial-intelligence-in-the-biomedical-sciences#series.

Nanobiotechnology and Artificial Intelligence in Gastrointestinal Diseases

Edited by
Vivek K Chaturvedi
Department of Gastroenterology, Institute of Medical Sciences, Banaras Hindu University, Varanasi, Uttar Pradesh 221005, India

Anurag Kumar Singh
Department of Pharmaceutical Engineering and Technology-Indian Institute of Technology, Banaras Hindu University, Varanasi, Uttar Pradesh 221005, India

Cancer Biology Research and Training, Department of Biological Sciences, Alabama State University, 915 S Jackson Street, Montgomery AL 36101-0271, USA

Jay Singh
Department of Chemistry, Institute of Science, Banaras Hindu University, Varanasi, Uttar Pradesh 221005, India

Dawesh P Yadav
Department of Gastroenterology, Institute of Medical Sciences, Banaras Hindu University, Varanasi, Uttar Pradesh 221005, India

IOP Publishing, Bristol, UK

ISBN   978-0-7503-6134-7 (ebook)
ISBN   978-0-7503-6132-3 (print)
ISBN   978-0-7503-6135-4 (myPrint)
ISBN   978-0-7503-6133-0 (mobi)

DOI   10.1088/978-0-7503-6134-7

Version: 20240801

IOP ebooks

British Library Cataloguing-in-Publication Data: A catalogue record for this book is available from the British Library.

Published by IOP Publishing, wholly owned by The Institute of Physics, London

IOP Publishing, No.2 The Distillery, Glassfields, Avon Street, Bristol, BS2 0GR, UK

US Office: IOP Publishing, Inc., 190 North Independence Mall West, Suite 601, Philadelphia, PA 19106, USA

*To those who care, conserve, and protect but do not destroy the beauty
and unique characteristics of
Kshit (Earth)
Jal (Water)
Pawak (Fire)
Gagan (Sky)
and
Sameera (Air).*

Contents

4   Novel drug delivery systems for inflammatory bowel disease   4-1
Ashutosh Kumar, Pratistha Singh, Rajesh Kumar and Sunil Dutt

5   Nanotechnology in gastrointestinal endoscopy   5-1
Rajesh Kumar, Sunil Dutt, Ankush Goyal, Ashutosh Kumar
and Brijesh Kumar

6 Nano-biotechnology in gastrointestinal cancer   **6-1**
Mohammad Zafaryab, Mazharul Haque and Komal Vig

7 Role of nanoparticles for the treatment of gastric cancer 7-1

Ravi Kumar Yadav, Shefali Singh, Zeba Azim, Niraj Kumar Goswami and Navneet Yadav

8   Artificial intelligence in hepatitis and chronic liver disease

8-1

Akbar Hamid, Gira Sulabh and Vinod Kumar

12 Artificial intelligence (AI) based colonoscopy   12-1

Akbar Hamid, Rajesh Kumar, Vivek K Chaturvedi, Sunil Dutt, Gira Sulabh, Vinod Kumar and D P Yadav

Preface

Nanotechnology and artificial intelligence (AI) has transformed numerous fields of research as well as daily life spans during the past 20 years. It has shown a promising ability to treat the majority of medical complications, including gastrointestinal (GI), infectious, cancer, genetic, and neurological diseases. One of the most promising fields in nanotechnology and AI-based personalized nanomedicine systems is defined as a highly specialized medical intervention for the diagnosis, prevention, and treatment of GI diseases, which helps medical practitioners increase the level of diagnostic accuracy and efficiency. The diagnosis and treatment of gastroenterological illnesses are expected to be significantly impacted by the combination of nanotechnology and AI. The essential aspect of AI-based nano-medicine is 'drug delivery,' which is one of the most exciting applications of nanotechnology and can manipulate molecules and supramolecular structures to make devices with pre-programmed functionality. The present drug delivery methods are divided into nano- and microscale systems, which primarily make use of nanoparticles, liposomes, polymeric micelles (nanovehicles), dendrimers, nanocrystals, microchips, microtherapeutic systems, and innovative 100 nm-sized microparticles. Future advancements in these technologies will create effective nano/microdrug delivery systems that will meet healthcare problems for the detection and treatment of infectious diseases, with a special focus on those microorganisms that are developing drug resistance. This book contains 13 chapters that are broadly focused on recent developments in nanotechnology and AI-based drug delivery systems, diagnosis, and the role of various nanomaterials in the management of GI, such as abdominal pain, bowel obstruction, diarrhoea, pancreatitis, upper gastro-intestinal bleeding (UGIB), non-alcoholic fatty liver diseases (NAFLD), intestinal tuberculosis (ITB), celiac disease, and duodenal ulcer. The role of nanotechnology and AI in GI illnesses is covered in chapter 1 as a breakthrough advancement in the fields of drug delivery, disease diagnostics, and treatment. The use of various nano-biosensors for the diagnosis and treatment of gastrointestinal tract illnesses is covered in chapter 2. Chapter 3 focuses on the role of nanoscience in controlled drug delivery in the GI tract, and management of GI disorders. Chapter 4 emphasizes one of the most emerging fields of GI tract-based novel drug delivery systems for inflammatory bowel disease. The use of nanotechnology in GI endos-copy is examined in chapter 5. Nowadays, superparamagnetic iron oxide nano-particles and other magnetic nanoparticles attract a great deal of attention from researchers all over the world due to their strong magnetic properties, which provide an added advantage when they are used in GI endoscopy. The contribution of nanobiotechnology to GI cancer and its use in drug delivery are discussed in chapter 6. The reader's comprehension of new ideas and the application of drug delivery carriers in GI delivery will be improved by a thorough explanation provided on the difficult barriers for drug delivery that combine the difficulties brought on by solid tumours, the physiologic environment of the GI tract, and the tight epithelial tissue barriers. Chapter 7 is also about the revolutionary applications of the role of nanoparticles for the treatment of gastric cancer as a future cancer theragnostic. Chapter 8 discusses the application of AI in chronic liver diseases, which is considered one of the most compelling medicinal platforms of AI-based systems. Artificial intelligence (AI) particularly in deep learning, has made it possible to extract clinically relevant information from complex and diverse clinical datasets of therapeutics, and also has great promise for improving the therapeutic index. Chapter 9 emphasizes the role of AI applications in clinical decision support. A detailed description of the idea of artificial intelligence (AI) based colonoscopy is provided in chapter 10, along with information on how it can be used to monitor systems that promise to improve colorectal polyp and cancer detection, classification, screening, and surveillance. Chapter 11 is dedicated to the utilization of nanomedicines for liver fibrosis. Chapter 12 covers various aspects related to artificial intelligence in GI colonoscopy. Overall, the chapters in this book are quite useful because they were authored by one or more professionals who are knowledgeable about the subject matter. In this way, we hope to provide a comprehensive resource for clinicians, scientists working in the area, undergraduate and graduate students studying a variety of fields, including gastroenterology, biotechnology, nanotechnology, pharmaceutical biotechnology, pharmacology, pharmaceutics, nanomedicine, tissue engineering, biomaterials, etc, and allied subjects. Also, this book is beneficial for those who work for numerous regulatory agencies, businesses, and nanotechnological groups. We would like to express our gratitude to all the contributors for their extraordinary efforts to present up-to-date knowledge on the topics covered in their chapters.

Vivek K Chaturvedi
Anurag Kumar Singh
Jay Singh
Dawesh P Yadav

Acknowledgements

It gives us immense pleasure to acknowledge Bharat Ratna Mahamana Pt. Madan Mohan Malviya Ji, founder of the Banaras Hindu University, Varanasi, Uttar Pradesh, India.

Vivek K Chaturvedi gratefully acknowledges the Department of Health Research (DHR), Ministry of Health and Family Welfare, Government of India, for support through the Young Scientist Fellowship Grant R.12014/56/2022-HR.

Anurag Kumar Singh would like to acknowledge the Indian Council of Medical Research (ICMR), Government of India, for support through the Research Associate (ICMR-RA) Award (No.: 3/1/2/110Neuro/2019-NCD-I).

Jay Singh and Dawesh P Yadav would like to acknowledge Institutes of Eminence (IoE)-BHU Grant, Ministry of Education, India, for providing constant assistance in all possible ways.

It is also our great pleasure to acknowledge and express our enormous debt to all the contributors who have provided quality material to prepare this book. We are grateful to our beloved family members, who joyfully supported and stood with us in the many hours of our absence to finish this book project. We are also grateful to our friends and colleagues who offered their support and encouragement throughout the writing process. I would also like to acknowledge the publishing team at IOP Press for their professionalism, enthusiasm, and belief in this project. Their expertise in design, production, and marketing has been essential in bringing this book to life.

Vivek K Chaturvedi
Anurag Kumar Singh
Jay Singh
Dawesh P Yadav

Editor biographies

Vivek Kumar Chaturvedi

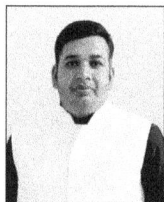

Dr Vivek Kumar Chaturvedi is a Young-Scientist Fellow (Department of Health Research, Ministry of Health and Family Welfare) at Institute of Medical Sciences, Banaras Hindu University, Varanasi, India. Before joining the laboratory as a Young Scientist Fellow, He worked as a Postdoctoral research associate at the Department of Gastroenterology, IMS-BHU, Varanasi. He earned his PhD degree in Biotechnology from University of Allahabad (a central university), Prayagraj, India. He received his BSc degree in biological sciences and MSc degree in Biochemistry from Veer Bahadur Singh Purvanchal University, Jaunpur, India. Dr Chaturvedi's research interests include the synthesis and functionalization of nano-biomaterials as well as their fabrication for the development of various biosensors that may be useful for the early detection and treatment of cancer and gastrointestinal diseases. Besides these, he has published many original articles in peer-reviewed high-impact journals along with many internationally edited and authored books.

Anurag Kumar Singh

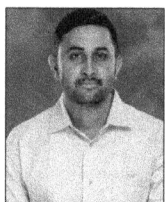

Dr Anurag Kumar Singh is currently working as a Research Associate (ICMR-RA) in Department of Pharmaceutical Engineering and Technology, Indian Institute of Technology (Banaras Hindu University), Varanasi, India. Previously he has worked as a Postdoctoral Research Assistant in Cancer Biology Research and Training at the Department of Biological Sciences, Alabama State University (USA) and Institute of Nanotechnology and Advanced Materials, Department of Chemistry, Faculty of Exact Science, Bar-Ilan University, Israel. He has more than 1.5 years postdoctoral research experience to date. He has completed his doctoral degree from the Centre of Experimental Medicine and Surgery, Institute of Medical Sciences, Banaras Hindu University, Varanasi, Uttar Pradesh, India. He earned MPharm degree from the School of Chemical Sciences and Pharmacy, Central University of Rajasthan, Ajmer, Rajasthan, India. His scholarly interests range from developing novel nano-particulate systems for chronic pain, neurodegenerative disorders, brain-targeted drug delivery, including dendrimer, nanoporous silica/silicon materials, and polymeric-based nano-particles for controlled drug delivery to diagnostics and therapy. His research interests include the development of nanoparticles/nanomedicines for biomedical and health-care applications and building a bridge between engineering, pharmaceutical, and medical research. He has published several research papers, including reviews, and journal editorials in various peer-reviewed national and international journals. He has more than two edited/authored books and has authored more than ten book chapters of internationally reputed press for publications.

Jay Singh

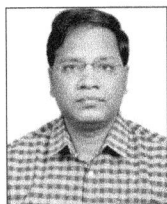

Dr Jay Singh is currently working as an Assistant Professor at the Department of Chemistry, Institute of Sciences, Banaras Hindu University, Varanasi, Uttar Pradesh, since 2017. He received his PhD degree in Polymer Science from Motilal Nehru National Institute of Technology in 2010 and obtained his MSc and BSc from Allahabad University, Uttar Pradesh, India. He has held postdoctoral fellowships at the National Physical Laboratory, New Delhi, Chonbuk National University, South Korea, and Delhi Technological University, Delhi. Dr Jay has been honoured with prestigious fellowships such as CSIR (RA), DST-Young Scientist Fellowship, and DST-INSPIRE Faculty Award. His research focuses on the development of chemically and biologically synthesized nanomaterials and their nanobiocomposites, conducting polymers, and self-assembled monolayers. He is dedicated to creating clinically significant biosensors and sensors for the estimation of various bioanalytes based on enzymes, antibodies, DNA, and toxic chemicals and gases. With over 140 international research papers published and a total citation count exceeding 5000, Dr Jay possesses an h-index of 42. He has successfully completed or is currently running various research projects funded by different agencies. Moreover, he has authored/edited more than 17 books and contributed over 50 book chapters for internationally renowned publishers such as Elsevier, Springer Nature, IOP, Wiley, and CRC. Dr Jay has also handled special issues in esteemed journals for Elsevier, Wiley, Springer, MDPI, and Frontiers. Currently, his active research involves the fabrication of sustainable metal oxide-based biosensors for clinical diagnosis, food packaging applications, drug delivery, and tissue engineering. His work has significantly contributed to the understanding of interfacial charge transfer processes and sensing capabilities of metal nanoparticles.

Dawesh Prakash Yadav

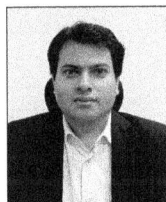

Dr Dawesh Prakash Yadav is presently working as Associate Professor of Gastroenterology at Banaras Hindu University, Varanasi (India). He did his MBBS and MD (General Medicine) from Institute of Medical Sciences (IMS), BHU Varanasi, India. He is the Member of Indian National Association for the Study of the liver (INASL), the Indian Society of Gastroenterology and received many other prestigious awards. Dr Yadav worked as a senior resident in All India Institute of Medical Sciences (AIIMS), New Delhi from 2013 to 2017. He joined as an Assistant Professor in IMS, BHU in 2017. In 2019 he was promoted to associate professor in the Department of Gastroenterology; IMS-BHU. Dr Yadav has been carrying out his research on various aspects of inflammatory bowel disease, liver cirrhosis and nanobiotechnology over the last decade. He has published more than 45 research papers and book chapters in peer-reviewed high-impact journals along with many international book chapters. He has currently edited three editorial books in Bentham Sciences. He has been serving as an editorial board member of many reputed journals.

Short description about chapters

Chapter 1

Nanotechnology and artificial intelligence

Anshu Singh[1], Vivek K Chaturvedi[2], Anurag K Singh[3,4], Jay Singh[1,*], Kshitij R B Singh[5] and Dawesh P Yadav[2]

[1]Department of Chemistry, Institute of Science, Banaras Hindu University, Varanasi, India

[2]Department of Gastroenterology, Institute of Medical Sciences, Banaras Hindu University, Varanasi, India

[3]Department of Pharmaceutical Engineering and Technology-IIT, BHU, Varanasi, India

[4]Cancer Biology Research and Training, Department of Biological Sciences, Alabama State University, 915 S Jackson Street, Montgomery AL 36101-0271, USA

[5]Graduate School of Life Science and Systems Engineering, Kyushu Institute of Technology, Kitakyushu, Japan

*Corresponding author (jaysingh.chem@bhu.ac.in) (Phone +918920993654)

The convergence of nanotechnology and artificial intelligence (AI) in medical science heralds a transformative era, promising groundbreaking innovations in diagnostics, therapeutics, and personalized medicine. Nanotechnology, operating at the scale of individual atoms and molecules, facilitates the design of advanced materials with unique properties, enabling precise drug delivery, diagnostic imaging, and theranostics. On the other hand, AI, with its prowess in machine learning and data analysis, enhances medical decision-making, diagnostic accuracy, and patient care. This chapter explores the revolutionary synergy between nanotechnology and AI, examining their individual contributions and the synergistic effects when integrated. In the realm of nanotechnology, the utilization of nanomaterials for drug delivery systems is explored, showcasing their ability to enhance targeting, reduce side effects, and revolutionize treatment, with a particular focus on successful applications in cancer therapy. Additionally, the development of nanosensors for diagnostics is discussed, emphasizing their role in early disease detection, real-time monitoring, and imaging.

Chapter 2

Nano-biosensors for diagnosis of gastrointestinal diseases

Mazharul Haque[1]*, Mohammad Zafaryab[1] and Komal Vig[1]

[1]School of Biological Sciences, Alabama State University, USA

*Correspondence author (mazharcirbsc@gmail.com)

The alteration in the gastrointestinal (GI) tract leads to the various gastrointestinal diseases. The common GI ailments include indigestion, irritable bowel syndrome (IBS), acid reflux, hemorrhoids and colon cancer etc. The affected population was estimated as 3.7% of the population worldwide in 2016 (a 23%

increase from 1990) and still elevation in these figures is the prime focus of concern. The unprecedented burden due to intestinal and intestine-originated disorders has been primary concern for researchers and clinicians. In this chapter we will address the application of nano-biosensors for detection and diagnosing gastrointestinal related diseases and point out the utmost importance of combining diagnosis and treatment. The future application of nano-biosensors in detecting GI related biomarkers for early diagnosis and expect to integrate material science and medical fields will be also addressed. Recent advances in nanotechnology have opened new dimensions in the diagnosis and treatment of GI derived disorders. The advancement due to integration of these fields may prove as an important mediator in improving the clinical translation. The technology based on Nanoparticle improves the precision of diagnosis when combined with biosensor with limited side effects and advanced diagnosis and therapy of gastrointestinal (GI) disorders. Currently, focus towards development of nano-biosensor by the researchers from the various fields has shown considerable interest to achieve advancement in applications in order to improve the sensitivity and specificity. The introduction of nano materials based sensors which is commonly known as nano-biosensors is currently most widely investigated method since last decades for the various applications in healthcare. These nano-biosensors have been employed for detection of numerous target analytes includes, microorganisms, virus, nucleic acids, peptides, proteins for the early diagnosis of pathogens causing pathogenesis. These nano based biosensors enabled us to detect the target analytes very quickly and efficiently in the system. The nano materials are very reactive in nature which enhances the catalytic, physical as well as chemical characteristic of the biosensor give rise to enhanced sensitivity and specificity. The new techniques have been proved as breakthrough in improving the sensitive detection and quantification of certain parameters. These nano-biosensors have emerged with many possibilities due to unique properties such as sensitivity, simplicity, robustness and cost effectiveness providing the bridge between diagnosis and treatment.

Chapter 3

Nanoscience in controlled drug release in the gastrointestinal tract

Ritu[1], Bharmjeet[1], Nida-e-Falak[1], Asmita Das[1], Rahul Gupta[2] and Prakash Chandra[1*]

[1]Department of Biotechnology, Delhi Technological University, New Delhi 110042, India

[2]Department of Information Technology, Delhi Technological University, New Delhi 110042, India

*Corresponding author (prakashchandra@dtu.ac.in) (Phone number+917782020444)

The use of nanotechnology in drug delivery has the potential to revolutionize the field by improving the efficacy, safety, and convenience of therapeutic interventions. However, the complexity of the gastrointestinal (GI) tract presents unique challenges that require sophisticated and precise drug release strategies. In recent years, artificial intelligence (AI) has emerged as a powerful tool for optimizing drug delivery systems. Machine learning algorithms can be used to analyze large amounts of data and predict how drugs will behave in different physiological conditions, allowing for the development of more accurate and personalized drug delivery systems. Moreover, AI can be combined with nanoscience to create intelligent drug delivery systems that respond to the needs of the patient in real-time. This book chapter will explore the latest advances in the field of nanoscience and AI for controlled drug release in the GI tract and different types of nanomaterials that can be used for drug delivery will be discussed, including liposomes, polymeric nanoparticles, and dendrimers. Also, various methods for controlling drug release will also be covered, including pH-sensitive systems, enzyme-sensitive systems, and stimuli-responsive systems. The use of AI in the development of intelligent drug delivery systems, such as microrobots and smart capsules, will also be discussed. In conclusion, the combination of nanoscience and AI has the potential to revolutionize drug delivery in the GI tract, leading to more effective, personalized, and safe therapies. This book chapter will provide an in-depth review of the latest advances in the field and will be of interest to researchers and practitioners in nanoscience, drug delivery, and AI.

Chapter 4

Novel drug delivery systems for inflammatory bowel disease

Ashutosh Kumar[1], Pratistha Singh[1], Rajesh Kumar[2] and Sunil Dutt[2]

[1]Department of Ophthalmology, University of California Los Angeles, California-90095, USA

[2]Maharaja Agrasen School of Pharmacy, Maharaja Agrasen University, Atal Shiksha Kunj, Solan, Himachal Pradesh 174103, India

Corresponding author (rajdhiman60@gmail.com) (Phone +919817893170)

Crohn's disease and ulcerative colitis constitute the majority of the chronic and recurrent inflammatory disorder known as inflammatory bowel disease (IBD). These are incurable and complex disease states. The treatment of IBD is complex because of GI tract inflammation and epithelium damage. Several approaches have been used to treat this chronic illness. To treat the inflamed region of the GI tract selective and site-specific drug delivery methods continue to be important. Antibiotics, steroids, immunosuppressive and high non-steroidal anti-inflammatory drugs have used for the treatment of IBD. Targeted drug delivery to the specific inflammatory area of the bowl increases therapeutic efficacy and allows for localized treatment, which lowers systemic toxicity. Some drug formulations have been formulated as targeted delivery to reduce the early signs of inflammation. Drugs made from nanoparticles (NPs) have recently received a lot of attention due to their potential to address these issues. There is various type of nanodrug delivery system, which can deliver the drug into the inflamed or targeted area of the gut for the prolonged and desired action. Some novel drug delivery has been developed for targeting the inflamed area of the gut. These novel drug delivery systems are now frequently employed to deliver medications, proteins, DNA, RNA, genes, polypeptides, medicines, and even vaccinations. Enteric-coated pills, prodrugs and hybrid drug delivery systems are the examples of some novel drug delivery systems. A stable and functionally developed novel drug delivery system is required in order to deliver the drugs specifically to the disease site, increase the duration of the drug's residence time, and reduce systemic effects. This chapter will discuss the type and the role of novel drug delivery system in the treatment of IBD along with challenges and future aspects in the treatment of IBD.

Chapter 5

Nanotechnology in gastrointestinal endoscopy

Rajesh Kumar[1], Sunil Dutt[1], Ankush Goyal[1], Ashutosh Kumar[2] and Brijesh Kumar[3*]

[1]Maharaja Agrasen School of Pharmacy, Maharaja Agrasen University, Atal Shiksha Kunj, Solan, Himachal Pradesh 174103, India

[2]Department of Ophthalmology, University of California, Los Angeles, USA

[3]Department of Pharmacology, Institute of Medical Sciences, Banaras Hindu University, Varanasi, India

*Corresponding author (rajdhiman60@gmail.com, asthwal@rediffmail.com)

Nanotechnology is a field which deals with the development of intentional design and characterizations of nanoscale particles (1–100 nm) for the diagnosis, treatment, mitigation of illnesses as well as other desirable uses. These engineered devices are controlled by their size and shape through physical characteristics to produce the intended impact at subcellular and molecular level with unique attributes. These nanoparticles, which can cross the blood–brain barrier and have the capacity to avoid immune system interception, have a longer half-life than microparticles, making them suitable for use as drug delivery vehicles. Quantum dot and cadmium selenide semiconductor nanoparticles are two diagnostic techniques that may simultaneously scan a blood sample for various proteins, viruses, and other desirable compounds. Environmental nanoparticles can reach the human body through several pathways, including the gastrointestinal tract. As soon as anything is consumed, it easily passes through the mucus layer and interacts with the enterocytes. Nanopowder as hemostatic agent in gastric ulcer bleed, prevention of clogging of plastic stents, nano-based capsule-endoscopy, molecular imaging and optical biopsy, bio-sensing and maneuvering technology, nanorobots are some tools used in the diagnostic and therapeutic endoscopy such as the endoscopic hemostasis of peptic ulcer bleeding, prevention of clogging of plastic stent and advance capsule endoscopy. These nanoparticles, which are either approved for clinical use or are undergoing clinical trials, have technical challenges and potential adverse reactions like back pain, vasodilatation and acute urinary retention, fever, cytopenia, mild renal toxicity, and peripheral sensory neuropathy because of their diverse range. Hence, toxicity investigations and quality control studies for these nanoparticles will serve as a benchmark for the unfulfilled potential of nanotechnology in the diagnostic and therapeutic fields, along with endoscopy.

Chapter 6

Nano-biotechnology in gastrointestinal cancer

Mohammad Zafaryab[1*], Mazharul Haque[1] and Komal Vig[1]

[1]School of Biological Sciences, CNBR, Alabama State University, USA

*Corresponding author (zafar.cirbsc@gmail.com)

The incident of Gastrointestinal cancer worldwide is 26% with all cancer related death is 35% as per Globocan database. Gastrointestinal cancer, which includes tumors of the stomach, esophagus, liver, biliary system, pancreas, and colon, is one of the most common cancers and the largest cause of cancer-related death worldwide. Gastrointestinal related cancer has same weightage in term of diagnosis and therapeutic as well. Developments in nanotechnology have explored new edges in the diagnosis and treatment of cancer. Nano-biotechnology is emerging field that utilize the optimized nanoscale system to overcome, issue in related to diagnostic and therapeutic of cancer. As far as diagnosis of Gastroinstestinal cancer is concern, the routine systematic imaging like Magnetic resonance image, Computational tomography (CT) and positron emission tomography, local imaging that convers endoscopy and ultrasound is also have large apprehension. Conventional use of contrast agent in this imaging system has low specificity, quick maintenance time period, severe side effect as well. Currently, the advancements in field of nano-technology, contributed the nanoparticles like quantum dot, gold nanoparticles and iron oxide nanoparticles, have presented many aids in Gastroinstinal cancer imaging as bearing nano size, manipulative surface properties and having good retention time in body. There is search going on to combined the existing traditional diagnostic method with nanoparticles significantly improving the imaging of digestive track to early diagnosis and predict the accuracy of cancer stages. Traditional drug has large number of side effect due low to its low specificity and non-targeted delivery. However, there is huge study demonstrated that nanosized drug were found effective against the gastrointestinal cancer as its optimized nano system in order to improve specificity, targeted delivery and reduce the toxicity as well. Here, we discuss the most recent research on the application of nanoparticles to the detection and treatment of gastrointestinal cancer.

Chapter 7

Role of nanoparticles for the treatment of gastric cancer

Ravi Kumar Yadav[1*], Shefali Singh[1], Zeba Azim[2], Niraj Kumar Goswami[3] and Navneet Yadav[4]

[1]Department of Botany, Kashi Naresh Government Post Graduate, College, Gyanpur, Bhadohi, U.P. 221304, India

[2]Department of Botany, University of Allahabad, Prayagraj 211002, India

[3]Mahant Avaidyanath Government Degree College, India

The second-leading cause of cancer-related fatalities worldwide is gastric cancer. The advancement in medicine will probably be linked to the research of cancer biology, followed by the formation of a customized and molecular-based method for the administration of anticancer medications. Proper medications for cancerous diseases rely highly on their timely diagnosis for which *in vivo* molecular imaging technique is popular but a trend for a more feasible approach is seen as molecular imaging requires specialized molecular probes. The use of nanoparticles (NPs) is the current paradigm for diagnosing and treating gastric cancer. With the advent of extensive explorations in the field of nanotechnology, NPs have been realized to have proficient curative properties for gastric cancer. Since the past decade, extensive research work has been allocated to applications of NPs in the direction of therapeutics and diagnosis. Several reports have documented that NPs-based therapeutic agents overcome problems associated with conventional therapy. But, it seems that perusal of the characteristics of NPs and their interactive efficacies with biological entities is vital to analyze the potential of NPs-based nanomedicines and NPs-based diagnostic protocols. Now-a-days green synthesized NPs are also used as a potential agent for gastric cancer treatment. This study is significant since NPs might also pose certain side effects and toxicity and these aspects should be well addressed prior to the utilization of NPs in biological systems. This chapter will encompass the diverse purview of NPs and how this can be a plausible alternative in the diagnosis and therapeutic treatment of gastric cancer.

Chapter 8

Artificial intelligence in hepatitis and chronic liver disease

Akbar Hamid[1], Gira Sulabh[2] and Vinod Kumar[3]*

[1]Department of Gastroenterology, Sanjay Gandhi Postgraduate Institute of Medical Sciences, Lucknow, Uttar Pradesh 226014, India

[2]Department of Pharmacology, Heritage Institute of Medical Sciences (HIMS), Varanasi-221311, India

[3]Department of Gastroenterology, Institute of Medical Sciences, Banaras Hindu University, Varanasi, Uttar Pradesh 221005, India

*Corresponding author (vinodkumarchief@gmail.com)

Artificial Intelligence (AI) is a well-developing field of computer science that imitates human technical thinking to solve problems. The use of different AI models in hepatology is a recent development in the medical field for better diagnostics. Conventional diagnostic methods are being integrated with modern AI to enhance the performance of treatment. AI's ability to miming the data in human parameters, and forecast the occurrence of hepatitis and other chronic liver diseases. Classifying the different stages of hepatitis, fatty liver disease and hemochromatosis are possible along with the diagnosis and screening. Early disease prediction, complications and mortality can be studied using the algorithms such as regression models, since hepatitis early diagnosis is clinically limited in early stages. AI can predict the risk related to the vascular invasion of hepatocellular carcinoma and hepatitis related to cirrhosis. It also calculates the liver failure rate in HCC patients. Ultimately AI will eventually help in reducing medical errors and managing the patient clinical output.

Chapter 9

Artificial intelligence applications for clinical decisions support

Bhaskar Sharma[1*], Renu Negi[2], Anjali Yadav[1], Yogesh Sharma[1] and Vivek K Chaturvedi[3]

[1]Neurobiology Laboratory, Department of Anatomy, All India Institute of Medical Sciences, New Delhi 110029, India

[2]Systems Toxicology Group, CSIR-Indian Institute of Toxicology Research Vishvigyan Bhavan, 31, Mahatma Gandhi Marg, Lucknow, Academy of Scientific and Innovative Research (AcSIR), Ghaziabad, Uttar Pradesh 201002, India

[3]Department of Gastroenterology, Institute of Medical Sciences, Banaras Hindu University, Varanasi, India

*Corresponding author (sharma.bhaskar003@gmail.com)

Clinical Decision Support (CDS) systems represent a groundbreaking advancement in healthcare, fundamentally changing how clinicians make critical decisions by offering evidence-based guidance and knowledge directly at the point of care. By seamlessly integrating with electronic health record (EHR) systems, these platforms harness extensive patient data, medical literature, and best practice guidelines, empowering clinicians with the insights needed for informed decision-making. Through sophisticated analysis of large datasets, CDS systems uncover nuanced patterns and insights that enable early intervention and optimize resource allocation, thereby enhancing patient care outcomes. Despite the transformative potential of CDS, concerns persist regarding algorithm bias, data privacy, and stakeholder engagement, necessitating careful consideration and ongoing refinement. Case studies underscore the tangible impact of CDS, demonstrating its ability to enhance adherence to clinical standards, reduce hospital readmissions, and elevate patient satisfaction levels. Furthermore, the integration of artificial intelligence (AI) technologies bolsters the capabilities of CDS systems across various domains, including medical imaging analysis, virtual patient care, medication safety assurance, diagnostic support, medical research facilitation, and rehabilitation. Administrative applications of AI within CDS systems streamline essential tasks such as claims processing and clinical documentation, driving operational efficiency and alleviating administrative burdens on healthcare professionals. In summary, CDS systems play a pivotal role in revolutionizing healthcare delivery by equipping clinicians with actionable insights, improving clinical decision-making, and ultimately leading to better patient outcomes.

Chapter 10

Role of artificial intelligence in an early diagnosis and prediction of gastric cancer as an advanced therapeutic technique

Juhi Singh[1] and Vinod Kumar Dixit[1*]

[1]Department of Gastroenterology, Institute of Medical Sciences, Banaras Hindu University, Varanasi 221005, India

*Corresponding author (drvkdixit@gmail.com, vkdixit@bhu.ac.in) (Phone number: 8601100564)

One of the most prevalent malignant tumours with a high fatality rate is gastric cancer (GC). Human professionals' meticulous assessments of medical pictures are crucial for making accurate diagnoses and treatment choices for GC. This ailment has historically proven difficult to diagnose. Furthermore, the imaging settings, limited expertise, objective criteria, and inter-observer inconsistencies impede the development of accuracy. Healthcare research has advanced thanks to artificial intelligence (AI). Applications that help with cancer diagnosis and prognosis have been developed as a result of the accessibility of open-source healthcare statistics. Accurate evaluation, diagnosis, and treatment of stomach malignant growth and helicobacter pylori bacteria can be achieved with AI-assisted image analysis; links between these sub-fields can give more information than traditional analysis. AI-assisted categorization of genomic, epigenetic, and metagenomic data may lead to improved personalised therapy recommendations for gastrointestinal malignancies. In a number of therapeutic settings, including GC, researchers are looking at the extensive uses of artificial intelligence (AI). With endoscopic inspection and pathologic evidence during GC screening, AI can identify precancerous conditions and help with early cancer identification. AI can help TNM staging and subtype categorization in the diagnosis of GC. AI can assist with prognosis prediction and surgical margin estimation for treatment options. Here, we include some AI methods for early stomach cancer prediction. Even though several methods advocated in various texts have shown excellent prediction outcomes, cancer mortality has not decreased. As a result, a further in-depth study is needed in the field of cancer prediction in relation to AI that may be applied as a therapy.

Chapter 11

Nanomedicines in liver fibrosis

Saras Tiwari[1], Bhaskar Sharma[2], Jugasmita Deka[3], Prabhakar Singh[4*] and Vivek K Chaturvedi[5]

[1]Department of Cellular and Molecular Medicine, Faculty of Medicine, University of Ottawa, Canada

[2]Neurobiology Laboratory, Department of Anatomy, All India Institute of Medical Sciences, New Delhi 110029, India

[3]State University of New York Upstate Medical University, USA

[4]Electron Microscopy Facility, All India Institute of Medical Sciences, New Delhi 110029, India

[5]Department of Gastroenterology, Institute of Medical Sciences, Banaras Hindu University, Varanasi, India

*Corresponding author (prabhakar.singh@aiims.edu)

Chronic infection of liver cells causes scarring on liver tissue, resulting in Liver Fibrosis (LF), which is now a major global health concern. Hepatitis C, Hepatitis B, and alcohol abuse are the leading causes of liver damage, which results in the deposition of Extracellular cell matrix (ECM) and liver fibrosis. Ultrasonography and magnetic resonance imaging are commonly used as non-invasive diagnostic methods for hepatic fibrosis. The conventional therapy used to treat liver diseases is ineffective because it does not deliver a sufficient amount of drug concentration in the liver and is imprecise. Several clinical and preclinical Study has shown that the utilisation of nanotechnology to deliver therapeutic agents including drug molecules, and nucleic acids, in adequate amount and to target specifically the HSC (hepatic stellate cells) could be the future treatment to cure Liver diseases caused by LF. According to research, nanomedicines can reverse premature hepatic fibrosis. Many nanoparticulate systems (NPs) such as Liposomes, Inorganic NPs, and Nano-micelles have been studied because of their diverse properties for drug delivery and in addition to some therapeutic moieties. Out of these, Liposomal NPs have shown very promising results in clinical trials and are being considered as an extremity for the treatment of hepatic fibrosis. This book chapter discusses the causes, pathogenesis, diagnosis, and nanoparticulate systems used in the treatment of chronic liver diseases.

Chapter 12

Artificial intelligence (AI) based colonoscopy

Akbar Hamid[1#], Rajesh Kumar[2#], Vivek K Chaturvedi[3], Sunil Dutt[2], Gira Sulabh[3], Vinod Kumar[4*] and D P Yadav[4*]

[1]Department of Hepatology, Sanjay Gandhi Post Graduate Institute of Medical Sciences, Lucknow, India
[2]Maharaja Agrasen School of Pharmacy, Maharaja Agrasen University, Atal Shiksha Kunj, Solan, Himachal Pradesh, India
[3]Department of Pharmacology, Heritage Institute of Medical Sciences (HIMS), Varanasi-221311, India
[4]Department of Gastroenterology, Institute of Medical Sciences, Banaras Hindu University, Varanasi, India

#Sharing co-first author

*Corresponding author (vinodkumarchief@gmail.com; devesh.thedoc@gmail.com)

With the increase in the world population and development, a number of health-related issues are also increasing in gastrology. One of the major causes is poor food habits. To deal with this constant advancement is required in the field of medical sector which will not only help in easy and earlier diagnosis of the underlying health issue but also in accurate diagnosis. In this chapter advancement and collaboration of artificial intelligence with the medical sector are discussed below. How one technique helps is the accurate detection of colorectal cancer as well as other disease such as IBD or any other abnormalities in the colon. A different version of colonoscopy has been developed along with artificial intelligence discussed in this chapter with the future aspect and advancement.

List of contributors

Zeba Azim
Department of Botany, University of Allahabad, Prayagraj 211002, India

Bharmjeet
Department of Biotechnology, Delhi Technological University, New Delhi 110042, India

Prakash Chandra
Department of Biotechnology, Delhi Technological University, New Delhi 110042, India

Vivek K Chaturvedi
Department of Gastroenterology, Institute of Medical Sciences, Banaras Hindu University, Varanasi, Uttar Pradesh 221005, India

Asmita Das
Department of Biotechnology, Delhi Technological University, New Delhi 110042, India

Jugasmita Deka
State University of New York Upstate Medical University, USA

Vinod Kumar Dixit
Department of Gastroenterology, Institute of Medical Sciences, Banaras Hindu University, Varanasi 221005, India

Sunil Dutt
Maharaja Agrasen School of Pharmacy, Maharaja Agrasen University, Atal Shiksha Kunj, Solan, Himachal Pradesh 174103, India

Niraj Kumar Goswami
Mahant Avaidyanath Government Degree College, Jungle Kaudia, Gorakhpur, India

Ankush Goyal
Maharaja Agrasen School of Pharmacy, Maharaja Agrasen University, Atal Shiksha Kunj, Solan, Himachal Pradesh 174103, India

Rahul Gupta
Department of Information Technology, Delhi Technological University, New Delhi 110042, India

Akbar Hamid
Department of Hepatology, Sanjay Gandhi Postgraduate Institute of Medical Sciences, Lucknow, Uttar Pradesh 226014, India

Mazharul Haque
School of Biological Sciences, CNBR, Alabama State University, USA

Ashutosh Kumar
Department of Ophthalmology, University of California Los Angeles, California-90095, USA

Brijesh Kumar
Department of Pharmacology, Institute of Medical Sciences, Banaras Hindu University, Varanasi 221005, India

Rajesh Kumar
Maharaja Agrasen School of Pharmacy, Maharaja Agrasen University, Atal Shiksha Kunj, Solan, Himachal Pradesh 174103, India

Vinod Kumar
Department of Gastroenterology, Institute of Medical Sciences, Banaras Hindu University, Varanasi, Uttar Pradesh 221005, India

Renu Negi
Systems Toxicology Group, CSIR-Indian Institute of Toxicology Research Vishvigyan Bhavan, 31, Mahatma Gandhi Marg, Lucknow, Academy of Scientific and Innovative Research (AcSIR), Ghaziabad, Uttar Pradesh 201002, India

Nida-e-Falak
Department of Biotechnology, Delhi Technological University, New Delhi 110042, India

Ritu
Department of Biotechnology, Delhi Technological University, New Delhi 110042, India

Bhaskar Sharma
Neurobiology Laboratory, Department of Anatomy, All India Institute of Medical Sciences, New Delhi 110029, India

Yogesh Sharma
Neurobiology Laboratory, Department of Anatomy, All India Institute of Medical Sciences, New Delhi 110029, India

Anshu Singh
Department of Chemistry, Institute of Science, Banaras Hindu University, Varanasi 221005, India

Anurag K Singh
Department of Pharmaceutical Engineering and Technology-Indian Institute of Technology, BHU, Varanasi, India

Cancer Biology Research and Training, Department of Biological Sciences, Alabama State University, 915 S Jackson Street, Montgomery AL 361010271, USA

Jay Singh
Department of Chemistry, Institute of Science, Banaras Hindu University, Varanasi 221005, India

Juhi Singh
Department of Gastroenterology, Institute of Medical Sciences, Banaras Hindu University, Varanasi 221005, India

Kshitij R B Singh
Graduate School of Life Science and Systems Engineering, Kyushu Institute of Technology, Kitakyushu, Japan

Prabhakar Singh
Electron Microscopy Facility, All India Institute of Medical Sciences, New Delhi 110029, India

Pratistha Singh
Department of Ophthalmology, University of California Los Angeles, California 90095, USA

Shefali Singh
Department of Botany, Kashi Naresh Government Post Graduate, College, Gyanpur, Bhadohi, U.P. 221304, India

Gira Sulabh
Department of Pharmacology, Heritage Institute of Medical Sciences (HIMS), Varanasi-221311, India

Saras Tiwari
Department of Cellular and Molecular Medicine, Faculty of Medicine, University of Ottawa, Canada

Komal Vig
School of Biological Sciences, CNBR, Alabama State University, USA

Anjali Yadav
Neurobiology Laboratory, Department of Anatomy, All India Institute of Medical Sciences, New Delhi 110029, India

Dawesh P Yadav
Department of Gastroenterology, Institute of Medical Sciences, Banaras Hindu University, Varanasi 221005, India

Navneet Yadav
Department of Mechanical Engineering, Faculty of Science and Engineering, Swansea University, Swansea SA1 8EN, United Kingdom

Ravi Kumar Yadav
Department of Botany, Kashi Naresh Government Post Graduate, College, Gyanpur, Bhadohi, U.P. 221304, India

Mohammad Zafaryab
School of Biological Sciences, CNBR, Alabama State University, USA

Introduction

Nanotechnology and artificial intelligence (AI) have the potential to transform the existing treatment and diagnosis choices for gastrointestinal (GI) disorders. Several studies have shown that GI diseases can be early diagnosed and successfully treated using nanomaterials associated with AI applications. The GI tract has become a considerable target system for nanotechnology and AI, and it contains a wide range of substances, such as water, nutrients, or therapeutics that are absorbed in the GI tract when transported through the digestive tract. The behaviour of nanotechnology employed for GI disease diagnosis or therapy can be controlled depending on the pH, pressure, transit duration, and bacterial concentration of each specific nanomaterial. Because of their adjustable interactions with macrophages, M cells, immune cells and intestinal epithelial cells nanoparticles have demonstrated considerable promise in gastroenterology and may become a potential delivery system for vaccines. The use of AI-based advanced machines for GI surgery as well as in the study of medicine is expanding quickly. AI within the diagnostic process supports medical specialists to improve the level of diagnostic accuracy and efficiency, thus providing emergent digitalized healthcare services. Nanotechnology with AI is anticipated to have a significant impact on how GI disorders are diagnosed and treated. In terms of effectiveness, dependability, and practicality, several of the medicines and diagnostics based on AI described here outperform traditional materials. In the future, GI problems may be successfully treated using AI-based machines and their intricate mixes, which may include therapeutic substances. This book explains how the most recent advances in applications of novel biomaterials, nanotechnology and AI have paved the way for breakthroughs in drug delivery. This book demonstrates present and future applications in a setting where it is essential to provide effective, patient-centered, and long-lasting healthcare systems. This book provides an overview of the technological approaches mainly focused on the role of AI and their implications in GI disorders such as abdominal pain, bowel obstruction, diarrhoea, pancreatitis, upper gastrointestinal bleeding (UGIB), non-alcoholic fatty liver diseases (NAFLD), intestinal tuberculosis (ITB), celiac disease, and duodenal ulcer as well as include the role of nanotechnology and AI in GI illnesses. Due to its high calibre material, the book will appeal to a wide range of readers, including academics, students, researchers and medical students as well as practitioners. It would be particularly interesting to readers interested in health, business, and research linked to the biomedical sciences. The main marketing and differentiating factors are the numerous libraries operating in numerous reputable private and governmental institutions or organizations.

IOP Publishing

Nanobiotechnology and Artificial Intelligence in Gastrointestinal Diseases

Vivek K Chaturvedi, Anurag Kumar Singh, Jay Singh and Dawesh P Yadav

Chapter 1

Nanotechnology and artificial intelligence

Anshu Singh, Vivek K Chaturvedi, Anurag K Singh, Jay Singh, Kshitij R B Singh and Dawesh P Yadav

The convergence of nanotechnology and artificial intelligence (AI) in medical science heralds a transformative era, promising groundbreaking innovations in diagnostics, therapeutics, and personalized medicine. Nanotechnology, operating at the scale of individual atoms and molecules, facilitates the design of advanced materials with unique properties, enabling precise drug delivery, diagnostic imaging, and theranostics. On the other hand, AI, with its prowess in machine learning (ML) and data analysis, enhances medical decision-making, diagnostic accuracy, and patient care. This chapter explores the revolutionary synergy between nanotechnology and AI, examining their individual contributions and the synergistic effects when integrated. In the realm of nanotechnology, the utilization of nanomaterials for drug delivery systems is explored, showcasing their ability to enhance targeting, reduce side effects, and revolutionize treatment, with a particular focus on successful applications in cancer therapy. Additionally, the development of nanosensors for diagnostics is discussed, emphasizing their role in early disease detection, real-time monitoring, and imaging.

1.1 Introduction

The convergence of nanotechnology and AI in the field of medical science marks a paradigm shift that holds the promise of revolutionizing healthcare on an unprecedented scale. This groundbreaking synergy combines the precision and versatility of nanoscale technologies with the analytical prowess of intelligent algorithms, paving the way for transformative advancements in diagnostics, treatment modalities, and overall patient care. Nanotechnology, operating at the scale of individual atoms and molecules, allows for the precise engineering of materials and devices with novel properties. This capability has given rise to a myriad of applications, ranging from

doi:10.1088/978-0-7503-6134-7ch1

targeted drug delivery systems to highly sensitive diagnostic tools [1–5]. Concurrently, AI, with its capacity to analyze vast datasets, identify patterns, and make real-time decisions, has emerged as a powerful tool in various fields, including healthcare [6–10]. At the crossroads of these two cutting-edge fields, the convergence of nanotechnology and AI presents a unique opportunity to address the complex challenges in contemporary medical science. The ability to manipulate matter at the nanoscale offers unparalleled control over biological systems, enabling the development of innovative solutions for diseases that have proven elusive to traditional treatment approaches. Simultaneously, the integration of AI augments the capabilities of healthcare technologies by providing intelligent data analysis, pattern recognition, and decision-making, thereby enhancing the overall efficacy and efficiency of medical interventions [6–8]. Furthermore, the convergence of nanotechnology and AI in medical science marks a groundbreaking synergy that holds immense promise for the diagnosis and treatment of various gastrointestinal (GI) disorders [11, 12]. For instance, nano-biosensors offer sensitive and specific detection of biomarkers associated with GI diseases, facilitating early diagnosis and intervention [13–17]. These biosensors hold immense potential for the non-invasive detection of conditions such as inflammatory bowel disease (IBD) [18]. This fusion of cutting-edge technologies has paved the way for innovative approaches in controlled drug release, targeted drug delivery, and advanced diagnostic methods. In this realm, the intersection of nanoscience and AI has become particularly impactful, addressing challenges in the GI tract, liver diseases, and various cancers [19]. The intricate interplay between nanotechnology and AI in addressing these challenges will be dissected, unveiling the potential applications and transformative impact on patient outcomes. Additionally, AI-based colonoscopy has emerged as a transformative tool for early detection and diagnosis of GI disorders [20]. The combination of AI and nanotechnology offers the potential for highly sensitive and specific imaging, enabling more accurate identification of abnormalities during endoscopic procedures [21–28]. In the field of liver diseases, nanomedicines have shown promise in treating conditions such as liver fibrosis. The targeted delivery of therapeutic agents to specific liver cells, facilitated by nanotechnology, enhances treatment outcomes [29–31]. Integrating AI into the management of chronic liver diseases allows for predictive modelling, early diagnosis, and personalized treatment strategies. Further, the role of nanoparticles in the treatment of gastric cancer is another compelling aspect of this convergence. Nanoparticles, engineered for specific drug delivery to cancerous cells, demonstrate the potential to enhance the efficacy of anticancer treatments [32–34]. AI complements this by contributing to early diagnosis, prediction of disease progression, and the development of advanced therapeutic techniques for gastric cancer [35–37]. Also, nanotechnology is reshaping the landscape of GI endoscopy. The development of miniaturized devices and sensors at the nanoscale, integrated with AI algorithms, enhances the precision and diagnostic capabilities of endoscopic procedures [38–40]. In this exploration of the convergence of nanotechnology and AI in medical science, we delve into the revolutionary synergy that is transforming the landscape of diagnosis, treatment, and monitoring of GI disorders. The integration of these cutting-edge technologies holds the potential to usher in a new era of precision medicine, where tailored therapeutic interventions and early detection strategies become commonplace in the quest for improved patient outcomes. The present chapter aims to delve deeper into the synergistic implications of nanotechnology and AI in revolutionizing the field of medical science. By exploring the intersection of these cutting-edge technologies, we uncover a wealth of opportunities for transformative innovation across various domains of healthcare. From enhanced diagnostics and targeted therapeutics to personalized medicine and predictive analytics, the integration of nanotechnology and AI offers unprecedented capabilities to address complex medical challenges. Through comprehensive analysis and synthesis of existing research, this chapter seeks to elucidate the synergistic interactions between nanotechnology and AI, shedding light on their combined potential to redefine the landscape of medical science and improve patient outcomes worldwide.

1.2 Nanotechnology in medical science

1.2.1 Nanomaterials in drug delivery

Nanomaterials have emerged as a revolutionary platform for drug delivery, offering precise control over therapeutic payloads and their release kinetics. At the nanoscale, drug delivery systems can encapsulate medications within nanocarriers, such as inorganic nanoparticle, organic nanoparticle, polymeric nanoparticles, liposomes, dendrimers, carbon nanotubes, etc (as shown in figure 1.1) allowing for targeted delivery to specific tissues or cells [41–49]. These nanocarriers can bypass biological barriers, penetrate deep into tissues, and accumulate at sites of disease, thereby

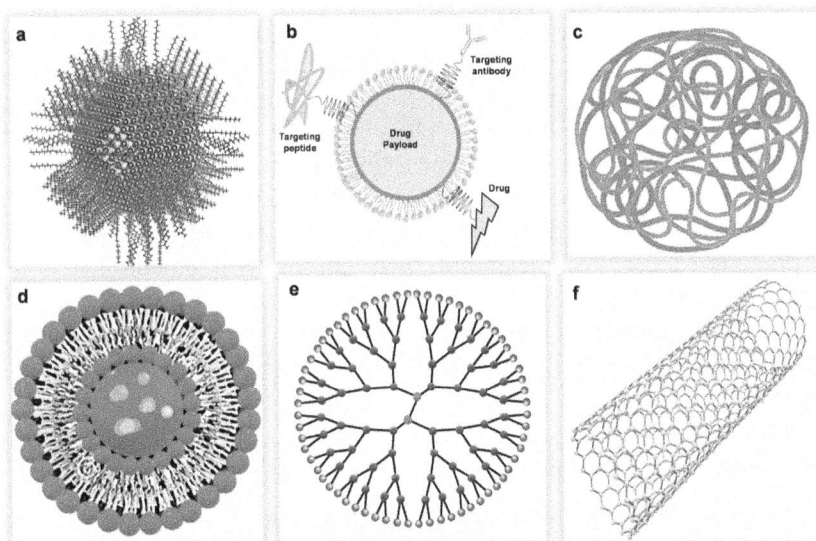

Figure 1.1. Different types of nanomaterials used in biomedical research and drug delivery (a) inorganic nanoparticle, (b) organic nanoparticle, (c) polymeric nanoparticle, (d) liposome, (e) dendrimer, and (f) carbon nanotube.

enhancing drug efficacy while minimizing systemic toxicity [50]. By exploiting the unique properties of nanomaterials, such as their high surface area-to-volume ratio and tuneable surface chemistry, drug delivery systems can achieve enhanced targeting and reduced side effects compared to conventional formulations [51, 52]. One notable example of successful application in cancer treatment is the use of liposomal formulations of chemotherapeutic agents, such as Doxil (liposomal doxorubicin), which has demonstrated improved tumor targeting and reduced cardiotoxicity in patients with various malignancies [52–56]. Similarly, nanoparticle-based drug delivery systems, such as Abraxane (albumin-bound paclitaxel), have shown efficacy in treating metastatic breast cancer and pancreatic cancer, offering superior pharmacokinetics and reduced risk of hypersensitivity reactions compared to conventional formulations [57–60]. These examples underscore the transformative potential of nanomaterials in drug delivery, paving the way for safer and more effective therapies in oncology and beyond.

1.2.2 Use of nanomaterials in designing diagnostic nanosensors

The development of nanoscale sensors has revolutionized early disease detection by offering unprecedented sensitivity and specificity in detecting biomarkers indicative of various pathologies. These miniature devices, often composed of nanomaterials such as carbon nanotubes, quantum dots, or metallic nanoparticles, can detect subtle changes in biological molecules, enabling the diagnosis of diseases at their earliest stages [61–63]. One compelling example of nanosensor application is in the detection of circulating tumor cells (CTCs) for cancer diagnosis and monitoring. By functionalizing nanoparticles with antibodies specific to tumor-associated antigens, nanosensors can selectively capture CTCs from blood samples with remarkable efficiency [64]. This approach allows for the non-invasive detection of cancer metastasis and monitoring of disease progression in real-time, facilitating timely intervention and personalized treatment strategies. Furthermore, nanosensors can be integrated into imaging modalities, such as magnetic resonance imaging (MRI) or positron emission tomography (PET), enabling precise localization of tumors and assessment of treatment response [65]. Case studies have demonstrated the clinical utility of nanosensor-based diagnostics in various cancer types, including breast cancer, prostate cancer, and melanoma, highlighting their potential to transform cancer care by enabling early detection and personalized management strategies. Overall, nanoscale sensors represent a promising frontier in medical diagnostics, offering unparalleled sensitivity and versatility for early disease detection and real-time monitoring.

1.2.3 Nanomaterials as theranostics

Theranostics represents a groundbreaking approach that seamlessly integrates diagnostics and therapy, offering a multifaceted solution for precision medicine. At the heart of theranostics lies the utilization of nanoparticles, which serve dual roles as both diagnostic agents and therapeutic carriers. These nanoparticles can be engineered to carry therapeutic payloads, such as drugs or genetic material, while simultaneously bearing imaging moieties that enable real-time visualization of disease sites. This unique combination enables clinicians to not only diagnose diseases with high accuracy but also deliver targeted treatments directly to the affected tissues, thereby maximizing therapeutic efficacy while minimizing systemic side effects [66, 67]. Moreover, theranostics holds immense promise in advancing personalized medicine by tailoring treatments to individual patient profiles. By leveraging imaging data to guide treatment selection and monitor therapeutic response, clinicians can optimize treatment regimens and adapt interventions based on real-time feedback, leading to improved outcomes and enhanced patient care [68, 69]. The advent of theranostic nanoparticles represents a paradigm shift in healthcare, offering a holistic approach to disease management that transcends traditional boundaries between diagnostics and therapy, ultimately empowering clinicians with the tools they need to deliver precise, personalized treatments to patients.

1.3 Artificial intelligence in medical science

The integration of AI in healthcare is revolutionizing how medical data is utilized for diagnosis, treatment, and research. One significant challenge in leveraging medical data stems from the diverse nature of information sources, particularly the distinction between structured and unstructured data [70]. Structured data, such as imaging, genetic, and electrophysiological (EP) data, are relatively straightforward for AI analysis as they are typically in a format that can be easily processed by algorithms. These data types provide quantifiable measurements or observations, making them amenable to ML techniques. ML algorithms can analyze structured data to identify patterns, cluster patient traits, predict disease outcomes, or assist in decision-making processes [71]. On the other hand, unstructured data sources like clinical notes and medical journals contain narrative texts that are rich in information but challenging for traditional algorithms to interpret directly. Natural language processing (NLP) methods address this challenge by extracting relevant information from unstructured text and transforming it into machine-readable structured data [72], which can then be analyzed using ML techniques. This integration of NLP and ML enables AI applications to mine insights from vast amounts of textual data, supplementing and enriching structured medical data. For example, researchers like Karakülah *et al* [69] have employed AI technologies to extract phenotypic features from clinical notes and case reports, enhancing the accuracy of diagnosis, particularly in the context of congenital anomalies. By converting unstructured clinical narratives into structured electronic medical records (EMRs) [73], AI systems can facilitate more comprehensive analyses, leading to improved patient care and outcomes. The flowchart depicted in figure 1.2 outlines the sequential process starting from the generation of clinical data, progressing through the enrichment of this data via NLP, and culminating in the analysis of the data using ML techniques to facilitate clinical decision-making.

Thus, AI devices in healthcare primarily fall into two major categories: ML techniques for analyzing structured data and NLP methods for extracting information from unstructured data. The synergy between these approaches holds great

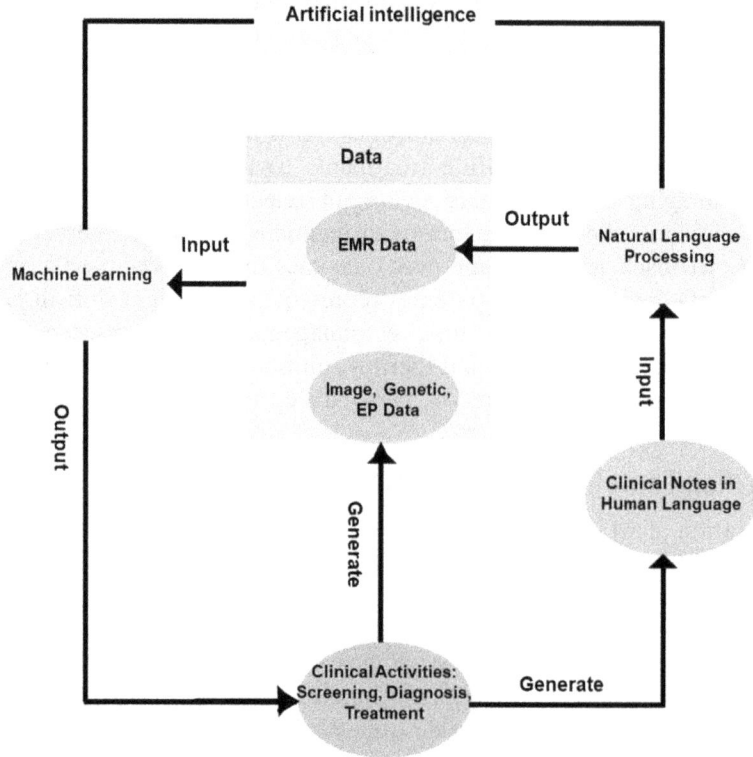

Figure 1.2. Flow chart illustrating the roadmap from the generation of clinical data to the enrichment of this data through NLP, followed by the analysis of the data using ML techniques, leading to clinical decision-making.

promise for advancing medical research, diagnosis, and treatment by harnessing the full potential of diverse medical data sources.

1.3.1 Machine learning in diagnostics

ML algorithms have emerged as powerful tools in medical diagnostics, revolutionizing the way diseases are identified and treated. These algorithms encompass a wide range of techniques, including supervised learning, unsupervised learning, and deep learning, which enable computers to analyze vast amounts of data and extract meaningful patterns and insights. In the realm of medical imaging, ML algorithms excel at image recognition and pattern analysis, allowing for the rapid and accurate identification of disease-specific features [74, 75]. For example, in radiology, convolutional neural networks (CNNs) have been employed to analyze medical images, such as x-rays, MRIs, and CT scans, to detect abnormalities indicative of various conditions, including tumors, fractures, and cardiovascular disease [76–80]. By automating the diagnostic process, ML algorithms not only improve the accuracy of disease identification but also enhance the efficiency of healthcare delivery, enabling faster diagnosis and treatment initiation. Moreover, ML algorithms can learn from experience and adapt over time, continually improving their performance and staying abreast of the latest medical advancements. As a result, ML holds immense potential to transform medical diagnostics, empowering clinicians with the tools they need to make more informed decisions and deliver optimal patient care.

1.3.2 Natural language processing in healthcare

NLP has emerged as a powerful tool in healthcare, enabling the extraction of valuable insights from vast amounts of unstructured medical texts, such as electronic health records (EHRs), clinical notes, and biomedical literature. NLP applications in healthcare encompass a wide range of tasks, including information extraction, sentiment analysis, entity recognition, and summarization, among others [81, 82]. For example, NLP algorithms can analyze clinical notes to extract key information regarding patient diagnoses, treatments, and outcomes, facilitating data-driven clinical decision-making. Moreover, NLP techniques enable the aggregation and synthesis of information from disparate sources, allowing researchers to uncover new patterns, associations, and trends in medical data. By enhancing clinical decision-making and research capabilities, NLP has the potential to improve patient outcomes, streamline healthcare delivery, and advance medical knowledge. However, the use of NLP in healthcare also raises ethical considerations, particularly regarding patient privacy and data security. The handling of sensitive patient data requires strict adherence to privacy regulations, such as the Health Insurance Portability and Accountability Act (HIPAA), to ensure patient confidentiality and data protection. Additionally, there is a need for transparency and accountability in the development and deployment of NLP algorithms to mitigate biases and ensure fair and equitable outcomes for all patients. Despite these challenges, the transformative potential of NLP in healthcare is undeniable, offering unprecedented opportunities to harness the power of language to improve patient care and advance medical science.

1.3.3 Predictive analytics in patient care

Predictive analytics, powered by AI, has emerged as a cornerstone in modern patient care, offering invaluable insights into predicting and optimizing patient outcomes. Through sophisticated ML algorithms, predictive analytics harnesses vast amounts of patient data, including demographics, clinical history, and diagnostic results, to forecast disease progression, treatment response, and adverse events. By analyzing these data points, AI algorithms can identify patterns, risk factors, and predictive biomarkers, enabling clinicians to anticipate potential complications and tailor treatment strategies accordingly [83]. Moreover, the integration of predictive analytics with EHRs facilitates the development of personalized treatment plans by providing clinicians with real-time access to patient data and predictive models. This enables proactive interventions, timely adjustments to treatment regimens, and optimization of healthcare resources, ultimately leading to improved patient outcomes and quality of care. Case studies across various medical specialties, such as oncology, cardiology, and critical care, have demonstrated the successful implementation of predictive analytics in clinical practice [84, 85]. For instance, predictive models have been utilized to anticipate sepsis onset in hospitalized patients, identify individuals at high risk of heart failure exacerbation, and predict cancer recurrence following treatment. These case studies underscore the transformative potential of predictive analytics in patient care, paving the way for a future where healthcare delivery is not only proactive and personalized but also predictive and preventive.

1.4 Synergies between nanotechnology and AI and their application in the medical field

The intersection of nanotechnology and AI presents a remarkable synergy with transformative implications for healthcare. By combining nanoscale materials with AI-driven algorithms, medical applications are revolutionized across various fronts. Nanotechnology facilitates the creation of ultra-sensitive diagnostic tools, targeted drug delivery systems, and innovative imaging modalities at the molecular level. AI, on the other hand, provides powerful data analysis capabilities, enabling the interpretation of complex biological signals and the optimization of treatment strategies. Together, these technologies offer unprecedented opportunities for personalized medicine, early disease detection, precise surgical interventions, and accelerated drug discovery and development. The integration of nanotechnology and AI promises to reshape the landscape of healthcare, paving the way for more effective, efficient, and patient-centered approaches to diagnosis, treatment, and disease management.

1.4.1 Nanoscience in controlled drug release in the GI tract

Nanoscience has ushered in a paradigm shift in the realm of controlled drug release, particularly within the GI tract, presenting a realm of unparalleled precision, efficacy, and targeted delivery [86–88]. Through the utilization of nanoparticles, scientists are empowered to finely manipulate crucial drug properties such as solubility, stability, and bioavailability, thereby orchestrating enhanced therapeutic outcomes while concurrently mitigating adverse side effects [89, 90]. This revolutionary approach to drug delivery within the GI tract is multifaceted, offering a nuanced toolkit for optimizing treatment strategies. Firstly, nanoparticles serve as proficient carriers, adept at encapsulating hydrophobic drugs and consequently enhancing their solubility and bioavailability within the challenging milieu of the GI tract [91–93]. For instance, lipid-based nanoparticles such as liposomes or solid lipid nanoparticles (SLNs) provide a protective envelope for poorly water-soluble drugs, facilitating their efficient absorption across the intestinal epithelium. Moreover, the functionalization of nanoparticles with ligands further enhances their utility by enabling targeted delivery to precise sites within the GI tract. This targeted approach is particularly advantageous as it allows for the attachment of ligands that bind specifically to receptors overexpressed in diseased tissues, thereby amplifying drug accumulation at the desired site while concurrently minimizing systemic exposure and off-target effects [93]. Additionally, nanoparticles offer exquisite control over drug release kinetics, ensuring sustained therapeutic levels over prolonged durations. Strategies such as pH-responsive polymers or stimuli-responsive nanocarriers afford tailored control over drug release, aptly adapted to the dynamic physiological conditions encountered within distinct segments of the GI tract. Furthermore, nanoparticles provide a protective shield for encapsulated drugs, shielding them from degradation by enzymes or harsh pH environments within the GI tract [94, 95]. This protective barrier not only enhances drug stability but also prolongs its therapeutic efficacy, thereby augmenting patient outcomes. As an exemplary illustration, nanostructured lipid carriers (NLCs) stand as a testament to the potential of nanoparticle-based drug delivery in the GI tract. Comprising a blend of solid and liquid lipids, NLCs offer a versatile platform for oral drug delivery, boasting enhanced drug loading capacities, improved stability, and finely modulated release kinetics. By judiciously manipulating the composition and structure of NLCs, researchers can tailor drug release profiles to align seamlessly with specific therapeutic requirements, thus epitomizing the transformative potential of nanotechnology in revolutionizing drug delivery within the GI tract.

1.4.2 Novel drug delivery systems for inflammatory bowel disease

Inflammatory bowel disease, encompassing conditions like Crohn's disease and ulcerative colitis, presents a significant medical challenge characterized by chronic inflammation of the GI tract, often leading to substantial morbidity and a diminished quality of life for affected individuals. Conventional drug delivery methods frequently fall short in providing optimal therapeutic outcomes due to inherent limitations such as systemic side effects, poor bioavailability, and insufficient targeting of inflamed tissues. In response, novel drug delivery systems tailored specifically for IBD have emerged, aiming to surmount these obstacles by offering controlled release, targeted delivery, and enhanced efficacy [96]. One promising avenue lies in nanoparticle-based drug delivery systems, including liposomes, polymeric nanoparticles, and dendrimers. These nanocarriers present several advantages such as improved drug stability, controlled release kinetics, and targeted delivery to inflamed intestinal tissues [97]. For instance, mesalamine-loaded nanoparticles have been engineered to combat ulcerative colitis effectively. By encapsulating mesalamine within nanoparticles, targeted delivery to the inflamed intestinal mucosa is achieved, minimizing systemic exposure and mitigating the adverse effects commonly associated with conventional oral administration [98]. Another innovative approach involves pH-sensitive drug delivery systems, which exploit the pH variations along the GI tract to achieve site-specific drug release [99]. Enteric-coated formulations or pH-responsive polymers are employed in these systems, remaining intact in the acidic gastric environment but releasing the drug payload in the more alkaline conditions of the intestines. For example, enteric-coated formulations of corticosteroids like budesonide have been developed for the treatment of Crohn's disease. These formulations shield the drug from degradation in the stomach, facilitating targeted delivery to the inflamed regions of the intestines, thereby enhancing therapeutic efficacy while minimizing systemic side effects [100].

Additionally, colon-specific drug delivery systems represent a promising strategy, aiming to deliver drugs directly to the colon, where inflammation is most pronounced in IBD patients. These systems employ various approaches such as prodrugs, coatings, or formulations resistant to absorption in the small intestine but designed to release the active drug specifically in the colon [101]. Through these innovative approaches, tailored drug delivery systems for IBD offer immense potential in improving treatment outcomes, minimizing side effects, and enhancing the overall management of this debilitating condition.

1.4.3 Nanotechnology in gastrointestinal endoscopy

Nanotechnology has ushered in a new era in GI endoscopy, presenting a plethora of innovative tools and techniques for diagnosis, imaging, and therapy. Through the exploitation of the unique properties of nanoparticles, researchers have pioneered novel approaches to enhance the accuracy, sensitivity, and therapeutic outcomes of GI endoscopic procedures [102]. One pivotal application lies in nanoparticle-based contrast agents, which facilitate superior imaging of GI tract tissues, thereby enabling enhanced visualization of lesions, tumors, and inflammatory conditions during endoscopic examinations. These contrast agents can be intricately engineered, conjugated with targeting ligands for specific molecular imaging, or functionalized with imaging probes for multimodal imaging techniques [100]. For instance, iron oxide nanoparticles coated with polyethylene glycol (PEG) have emerged as robust contrast agents for MRI of the GI tract, exhibiting high sensitivity and specificity in detecting GI tumors and lesions [103]. Additionally, nanotechnology has propelled the development of advanced endoscopic imaging techniques boasting improved resolution, depth penetration, and real-time visualization capabilities. Nanoparticles can be seamlessly integrated into endoscopic devices or imaging probes to augment contrast, fluorescence, or spectroscopic properties during GI endoscopy. Quantum dots, semiconductor nanoparticles renowned for their unique optical properties, have been integrated into endoscopic imaging systems to enable real-time fluorescence imaging of GI tract lesions, offering high photostability and multiplexing capabilities for simultaneous visualization of multiple molecular targets [104]. Furthermore, nanoparticles serve as invaluable tools for targeted drug delivery to specific sites within the GI tract, thereby enhancing therapeutic efficacy while mitigating systemic side effects. Through functionalization with targeting ligands, nanoparticles exhibit selective binding to diseased tissues or cells, facilitating site-specific drug release. For instance, gold nanoparticles conjugated with antibodies targeting overexpressed receptors on tumor cells have been leveraged for targeted drug delivery in GI cancers, enabling localized chemotherapy delivery and thereby minimizing off-target effects while optimizing treatment outcomes [105]. Finally, the advent of therapeutic nanoparticle-based devices has opened up new frontiers for minimally invasive interventions in the GI tract. Nanoparticle-coated stents, drug-eluting capsules, and nanoparticle-based ablation therapies offer innovative approaches for the treatment of various GI diseases and disorders. Notably, nanoparticle-coated stents have been developed to address GI strictures and obstructions, releasing anti-inflammatory or antimicrobial agents to prevent restenosis and promote tissue healing following endoscopic placement. In essence, nanotechnology represents a paradigm shift in GI endoscopy, empowering clinicians with unprecedented precision, efficacy, and therapeutic versatility in the management of GI diseases and disorders.

1.4.4 Nano-biotechnology in gastrointestinal cancer

Nano-biotechnology has emerged as a groundbreaking approach in the realm of GI cancer, offering innovative solutions to address the challenges encountered with traditional therapies. By amalgamating the principles of nanotechnology and biotechnology, researchers have devised novel strategies aimed at improving early detection, refining targeted therapy, and circumventing drug resistance mechanisms in GI cancers [106]. In the domain of early detection and diagnosis, nanoparticles and nanostructured materials have been instrumental in enhancing imaging techniques and biomarker detection. For instance, gold nanoparticles functionalized with antibodies specific to cancer biomarkers enable highly sensitive detection of GI cancer cells in blood or tissue samples, thereby facilitating early diagnosis and ongoing disease monitoring. Moreover, nanoparticle-based drug delivery systems play a pivotal role in targeted therapy by delivering chemotherapeutic agents, immunotherapeutics, or gene therapies directly to tumor cells while minimizing systemic toxicity [107]. Lipid-based nanoparticles loaded with chemotherapy drugs can be engineered to selectively accumulate in GI tumors through passive or active targeting mechanisms, thereby enhancing therapeutic efficacy and reducing adverse effects on healthy tissues [108]. Additionally, nano-biotechnology strategies aim to overcome drug resistance mechanisms commonly observed in GI cancers by delivering combination therapies or surmounting barriers within the tumor microenvironment. For example, nanoparticle-mediated co-delivery of chemotherapy drugs and targeted therapy agents can synergistically inhibit multiple signaling pathways involved in cancer progression, thereby diminishing the likelihood of drug resistance development [109]. Furthermore, nanotechnology facilitates the development of personalized medicine approaches for GI cancer patients by enabling precise targeting of tumor-specific molecular alterations and tailoring therapies based on individual patient characteristics. Nanoparticle-based platforms for liquid biopsy allow non-invasive monitoring of tumor-specific mutations and molecular signatures in circulating tumor DNA or exosomes, enabling clinicians to make informed treatment decisions and monitor treatment response in real-time. In essence, nano-biotechnology holds immense promise in revolutionizing the diagnosis, treatment, and management of GI cancers, offering a multifaceted approach to combat this formidable disease.

1.5 Role of nanoparticles for the treatment of gastric cancer

Nanoparticles are playing a pivotal role in revolutionizing the treatment landscape for gastric cancer, offering targeted drug delivery, enhanced therapeutic efficacy, and reduced systemic side effects. Gastric cancer, a leading cause of cancer-related mortality worldwide, presents a pressing need for effective treatment strategies. Nanoparticle-based therapies have emerged as promising approaches to tackle the challenges associated with conventional treatments. Firstly, nanoparticles can be intricately engineered to deliver chemotherapeutic agents directly to gastric cancer cells, thus minimizing off-target effects and improving drug efficacy [110]. For instance, polymeric nanoparticles functionalized with ligands targeting overexpressed receptors on gastric cancer cells, such as epidermal growth factor receptor (EGFR) or human epidermal growth factor receptor 2 (HER2), facilitate targeted drug delivery [111]. Notably, nanoparticle-bound docetaxel has demonstrated selective accumulation in gastric tumor tissues, leading to significantly enhanced therapeutic outcomes. Additionally, nanoparticles offer a means to overcome drug resistance mechanisms commonly encountered in gastric cancer by delivering combination therapies or targeting multiple signaling pathways involved in cancer progression. Multifunctional nanoparticles capable of co-delivering chemotherapeutic drugs and targeted therapy agents, such as tyrosine kinase inhibitors like trastuzumab, have shown promising results in preclinical studies, potentially offering a solution to resistance and holding potential for clinical translation. Furthermore, nanoparticle-based contrast agents and imaging probes enable improved visualization of gastric tumors, facilitating early detection and accurate diagnosis. Superparamagnetic iron oxide nanoparticles (SPIONs) coated with biocompatible polymers, for instance, serve as contrast agents for MRI of gastric tumors, providing high-resolution imaging crucial for surgical planning and disease staging [112]. Lastly, nanoparticles can be engineered to release therapeutic agents directly at the tumor site, minimizing systemic exposure and reducing adverse effects on healthy tissues. Thermosensitive liposomes loaded with chemotherapeutic drugs represent a prime example of this localized therapy approach, selectively releasing the payload within gastric tumor tissues upon external stimuli such as mild hyperthermia. In essence, nanoparticles hold immense promise in reshaping the treatment paradigm for gastric cancer, offering targeted, efficient, and minimally invasive therapeutic options to improve patient outcomes and quality of life.

1.6 Artificial intelligence in hepatitis and chronic liver disease

AI has emerged as a transformative tool in the management of hepatitis and chronic liver disease (CLD), offering innovative solutions for early diagnosis, personalized treatment planning, and disease monitoring. With hepatitis, encompassing both viral (e.g., hepatitis B and C) and non-viral causes (e.g., alcoholic liver disease, non-alcoholic fatty liver disease), along with CLD, representing significant global health burdens, effective strategies for prevention, diagnosis, and management are imperative. AI algorithms leverage complex datasets, including patient demographics, clinical history, laboratory tests, imaging studies, and genetic information, to identify individuals at risk of developing hepatitis or CLD and predict disease progression [113]. For instance, ML models trained on EHRs accurately predict the risk of liver fibrosis progression in patients with non-alcoholic fatty liver disease (NAFLD) based on clinical parameters such as age, body mass index (BMI), liver enzymes, and imaging findings, enabling early intervention and personalized management strategies [114, 115]. Additionally, AI-powered image analysis techniques, such as deep learning algorithms, enhance the interpretation of radiological imaging studies, including ultrasound, computed tomography (CT), and MRI, aiding in the diagnosis and staging of hepatitis and CLD. These technologies improve diagnostic accuracy, treatment optimization, and disease monitoring, ultimately leading to better patient outcomes and quality of life. Furthermore, AI-driven decision support systems assist healthcare providers in selecting the most appropriate treatment strategies based on individualized risk profiles, treatment response predictions, and therapeutic guidelines, thus optimizing therapy and improving patient outcomes. Lastly, AI technologies enable continuous monitoring of disease progression and treatment response through real-time analysis of clinical data and patient-reported outcomes, facilitating proactive interventions and personalized medicine approaches in the management of hepatitis and CLD.

1.7 Artificial intelligence applications for clinical decisions support

AI applications for clinical decision support (CDS) have transformed healthcare by furnishing clinicians with invaluable insights, evidence-based recommendations, and personalized treatment strategies to enhance patient outcomes. CDS systems harness AI algorithms to sift through extensive patient data, medical literature, and clinical guidelines, empowering healthcare providers to make well-informed decisions directly at the point of care [115]. One pivotal role of AI in CDS lies in aiding diagnosis and predicting patient outcomes by scrutinizing diverse patient datasets, spanning medical history, laboratory results, imaging studies, and genetic information. For instance, IBM Watson for Oncology exemplifies an AI-driven CDS system adept at analyzing patient data and medical literature to furnish evidence-based treatment recommendations for cancer patients. By amalgamating clinical and molecular data, Watson for Oncology guides oncologists in tailoring treatment options to each patient's unique tumor characteristics and genetic mutations [116]. Moreover, AI-powered CDS systems play a crucial role in treatment planning and optimization by synthesizing patient data and clinical guidelines to craft personalized treatment plans and refine therapeutic interventions. ClosedLoop.ai is a notable example, leveraging predictive analytics and ML to optimize treatment plans for patients with chronic diseases like diabetes, hypertension, and heart failure. By analyzing real-time patient data and identifying trends, ClosedLoop.ai aids clinicians in adjusting medication dosages, recommending lifestyle modifications, and averting disease complications [117]. Additionally, AI-based CDS systems support medication management by identifying potential drug interactions, adverse drug reactions, and medication errors, thereby enhancing patient safety and adherence. Platforms like Dosis analyze patient data comprehensively to provide real-time recommendations for medication dosing and adjustments, taking into account individual factors such as renal function, liver function, and comorbidities to prescribe medications safely and prevent adverse events. Furthermore, AI-enabled CDS systems streamline clinical workflows, mitigate administrative burden, and boost efficiency by automating routine tasks, prioritizing patient care activities, and fostering communication among healthcare team members. Epic's AI-driven virtual assistant, the Epic AI Assistant, seamlessly integrates with EHR systems to furnish clinicians with contextual information and actionable insights during patient encounters, aiding in documentation, test ordering, and treatment plan review. In essence, AI in CDS holds immense promise in augmenting clinical decision-making, optimizing patient care, and advancing healthcare delivery.

1.8 Role of artificial intelligence in an early diagnosis and prediction of gastric cancer as an advanced therapeutic technique

AI serves as a pivotal tool in the early diagnosis and prediction of gastric cancer, ushering in innovative solutions to enhance patient outcomes through advanced therapeutic techniques. Gastric cancer, a leading cause of cancer-related mortality worldwide, underscores the critical importance of early detection and personalized treatment strategies. AI-driven approaches harness ML algorithms, deep learning techniques, and big data analytics to analyze diverse datasets, identifying patterns, biomarkers, and risk factors associated with gastric cancer development and progression [118, 119]. For early diagnosis, AI algorithms scrutinize comprehensive datasets encompassing patient demographics, medical history, symptoms, laboratory tests, imaging studies, and histopathological findings, facilitating timely detection of gastric cancer lesions. Notably, systems like EndoBRAIN, an AI-based diagnostic system developed by Olympus, employ deep learning algorithms to analyze endoscopic images, accurately detecting early-stage gastric cancer lesions by discerning subtle abnormalities such as mucosal changes and dysplastic lesions [120]. Furthermore, AI-driven risk prediction models integrate individual patient characteristics, genetic predisposition, environmental factors, and lifestyle habits to stratify patients based on their likelihood of developing gastric cancer. A notable example is an ML model developed to predict gastric cancer risk using demographic, clinical, and lifestyle factors, enabling targeted screening and preventive measures for high-risk individuals. In the realm of precision medicine, AI algorithms delve into molecular profiling data, genomic alterations, and tumor biomarkers to tailor treatment strategies, identifying optimal therapeutic options for gastric cancer patients. Platforms like IBM Watson for Genomics leverage AI to analyze genomic sequencing data, identifying actionable mutations and potential targeted therapy options, thus aiding oncologists in selecting personalized treatment regimens and optimizing patient outcomes [121]. Moreover, AI-driven decision support systems, exemplified by initiatives like CancerLinQ, aggregate real-world cancer data to provide oncologists with real-time insights and evidence-based recommendations, enhancing treatment decision-making and optimizing therapeutic interventions for patients with gastric cancer [122]. In essence, AI's integration into the early diagnosis, prediction, and treatment optimization of gastric cancer holds immense promise in revolutionizing patient care and improving clinical outcomes in the fight against this formidable disease.

1.9 Nanomedicines for liver fibrosis

Liver fibrosis, characterized by progressive scarring of liver tissue, is a significant consequence of chronic liver diseases like hepatitis B and C, non-alcoholic fatty liver disease (NAFLD), and alcoholic liver disease. This condition poses a substantial global health burden, often leading to liver dysfunction, cirrhosis, and eventual liver failure if not managed effectively. Nanomedicine, which involves the application of nanotechnology in medicine, presents promising avenues for the diagnosis, treatment, and management of liver fibrosis. One key aspect is the targeted delivery of therapeutics using nanoparticles, engineered to reach hepatic stellate cells (HSCs), pivotal in liver fibrogenesis [123]. For instance, lipid-based nanoparticles such as liposomes or SLNs, loaded with anti-fibrotic agents like pirfenidone or nintedanib, can specifically target activated HSCs within the fibrotic liver. By delivering therapeutic payloads directly to the site of fibrosis, nanoparticle-based drug delivery systems enhance drug efficacy while minimizing off-target effects [124]. Additionally, nanoparticles can encapsulate nucleic acid-based therapeutics such as small interfering RNA (siRNA) or microRNA (miRNA) to selectively target and downregulate genes involved in fibrogenesis and inflammation. For example, polymeric nanoparticles conjugated with siRNA targeting transforming growth factor-beta (TGF-β) or platelet-derived growth factor (PDGF) receptors can inhibit signaling pathways implicated in HSC activation and collagen deposition [125]. Nanoparticles also serve diagnostic purposes by acting as contrast agents for non-invasive imaging modalities like MRI and PET, allowing accurate assessment of liver fibrosis severity and disease progression monitoring. Moreover, theranostic nanoparticles integrate diagnostic and therapeutic functions into a single platform, enabling simultaneous imaging and treatment of liver fibrosis. These innovations in nanomedicine hold promise for advancing the management of liver fibrosis, potentially leading to improved patient outcomes and enhanced quality of life.

1.10 Artificial intelligence-based colonoscopy

AI-based colonoscopy is revolutionizing gastroenterology by significantly improving the accuracy, efficiency, and effectiveness of colorectal cancer (CRC) screening and surveillance. As CRC ranks among the most prevalent malignancies globally, early detection through colonoscopy is paramount in mitigating associated morbidity and mortality. AI technologies, leveraging ML and computer vision algorithms, analyze endoscopic images and videos to aid gastroenterologists in detecting colorectal lesions, characterizing their histology, and guiding real-time decision-making during procedures. For instance, the CADe-Net (Computer-Aided Detection Network), employs deep learning techniques to promptly detect and highlight suspicious lesions during colonoscopy, thereby enhancing adenoma detection rates and minimizing miss rates [126]. Furthermore, AI algorithms, like the CADx-Net (Computer-Aided Diagnosis Network) from the University of Tokyo, utilize CNNs to classify colorectal lesions based on their endoscopic appearance, providing gastroenterologists with immediate diagnostic assistance and improving diagnostic accuracy [127]. Additionally, AI-based decision support systems, exemplified by EndoBRAIN, an

AI-driven diagnostic system developed by Olympus, analyze endoscopic images and videos in real time, highlighting suspicious lesions, offering automated measurements, and providing decision support recommendations aligned with clinical guidelines [128]. By facilitating real-time decision-making, AI-based colonoscopy enhances the quality and efficiency of colonoscopy procedures, ultimately advancing CRC screening and surveillance efforts.

1.11 Clinical validation of artificial intelligence for gastrointestinal diseases

Clinical validation of AI for GI diseases involves rigorous assessment of AI algorithms in real-world clinical settings to ascertain their performance, accuracy, and clinical utility. GI diseases encompass a broad spectrum of conditions affecting the digestive tract, including IBD, gastroesophageal reflux disease (GERD), CRC, among others [129, 130]. AI technologies, leveraging ML and deep learning algorithms, are increasingly applied across various facets of GI disease management, spanning diagnosis, risk stratification, treatment optimization, and disease monitoring. Through clinical validation studies, the reliability and efficacy of AI-based tools are evaluated, aiming to enhance diagnostic accuracy, improve patient outcomes, and optimize healthcare delivery in gastroenterology practice. For instance, these studies assess AI algorithms' performance in diagnosing GI diseases, such as colorectal polyps and Barrett's esophagus, using endoscopic images and histopathological samples, demonstrating high sensitivity and specificity in detecting lesions [129]. Additionally, AI-based models are validated for predicting disease progression and treatment response, enabling personalized risk stratification and prognostication for patients with GI diseases like Crohn's disease. Furthermore, clinical validation evaluates the effectiveness of AI-driven decision support systems in optimizing treatment selection and monitoring, exemplified by studies showing improved medication adherence and clinical outcomes in patients with IBD. Moreover, AI technologies undergo validation for enhancing the efficiency and quality of care delivery in gastroenterology practice, streamlining clinical workflows, and reducing diagnostic errors, as evidenced by studies demonstrating improved colonoscopy performance metrics with AI-driven quality improvement programs. Through comprehensive clinical validation, AI holds the potential to revolutionize GI disease management, offering valuable tools for improving patient care and healthcare outcomes.

1.12 Summary and conclusions

The convergence of nanotechnology and AI in medical science represents a revolutionary synergy with profound implications for healthcare. Throughout this exploration, we have witnessed how the integration of nanomaterials and AI techniques has led to groundbreaking advancements across various domains, including diagnostics, drug delivery, disease management, and therapeutic interventions. Nanotechnology offers unprecedented capabilities in designing precise drug delivery systems, imaging agents, and therapeutic devices at the nanoscale, enabling targeted treatments with enhanced efficacy and reduced side effects. On the other hand, AI harnesses the power of data analytics, ML, and predictive modeling to extract valuable insights from complex medical datasets, enabling personalized medicine, clinical decision support, and predictive diagnostics. Together, the marriage of nanotechnology and AI unleashes a new era of precision medicine, where therapies are tailored to individual patients' needs, diseases are detected at their earliest stages, and treatments are delivered with unparalleled precision. This revolutionary synergy holds the promise of transforming healthcare by improving patient outcomes, optimizing healthcare delivery, and driving innovation across the entire medical landscape. However, realizing the full potential of this convergence requires interdisciplinary collaboration, investment in research and development, regulatory frameworks to ensure safety and efficacy, and equitable access to these transformative technologies. As we embark on this journey towards a future where nanotechnology and AI converge to revolutionize medical science, it is imperative to harness the collective potential of these disciplines to address pressing healthcare challenges and pave the way for a healthier, more sustainable future for all.

Acknowledgments

A K S would like to acknowledge Banaras Hindu University for providing BRIDGE GRANT under BHU, IoE scheme. V K C gratefully acknowledges DHR-MoHFW, Government of India, for support through Young Scientist fellowship Grant R.12014/56/2022-HR. D P Y extend their appreciation to the Seed Grand (6031), IoE, BHU, Varanasi.

References

[1] Farokhzad O C and Langer R 2006 Nanomedicine: developing smarter therapeutic and diagnostic modalities *Adv. Drug Deliv. Rev.* **58** 1456–9

[2] Liu Y, Miyoshi H and Nakamura M 2007 Nanomedicine for drug delivery and imaging: a promising avenue for cancer therapy and diagnosis using targeted functional nanoparticles *Int. J. Cancer* **120** 2527–37

[3] Kawasaki E S and Player A 2005 Nanotechnology, nanomedicine, and the development of new, effective therapies for cancer *Nanomed. Nanotechnol. Biol. Med.* **1** 101–9

[4] Chaturvedi V K, Sharma B, Tripathi A D, Yadav D P, Singh K R, Singh J and Singh R P 2023 Biosynthesized nanoparticles: a novel approach for cancer therapeutics *Front. Med. Technol.* **5** 1236107

[5] Murdoch T B and Detsky A S 2013 The inevitable application of big data to health care *JAMA* **309** 1351–2

[6] Kolker E, Özdemir V and Kolker E 2016 How healthcare can refocus on its super-customers (patients, $n = 1$) and customers (doctors and nurses) by leveraging lessons from Amazon, Uber, and Watson *OMICS* **20** 329–33

[7] Dilsizian S E and Siegel E L 2014 Artificial intelligence in medicine and cardiac imaging: harnessing big data and advanced computing to provide personalized medical diagnosis and treatment *Curr. Cardiol. Rep.* **16** 1–8

[8] Patel V L, Shortliffe E H, Stefanelli M, Szolovits P, Berthold M R, Bellazzi R *et al* 2008 The coming of age of artificial intelligence in *Artif. Intell. Med.* **46** 5–17

[9] Jha S and Topol E J 2016 Adapting to artificial intelligence: radiologists and pathologists as information specialists *JAMA* **316** 2353–4

[10] Health NIo, Health UDo, Services H 2009 *Opportunities and Challenges in Digestive Diseases Research: Recommendations of the National Commission on Digestive Diseases* (Bethesda, MD: National Institutes of Health)

[11] Haghiashtiani G and McAlpine M C 2017 Sensing gastrointestinal motility *Nat. Biomed. Eng.* **1** 775–6

[12] Traverso G and Langer R 2015 Perspective: special delivery for the gut *Nature* **519** S19–S

[13] Matzeu G, Florea L and Diamond D 2015 Advances in wearable chemical sensor design for monitoring biological fluids *Sens. Actuators* B **211** 403–18

[14] Gao W, Emaminejad S, Nyein H Y Y, Challa S, Chen K, Peck A *et al* 2016 Fully integrated wearable sensor arrays for multiplexed *in situ* perspiration analysis *Nature* **529** 509–14

[15] Xiao T, Wu F, Hao J, Zhang M, Yu P and Mao L 2017 *In vivo* analysis with electrochemical sensors and biosensors *Anal. Chem.* **89** 300–13

[16] Sciurti E, Signore M, Velardi L, Di Corato R, Blasi L, Campa A *et al* 2024 Label-free electrochemical biosensor for direct detection of Oncostatin M (OSM) inflammatory bowel diseases (IBD) biomarker in human serum *Talanta* **271** 125726

[17] Wu D, Lu J, Zheng N, Elsehrawy M G, Alfaiz F A, Zhao H *et al* 2024 Utilizing nanotechnology and advanced machine learning for early detection of gastric cancer surgery *Environ. Res.* **245** 117784

[18] Hassan C, Spadaccini M, Iannone A, Maselli R, Jovani M, Chandrasekar V T *et al* 2021 Performance of artificial intelligence in colonoscopy for adenoma and polyp detection: a systematic review and meta-analysis *Gastrointest. Endosc* **93** 77–85. e6

[19] Banerjee A, Chakraborty C and Rathi M Sr 2020 Medical imaging, artificial intelligence, internet of things, wearable devices in terahertz healthcare technologies *Terahertz Biomedical and Healthcare Technologies* (Amsterdam: Elsevier) pp 145–65

[20] Stübling E-M, Bauckhage Y, Jelli E, Heinrich A, Balzer J C and Koch M (ed) 2017 Robotic-based THz imaging system for freeform surfaces *2017 42nd Int. Conf. on Infrared, Millimeter, and Terahertz Waves (IRMMW-THz)* (Piscataway, NJ: IEEE)

[21] Stylianou A and Talias M A 2013 Nanotechnology-supported THz medical imaging *F1000Research* **2** 100

[22] Yngvesson S K, Peter B S, Siqueira P, Kelly P, Glick S, Karellas A *et al* (ed) 2012 Feasibility demonstration of frequency domain terahertz imaging in breast cancer margin determination *Optical Interactions with Tissue and Cells XXIII* (Bellingham, WA: SPIE)

[23] Zhang J, Xing W, Xing M and Sun G 2018 Terahertz image detection with the improved faster region-based convolutional neural network *Sensors* **18** 2327

[24] Yang X, Zhao X, Yang K, Liu Y, Liu Y, Fu W *et al* 2016 Biomedical applications of terahertz spectroscopy and imaging *Trends Biotechnol.* **34** 810–24

[25] Sim Y C, Park J Y, Ahn K-M, Park C and Son J-H 2013 Terahertz imaging of excised oral cancer at frozen temperature *Biomed. Opt. Express* **4** 1413–21

[26] Wahaia F, Kasalynas I, Venckevicius R, Seliuta D, Valusis G, Urbanowicz A *et al* 2016 Terahertz absorption and reflection imaging of carcinoma-affected colon tissues embedded in paraffin *J. Mol. Struct.* **1107** 214–9

[27] Silva C O, Pinho J O, Lopes J M, Almeida A J, Gaspar M M and Reis C 2019 Current trends in cancer nanotheranostics: metallic, polymeric, and lipid-based systems *Pharmaceutics* **11** 22

[28] Pucek A, Tokarek B, Waglewska E and Bazylińska U 2020 Recent advances in the structural design of photosensitive agent formulations using 'soft' colloidal nanocarriers *Pharmaceutics* **12** 587

[29] Wawrzyńczyk D, Cichy B, Zaręba J K and Bazylińska U 2019 On the interaction between up-converting NaYF$_4$: Er^{3+}, Yb^{3+} nanoparticles and Rose Bengal molecules constrained within the double core of multifunctional nanocarriers *J. Mater. Chem.* C **7** 15021–34

[30] Raju G S R, Pavitra E, Merchant N, Lee H, Prasad G L V, Nagaraju G P *et al* 2018 Targeting autophagy in gastrointestinal malignancy by using nanomaterials as drug delivery systems *Cancer Lett.* **419** 222–32

[31] Quader S and Kataoka K 2017 Nanomaterial-enabled cancer therapy *Mol. Ther.* **25** 1501–13

[32] Zhu R, Zhang F, Peng Y, Xie T, Wang Y and Lan Y 2022 Current progress in cancer treatment using nanomaterials *Front. Oncol* **12** 930125

[33] Xu Z, Broza Y, Ionsecu R, Tisch U, Ding L, Liu H *et al* 2013 A nanomaterial-based breath test for distinguishing gastric cancer from benign gastric conditions *Br. J. Cancer* **108** 941–50

[34] Zhu X, Su T, Wang S, Zhou H and Shi W 2022 New advances in nano-drug delivery systems: *Helicobacter pylori* and gastric cancer *Front. Oncol* **12** 834934

[35] Oyarzun-Ampuero F, Guerrero A, Hassan-Lopez N, O, Morales J, Bollo S, Corvalan A *et al* 2015 Organic and inorganic nanoparticles for prevention and diagnosis of gastric cancer *Curr. Pharm. Des* **21** 4145–54

[36] Chugh V, Basu A, Kaushik A, Bhansali S and Basu A K 2024 Employing nano-enabled artificial intelligence (AI)-based smart technologies for prediction, screening, and detection of cancer *Nanoscale* **16** 5458–86

[37] Zhu Z, Ng D W H, Park H S and McAlpine M C 2021 3D-printed multifunctional materials enabled by artificial-intelligence-assisted fabrication technologies *Nat. Rev. Mater.* **6** 27–47

[38] Qiu Y, Ashok A, Nguyen C C, Yamauchi Y, Do T N and Phan H P 2024 Integrated sensors for soft medical robotics *Small* **2024** 2308805

[39] Farokhzad O C and Langer R 2009 Impact of nanotechnology on drug delivery *ACS Nano* **3** 16–20

[40] Bangham A D, Standish M M and Watkins J C 1965 Diffusion of univalent ions across the lamellae of swollen phospholipids *J. Mol. Biol.* **13** 238–52

[41] Chaturvedi V K, Singh A, Singh V K and Singh M P 2019 Cancer nanotechnology: a new revolution for cancer diagnosis and therapy *Curr. Drug Metab* **20** 416–29

[42] Yatvin M, Kreutz W, Horwitz B and Shinitzky M 1980 pH-Sensitive liposomes: possible clinical implications *Science* **210** 1253–5

[43] Wankar J N, Chaturvedi V K, Bohara C, Singh M P and Bohara R A 2020 Role of nanomedicine in management and prevention of COVID-19 *Front. Nanotechnol.* **2** 589541

[44] Heath T D, Fraley R T and Papahdjopoulos D 1980 Antibody targeting of liposomes: cell specificity obtained by conjugation of F (ab′) 2 to vesicle surface *Science* **210** 539–41

[45] Chaturvedi V K, Tripathi A D, Minocha T, Singh V, Singh M P and Yadav D P 2023 *In vitro* cytotoxic assessment of functionalized multi-walled carbon nanotubes against cervical cancer *J. Clust. Sci.* **34** 3075–85

[46] Klibanov A L, Maruyama K, Torchilin V P and Huang L 1990 Amphipathic polyethyleneglycols effectively prolong the circulation time of liposomes *FEBS Lett.* **268** 235–7

[47] Gref R, Minamitake Y, Peracchia M T, Trubetskoy V, Torchilin V and Langer R 1994 Biodegradable long-circulating polymeric nanospheres *Science* **263** 1600–3

[48] Tabassum N, Singh V, Chaturvedi V K, Vamanu E and Singh M P 2023 A facile synthesis of flower-like iron oxide nanoparticles and its efficacy measurements for antibacterial, cytotoxicity and antioxidant activity *Pharmaceutics* **15** 1726

[49] Goldberg M, Langer R and Jia X 2007 Nanostructured materials for applications in drug delivery and tissue engineering *J. Biomater. Sci. Polym. Ed.* **18** 241–68

[50] Etheridge M L, Campbell S A, Erdman A G, Haynes C L, Wolf S M and McCullough J 2013 The big picture on nanomedicine: the state of investigational and approved nanomedicine products *Nanomed. Nanotechnol. Biol. Med.* **9** 1–14

[51] Franco Y L, Vaidya T R and Ait-Oudhia S 2018 Anticancer and cardio-protective effects of liposomal doxorubicin in the treatment of breast cancer *Breast Cancer* **10** 131–41

[52] Rivankar S 2014 An overview of doxorubicin formulations in cancer therapy *J. Cancer Res. Ther.* **10** 853–8

[53] Vyas M, Simbo D A, Mursalin M, Mishra V, Bashary R and Khatik G L 2020 Drug delivery approaches for doxorubicin in the management of cancers *Curr. Cancer Ther. Rev.* **16** 320–31

[54] Ngan Y H and Gupta M 2016 A comparison between liposomal and nonliposomal formulations of doxorubicin in the treatment of cancer: an updated review *Arch. Pharm. Prac* **7** 1–13

[55] Desai N 2016 Nanoparticle albumin-bound paclitaxel (Abraxane®) *Albumin in Medicine: Pathological and Clinical Applications* (Springer) pp 101–19

[56] Behl A and Chhillar A K 2023 Nano-based drug delivery of anticancer chemotherapeutic drugs targeting breast cancer *Recent Pat. Anti-cancer Drug Discov.* **18** 325–42

[57] Tan Y L and Ho H K 2018 Navigating albumin-based nanoparticles through various drug delivery routes *Drug Discov. Today* **23** 1108–14

[58] van Eerden R A, Mathijssen R H and Koolen S L 2020 Recent clinical developments of nanomediated drug delivery systems of taxanes for the treatment of cancer *Int. J. Nanomed.* **15** 8151–66

[59] Savaliya R, Shah D, Singh R, Kumar A, Shanker R, Dhawan A *et al* 2015 Nanotechnology in disease diagnostic techniques *Curr. Drug Metab.* **16** 645–61

[60] Mughal S S 2022 Diagnosis and treatment of diseases by using metallic nanoparticles-a review *Authorea Preprints* https://doi.org/10.22541/au.166401168.84305772/v1

[61] Rajasundari K and Ilamurugu K 2011 Nanotechnology and its applications in medical diagnosis *J. Basic Appl. Chem.* **1** 26–32

[62] Li W, Wang H, Zhao Z, Gao H, Liu C, Zhu L *et al* 2019 Emerging nanotechnologies for liquid biopsy: the detection of circulating tumor cells and extracellular vesicles *Adv. Mater.* **31** 1805344

[63] Kunjachan S, Ehling J, Storm G, Kiessling F and Lammers T 2015 Noninvasive imaging of nanomedicines and nanotheranostics: principles, progress, and prospects *Chem. Rev.* **115** 10907–37

[64] Gallamini A, Zwarthoed C and Borra A 2014 Positron emission tomography (PET) in oncology *Cancers* **6** 1821–89

[65] Lim E-K, Kim T, Paik S, Haam S, Huh Y-M and Leec K 2021 Nanomaterials for theranostics: recent advances and future challenges *Nanomaterials and Neoplasms* (CRC Press) pp 587–775

[66] Kalash R S, Lakshmanan V K, Cho C-S and Park I-K 2016 Theranostics *Biomaterials Nanoarchitectonics* (Amsterdam: Elsevier) pp 197–215

[67] Lee D Y and Li K C 2011 Molecular theranostics: a primer for the imaging professional *Am. J. Roentgenol* **197** 318–24

[68] Moldwin A, Demner-Fushman D and Goodwin T R 2021 Empirical findings on the role of structured data, unstructured data, and their combination for automatic clinical phenotyping *AMIA Jt. Summits Transl. Sci. Proc.* **2021** 445

[69] Darcy A M, Louie A K and Roberts L W 2016 Machine learning and the profession of medicine *JAMA* **315** 551–2

[70] Murff H J, FitzHenry F, Matheny M E, Gentry N, Kotter K L, Crimin K *et al* 2011 Automated identification of postoperative complications within an electronic medical record using natural language processing *JAMA* **306** 848–55

[71] Karakülah G, Dicle O, Koşaner Ö, Suner A, Birant Ç C, Berber T *et al* 2014 Computer based extraction of phenoptypic features of human congenital anomalies from the digital literature with natural language processing techniques *Stud. Health Technol. Inform.* **205** 570–4

[72] Sajda P 2006 Machine learning for detection and diagnosis of disease *Annu. Rev. Biomed. Eng.* **8** 537–65

[73] Nichols J A, Herbert Chan H W and Baker M A 2019 Machine learning: applications of artificial intelligence to imaging and diagnosis *Biophys. Rev.* **11** 111–8

[74] Xu S, Guo J, Zhang G and Bie R 2020 Automated detection of multiple lesions on chest x-ray images: classification using a neural network technique with association-specific contexts *Appl. Sci.* **10** 1742

[75] Singh C 2021 Medical imaging using deep learning models *Eur. J. Eng. Tech. Res.* **6** 156–67

[76] Soffer S, Ben-Cohen A, Shimon O, Amitai M M, Greenspan H and Klang E 2019 Convolutional neural networks for radiologic images: a radiologist's guide *Radiology* **290** 590–606

[77] Kumar Y, Koul A, Singla R and Ijaz M F 2023 Artificial intelligence in disease diagnosis: a systematic literature review, synthesizing framework and future research agenda *J. Ambient Intell. Humaniz. Comput* **14** 8459–86

[78] Hussain S, Mubeen I, Ullah N, Shah S S U D, Khan B A, Zahoor M *et al* 2022 Modern diagnostic imaging technique applications and risk factors in the medical field: a review *BioMed. Res. Int.* **2022** 5164970

[79] Hudaa S, Setiyadi D B P, Lydia E L, Shankar K, Nguyen P T, Hashim W *et al* 2019 Natural language processing utilization in healthcare *Int. J. Eng. Adv. Technol.* **8** 1117–20

[80] Zhou B, Yang G, Shi Z and Ma S 2022 Natural language processing for smart healthcare *IEEE Rev. Biomed. Eng* **17** 4–18

[81] Rana M S and Shuford J 2024 AI in healthcare: transforming patient care through predictive analytics and decision support systems *J. Artif. Intell. Gen. Sci. (JAIGS)* **1** https://doi.org/10.60087/jaigs.v1i1.30

[82] Parikh R B, Gdowski A, Patt D A, Hertler A, Mermel C and Bekelman J E 2019 Using big data and predictive analytics to determine patient risk in oncology *American Society of Clinical Oncology Educational Book* **vol 39** (ASCO) pp e53–e8

[83] Rumsfeld J S, Joynt K E and Maddox T M 2016 Big data analytics to improve cardiovascular care: promise and challenges *Nat. Rev. Cardiol.* **13** 350–9

[84] Mei L, Zhang Z, Zhao L, Huang L, Yang X-L, Tang J *et al* 2013 Pharmaceutical nanotechnology for oral delivery of anticancer drugs *Adv. Drug Deliv. Rev.* **65** 880–90

[85] Agrawal U, Sharma R, Gupta M and Vyas S P 2014 Is nanotechnology a boon for oral drug delivery? *Drug Discov. Today* **19** 1530–46

[86] Emeje M O, Obidike I C, Akpabio E I and Ofoefule S I 2012 Nanotechnology in drug delivery *Recent Advances in Novel Drug Carrier Systems* **vol 1** (Books on Demand) pp 69–106

[87] Xu M, Han X, Xiong H, Gao Y, Xu B, Zhu G *et al* 2023 Cancer nanomedicine: emerging strategies and therapeutic potentials *Molecules* **28** 5145

[88] Alshangiti D M, El-Damhougy T K, Zaher A and Madani M 2023 Revolutionizing biomedicine: advancements, applications, and prospects of nanocomposite macromolecular carbohydrate-based hydrogel biomaterials: a review *RSC Adv.* **13** 35251–91

[89] Tiwari P, Yadav K, Shukla R P, Gautam S, Marwaha D, Sharma M *et al* 2023 Surface modification strategies in translocating nano-vesicles across different barriers and the role of bio-vesicles in improving anticancer therapy *J. Control. Release* **363** 290–348

[90] Shahzaib A, Kamran L A and Nishat N 2023 The Biomolecule-MOF nexus: recent advancements in biometal-organic frameworks (Bio-MOFs) and their multifaceted applications *Mater. Today Chem.* **34** 101781

[91] Mhetre R M, Waghmode R V, Khyamgonde S S, Nilee R S, Sable V U and Jadhav R I 2023 Liposome: an advanced pharmaceutical carrier in novel drug delivery system *Int. J. Sci. Res. Arch* **10** 874–94

[92] Vora L K, Sabri A H, Naser Y, Himawan A, Hutton A R, Anjani Q K *et al* 2023 Long-acting microneedle formulations *Adv. Drug Deliv. Rev.* **201** 115055

[93] Ghosh S, Ghosh S, Sharma H, Bhaskar R, Han S S and Sinha J K 2023 Harnessing the power of biological macromolecules in hydrogels for controlled drug release in the central nervous system: a review *Int. J. Biol. Macromol.* **254** 127708

[94] Pu Y, Fan X, Zhang Z, Guo Z, Pan Q, Gao W *et al* 2023 Harnessing polymer-derived drug delivery systems for combating inflammatory bowel disease *J. Control. Release* **354** 1–18

[95] Wei J, Mu J, Tang Y, Qin D, Duan J and Wu A 2023 Next-generation nanomaterials: advancing ocular anti-inflammatory drug therapy *J. Nanobiotechnol.* **21** 282

[96] Kunchanur M, Mannur V K, Raghuwanshi L and Mastiholimath V 2023 Design characterization and stability studies of mesalamine loaded solid lipid nanoparticles *Res. J. Pharm. Technol.* **16** 4767–73

[97] Verkhovskii R A, Ivanov A N, Lengert E V, Tulyakova K A, Shilyagina N Y and Ermakov A V 2023 Current principles, challenges, and new metrics in pH-responsive drug delivery systems for systemic cancer therapy *Pharmaceutics* **15** 1566

[98] Dressman J 2023 Comparative dissolution of Budesonide from four commercially available products for oral administration: implications for interchangeablity *Dissolution Technol.* **30** 224–9

[99] Azehaf H, Benzine Y, Tagzirt M, Skiba M and Karrout Y 2023 Microbiota-sensitive drug delivery systems based on natural polysaccharides for colon targeting *Drug Discov. Today* **28** 103606

[100] Yue N-n, Xu H-m, Xu J, Zhu M-z, Zhang Y, Tian C-M *et al* 2023 Application of nanoparticles in the diagnosis of gastrointestinal diseases: a complete future perspective *Int. J. Nanomed.* **18** 4143–70

[101] Dhamija P, Mehata A K, Setia A, Priya V, Malik A K, Bonlawar J *et al* 2023 Nanotheranostics: molecular diagnostics and nanotherapeutic evaluation by photoacoustic/ultrasound imaging in small animals *Mol. Pharm.* **20** 6010–34

[102] Yang J, Feng J, Yang S, Xu Y and Shen Z 2023 Exceedingly small magnetic iron oxide nanoparticles for T1-weighted magnetic resonance imaging and imaging-guided therapy of tumors *Small* **19** 2302856
[103] Tan K F, In L L A and Vijayaraj Kumar P 2023 Surface functionalization of gold nanoparticles for targeting the tumor microenvironment to improve antitumor efficiency *ACS Appl. Bio Mater.* **6** 2944–81
[104] Mahaki H, Mansourian M, Meshkat Z, Avan A, Hossein Shafiee M, Mahmoudian R A *et al* 2023 Nanoparticles containing oxaliplatin and the treatment of colorectal cancer *Curr. Pharm. Des* **29** 3018–39
[105] Li C-H, Chan M-H, Chang Y-C and Hsiao M 2023 Gold nanoparticles as a biosensor for cancer biomarker determination *Molecules* **28** 364
[106] Lu Y, Pan X, Nie Q, Zhou Z, Dai X and Liu O 2023 Administration methods of lipid-based nanoparticle delivery systems for cancer treatment *Biomater. Sci.* **11** 3800–12
[107] Li M, Sun X, Yin M, Shen J and Yan S 2023 Recent advances in nanoparticle-mediated co-delivery system: a promising strategy in medical and agricultural field *Int. J. Mol. Sci.* **24** 5121
[108] Qu J, Yang J, Chen M and Zhai A 2023 Anti-human gastric cancer study of gold nanoparticles synthesized using *Alhagi maurorum Inorg. Chem. Commun.* **151** 109859
[109] Marques A C, Costa P C, Velho S and Amaral M H 2023 Lipid nanoparticles functionalized with antibodies for anticancer drug therapy *Pharmaceutics* **15** 216
[110] Rahman M 2023 Magnetic resonance imaging and iron-oxide nanoparticles in the era of personalized medicine *Nanotheranostics* **7** 424
[111] Gary P J, Lal A, Simonetto D A, Gajic O and de Moraes A G 2023 Acute on chronic liver failure: prognostic models and artificial intelligence applications *Hepatol. Commun.* **7** e0095
[112] D'Amico G, Colli A, Malizia G and Casazza G 2023 The potential role of machine learning in modelling advanced chronic liver disease *Dig. Liver Dis* **55** 704–13
[113] Yip T C-F, Lyu F, Lin H, Li G, Yuen P-C, Wong V W-S *et al* 2023 Non-invasive biomarkers for liver inflammation in non-alcoholic fatty liver disease: present and future *Clin. Mol. Hepatol* **29** S171
[114] Sai S, Gaur A, Sai R, Chamola V, Guizani M and Rodrigues J J 2024 Generative AI for transformative healthcare: a comprehensive study of emerging models, applications, case studies and limitations *IEEE Access* **12** 31078–106
[115] Stascvych M and Zvarych V 2023 Innovative robotic technologies and artificial intelligence in pharmacy and medicine: paving the way for the future of health care—a review *Big Data Cogn. Comput* **7** 147
[116] Wang Z, Liu Y and Niu X (ed) 2023 Application of artificial intelligence for improving early detection and prediction of therapeutic outcomes for gastric cancer in the era of precision oncology *Seminars in Cancer Biology* (Amsterdam: Elsevier)
[117] Stan-Ilie M, Sandru V, Constantinescu G, Plotogea O-M, Rinja E M, Tincu I F *et al* 2023 Artificial intelligence—the rising star in the field of gastroenterology and hepatology *Diagnostics* **13** 662
[118] Siripurapu S, Darimireddy N K, Chehri A, Sridhar B and Paramkusam A 2023 Technological advancements and elucidation gadgets for healthcare applications: an exhaustive methodological review-part-I (AI, big data, block chain, open-source technologies, and cloud computing) *Electronics* **12** 750
[119] Jagsi R, Suresh K, Krenz C D, Jones R D, Griffith K A, Perry L *et al* 2023 Health data sharing perspectives of patients receiving care in cancerlinq-participating oncology practices *JCO Oncol. Pract* **19** 626–36

[120] Chen Z, Jain A, Liu H, Zhao Z and Cheng K 2019 Targeted drug delivery to hepatic stellate cells for the treatment of liver fibrosis *J. Pharmacol. Exp. Ther.* **370** 695–702

[121] Salunkhe S A, Chitkara D, Mahato R I and Mittal A 2021 Lipid based nanocarriers for effective drug delivery and treatment of diabetes associated liver fibrosis *Adv. Drug Deliv. Rev.* **173** 394–415

[122] Bartneck M, Warzecha K T and Tacke F 2014 Therapeutic targeting of liver inflammation and fibrosis by nanomedicine *Hepatobil. Surg. Nutr.* **3** 364

[123] Kudo S e, Mori Y, Misawa M, Takeda K, Kudo T, Itoh H *et al* 2019 Artificial intelligence and colonoscopy: current status and future perspectives *Dig. Endosc.* **31** 363–71

[124] Suzuki K 2013 Pixel-based machine learning in computer-aided diagnosis of lung and colon cancer *Machine Learning in Healthcare Informatics* (Berlin: Springer) pp 81–112

[125] Chadebecq F, Lovat L B and Stoyanov D 2023 Artificial intelligence and automation in endoscopy and surgery *Nat. Rev. Gastroenterol. Hepatol.* **20** 171–82

[126] Owais M, Arsalan M, Choi J, Mahmood T and Park K R 2019 Artificial intelligence-based classification of multiple gastrointestinal diseases using endoscopy videos for clinical diagnosis *J. Clin. Med.* **8** 986

[127] Yin J, Ngiam K Y and Teo H H 2021 Role of artificial intelligence applications in real-life clinical practice: systematic review *J. Med. Internet Res.* **23** e25759

[128] Kröner P T, Engels M M, Glicksberg B S, Johnson K W, Mzaik O, van Hooft J E *et al* 2021 Artificial intelligence in gastroenterology: a state-of-the-art review *World J. Gastroenterol.* **27** 6794

[129] Berbís M A, Aneiros-Fernández J, Olivares F J M, Nava E and Luna A 2021 Role of artificial intelligence in multidisciplinary imaging diagnosis of gastrointestinal diseases *World J. Gastroenterol.* **27** 4395

[130] Halegoua-De Marzio D and Arastu S 2021 Gastrointestinal diseases: sex and gender evidence in liver lesions, gastroesophageal reflux, and inflammatory bowel disease *How Sex and Gender Impact Clinical Practice* (Amsterdam: Elsevier) pp 129–52

IOP Publishing

Nanobiotechnology and Artificial Intelligence in Gastrointestinal Diseases

Vivek K Chaturvedi, Anurag Kumar Singh, Jay Singh and Dawesh P Yadav

Chapter 2

Nano-biosensors for diagnosis of gastrointestinal diseases

Mazharul Haque, Mohammad Zafaryab and Komal Vig

Alteration in the gastrointestinal (GI) tract leads to the various GI diseases. The common GI ailments include indigestion, irritable bowel syndrome (IBS), acid reflux, hemorrhoids and colon cancer etc. The affected population was estimated as 3.7% of the population worldwide in 2016 (a 23% increase from 1990) and still elevation in these figures is the prime focus of concern. The unprecedented burden due to intestinal and intestine-originated disorders has been of primary concern for researchers and clinicians. In this chapter we will address the application of nano-biosensors for detection and diagnosing GI-related diseases and point out the utmost importance of combining diagnosis and treatment. The future application of nano-biosensors in detecting GI-related biomarkers for early diagnosis and the expectation of integrating material science and medical fields will be also addressed. Recent advances in nanotechnology have opened new dimensions in the diagnosis and treatment of GI-derived disorders. The advancement due to integration of these fields may prove an important mediator in improving the clinical translation. Technology based on nanoparticles improves the precision of diagnosis when combined with biosensors, with limited side effects and advanced diagnosis and therapy of GI disorders. Currently, focus towards development of nano-biosensors by researchers from the various fields has attracted considerable interest to achieve advancement in applications in order to improve sensitivity and specificity. The introduction of nanomaterials-based sensors, which are commonly known as nano-biosensors is currently a widely investigated method over recent decades for the various applications in healthcare. These nano-biosensors have been employed for detection of numerous target analytes including microorganisms, virus, nucleic acids, peptides, proteins for the early diagnosis of pathogens causing pathogenesis. These nano-based biosensors enable us to detect the target analytes very quickly and efficiently in the system. Nanomaterials are very reactive in Nature, which enhances the catalytic, physical as well as chemical characteristics of the biosensor giving rise to enhanced sensitivity and specificity. The new techniques have been proved as a breakthrough in improving sensitive detection and quantification of certain parameters. These nano-biosensors have emerged with many possibilities due to unique properties such as sensitivity, simplicity, robustness and cost-effectiveness, providing the bridge between diagnosis and treatment.

2.1 Introduction

Gastrointestinal diseases (GIDs) usually refer to diseases involving the GI tract. The most common organs affected due to GI illness are the esophagus, stomach, small intestine, large intestine and rectum along with associated accessory organs including liver, gallbladder, and pancreas as well. One study estimated about 88.99 million cases of GIDs in 2019, causing 2.56 million deaths worldwide because of GIDs [1]. In 2019 nearly 375 170 deaths were estimated due to GI-related diseases, accounting for 215 168 deaths in men, and 160 002 deaths in women in the United States. The increased cases due to GI-related diseases amounting to 46.19 million are mainly in low and middle income countries. Statistical projections indicate increase of GIDs-associated problems in the near future as a mortality rate depicted in figure 2.1.

GI refers to disorder of the digestive tract. GIDs affect our GI tract from mouth to anus. The affects are functional and structural. The common examples of GIDs are colitis, lactose intolerance, food poisoning and diarrhea. The most commonly observed symptoms include bloating, constipation, heartburn, incontinence, nausea,

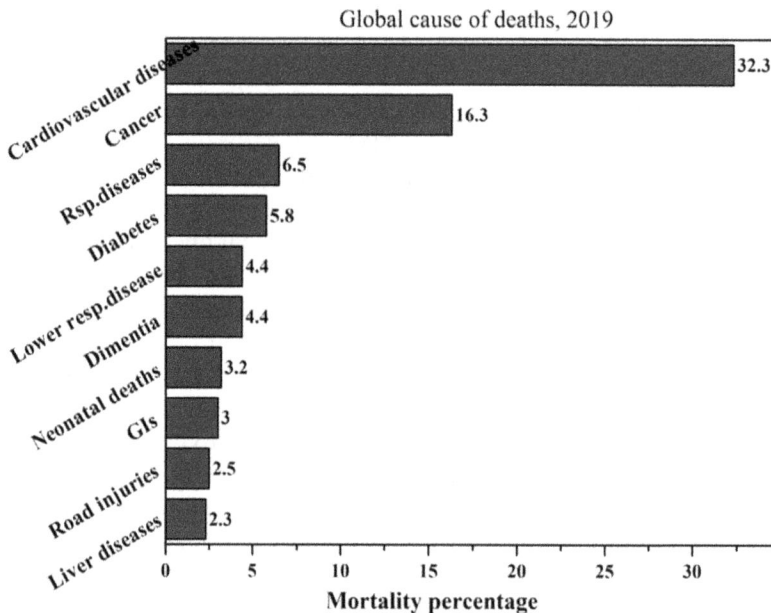

Figure 2.1. Global death burden due to various diseases.

and vomiting. Those affected experience abdominal pain and difficulties with swallowing. Men frequently present unusual symptoms in comparison to women and about 8 in 100 possess GID in comparison to 4 in 100 above the age of seventy five [2]. GID might give rise to physical, mental and social distress.

2.2 Causes

Most GIDs take place due to bacterial infections, inflammation, genetics, and mental distress. Various risk factors contribute to the development of various health conditions, including smoking, obesity, excessive alcohol use, overuse of specific medications, and a family history of such conditions [3]. There are other risk factors including old age, male gender and past GID history [4]. Many risk factors for GID can be potentially reduced such as smoking, obesity and lack of physical activity [5]. Smoking accounts for around 1.68%, whereas alcohol is responsible for 26.93% of GID [1]. The fundamental mechanism underlying GI disorders involves the perturbation of the GI tract's regular functioning, which encompasses the processes of digestion and absorption of ingested nutrients, as well as the elimination of waste products resulting from digestion [6]. There are various tests available for diagnosis such as endoscopy, ultrasound, CT scan and x-ray but there are a significant number of false positives [7].

2.3 Mechanism

GI issues frequently show identical symptoms and are commonly diagnosed solely on the basis of symptoms. To alleviate the signs of GI illnesses, numerous therapy methods have been developed. Few of them, however, may offer total relief from reflux symptoms, indigestion, abdominal pain, diarrhea, and constipation. The phenomenon of overlaps in GI disorders is likely attributed to several mechanisms, such as aberrant GI motility, visceral hypersensitivity, reduced GI mucosa barrier, and central nervous system variables. However, there is a scarcity of comprehensive investigations in this area, and the exact reasons of these overlaps remain unknown. Consequently, there are still unmet therapeutic needs and ambiguous criteria of non-neoplastic GI diseases. The continuous effectiveness of one Chinese formula, SNS, on GI disorders may offer a fresh perspective and a different angle. Traditional Chinese medicine (TCM) is used in this research of Si-Ni-San (SNS) synthesized data to validate the common causes behind digestive problems. The first conceivable explanation for the ostensibly higher incidence of overlaps in GI diseases may be 'reflux.' The regurgitation of the contents of the lower digestive tract into upper organs is one way to define 'reflux.' Functional dyspepsia and IBS were linked to disrupted motility, according to research. Numerous studies have also shown a direct link between gastrointestinal reflux disease (GERD) and ulcerative colitis, IBS, and functional dyspepsia. However, bacterial dysbiosis and migration may play a significant role in the pathogenesis of reflux illnesses. The upper GI bacteria are highlighted in the Walker review paper along with their links to conditions including IBS and celiac disease. The findings of Yang and colleagues also raise the question of whether microbiome dysbiosis may play a role in the etiology of GI illnesses associated with reflux. It is commonly recognized that several annulus muscles serve as 'gates' or 'check-points' for one-way passage in the GI tract. These muscles include the orbicularis oris, preventriculus, pylorus, oddi sphincters, ileocecal valve, aperture of the vermiform appendix, and anus. To prevent opening and effacement when pressed by lower contents, each of the 'gates' has smooth muscle or sphincter barriers fixed to them. When this is not done, instances of lower gut juice refluxing into the higher digestive tracts occur. One frequent approach relies on 'reflux' because these sphincters and smooth muscles are incapable of doing so. Instances of lower gut juice refluxing into the higher digestive tracts occur when this is not done. As a result of these sphincters' and smooth muscles' incapacity, one common mechanism depends on 'reflux'. Sphincters play a crucial role in GI processes. According to a manometric study, IBS patients had considerably lower esophageal sphincter pressures than controls with same ages and sexes. Other researches find that in patients with damaged sphincters and smooth muscles, GI hormones, glucose, and oxidative free radicals fluctuate. It is interesting to note that TCM formulas like SNS consistently work to maintain the sphincters' normal function, which means they can treat most reflux-related illnesses, if not all of them [8].

2.4 Diagnosis

The identification of GI disorders can be accomplished by the detection of several biomarkers in the bloodstream, encompassing symptoms such as dyspepsia and inflammatory bowel illnesses. A range of diagnostic biomarkers have been identified, encompassing serological, antibody-based, immunological, fecal, and genetic biomarkers. C-reactive protein (CRP) estimation from a blood test is considered to be most reliable [9]. The greater sensitivity and specificity make it preferable over other tests to examine GI problems. Meanwhile, the concentration of CRP in blood can be elevated by many folds in comparison to that of normal baseline value after initial symptoms appear for GI which reaches the maximum value. This unique characteristic of CRP marks it as as one of the earliest biomarkers for GID, which can allow it to be further utilized to confirm early diagnosis of GID onset. Therefore, the concentration of CRP in the bloodstream serves as a significant protein marker indicating the magnitude of CRP production, which in turn induces hepatocytes to selectively produce positive acute-phase proteins rather than negative-phase proteins [9]. Extensive research has been conducted on the topic of mucosal immunity, focusing specifically on the immunological features of IBD, with particular emphasis on the T-cell response. The available information indicates that the inherent decline in immune system function contributes to an inadequate reaction to intestinal inflammation in individuals with IBD. Nevertheless, it has been observed that certain immune regulatory mediators exhibit an elevation within the intestinal mucosa of individuals diagnosed with IBD.

2.5 Prognosis

The prognosis post GI differs significantly based on the degree and site of the GI damage, the progress and administration of complications. Prognosis rate is worst in older age, and socially isolated persons. The diagnostic evaluation typically focuses on the presenting symptoms of vomiting, weight loss, and anorexia, as well as the identification of specific indications such as melena, hematemesis, and abdominal discomfort. Several of these canine gastric mucosa exhibited symptoms indicative with GI preformation or peritonitis. The prescribed course of action involves either surgical intervention or medical care, which may encompass the administration of omeprazole, famotidine, sucralfate, or octreotide. Due to the frequent occurrence of metastases, the prognosis for recovery is often unfavorable.

2.6 Present methods of detection

Traditional methods for diagnosis of GIDs based on classical methods include x-ray, computed tomography scan (CT scan), magnetic resonance imaging (MRI), ultrasound and endoscopy depend on laboratory tests that may have long procedure from taking samples to receiving results [10]. A lot of work has gone into creating breakthrough diagnostic and treatment techniques to extend patient survival and improve quality of life. In order to substantially improve patient outcomes, advancements in image-based detection, personalized medicine distribution, and metastases ablation could be pursued. Traditional procedures sometimes fail to meet patients' expectations due to a lack of precision and insufficient patient categorization. There is a need for more specialized, highly targeted treatments. Nanotechnologies and nanodevices have been researched for their potential applications in advancing tailored therapy strategies in order to achieve this. A number of methods for various fabricated biosensors are reported as electrochemical (amperometric, potentiometric, conductometric), optical (fluorescence, refractive index, luminescence), capacitive biosensors, piezoelectric or calorimetric and field-effect transistor for quantification of various biomarkers. Biosensors may play a key responsibility as a substitute to classical methods of GIDs detection. They offer many advantages such as being rapid, robust, cost effective, user-friendly and having the ability for multi-analyte testing [11]. They do not require costly and time-consuming laboratory tests. Hence, the healthcare services cost can be reduced. The recent trend is to make use of nanomaterials having different morphology, size and composition of materials for biosensors owing to their unique properties including conductivity, high surface-to-volume ratio as well as good biocompatibility that leads to enhanced performance [12]. A number of nanomaterials such as those based on carbon (carbon nanotubes, graphene), metal nanoparticles (silver, gold, platinum, and copper), quantum dots of semiconductors (Cd, Ge, Te, Se), metal oxides (ZnO, SnO_2, TiO_2, CeO_2 and Al_2O_3) and silicon/gallium/indium etc, have been incorporated into biosensors for detection of various biomarkers [13]. Nanomaterials based on gold have been exploited for designing of different biosensors due to their exceptional electrical, optical as well as mechanical properties, however, high cost limits their use [14].

2.7 Biosensors

A biosensor can be defined as an analytical device, employed to detect any analyte (biomolecule), that combines a physico-chemical detector consisting of biological components [15]. The sensitive biological element is recognized when it interacts or binds with the target analyte. However, the target analyte may also interact directly with the transducer. The main function of the transducer or the detector component is to transform one signal to another resulting as the analyte interacts with the biological or the detector element directly, to easily detect and quantify. The biosensor has a reader device combined with a connected electronics or signal processors display so the output results in a user-friendly way [16]. The general aim in designing a biosensor is to provide quick, suitable point-of-care testing.

2.7.1 Components of biosensors

A biosensor is generally comprised of three parts depicted as in figure 2.2: the biological element as analyte viz. nucleic acids, enzymes, antibodies, cell receptors etc; a biorecognition site, transducer component; and a reader device that consists of the electronic system consisting of a signal amplifier, processor and display. Biomolecules expressed from organisms are used as receptors to interact with the target analyte acting as a recognition element known as a bioreceptor. The transducer measures output signal obtained from interaction which is proportional to the target analyte present in the sample.

Biosensors were divided into three generations: the first generation biosensors demonstrated the electrical response due to diffusion of the typical product of the involved reaction to the transducer; the second generation biosensors involved specific mediators between the transducer and the reaction towards production of improved response; and in the third generation biosensors there is no involvement of product or mediator, the reaction itself is the basis of the response.

2.7.2 Types of biosensors

Biosensors can be grouped on the basis of biorecognition components and type of transducer utilized. They can be electrochemical, optical and piezoelectric depending on the type of transducer that is used. The biosensor could be referred as an immunosensor (antibody, antigens, and biomarkers), enzymatic, DNA or RNA biosensor, microbial biosensor and whole-cell sensor etc, based on the biorecognition elements, as shown in figure 2.3.

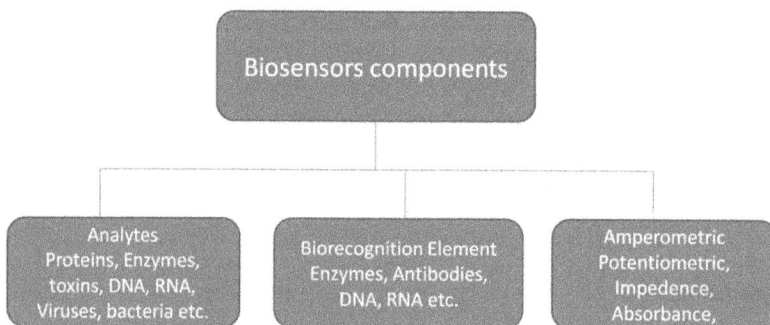

Figure 2.2. Main components of a biosensor.

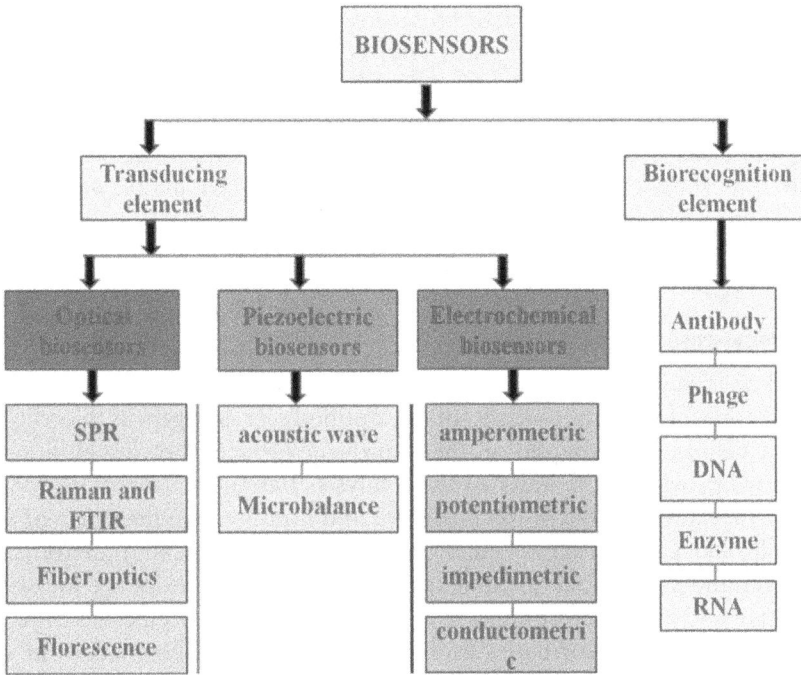

Figure 2.3. Types of biosensors.

2.7.3 Enzyme based biosensors

Enzymes are proteins which act as catalysts in chemical or biological processes. An enzyme catalyzes and enhances the rate of chemical or biological reaction at all chemical changes without contributing to the reaction. The enzyme converts initially a substrate into new products. The enzymes are immobilized on the surface of the transducer in an enzymatic biosensor, which produces an output signal during the reaction with the target analyte. The enzymatic biosensors convert output signal produced from enzymatic reaction into measurable signal in the form of optical, colorimetric, piezoelectric and electrochemical etc. The enzyme-based biosensors have been employed to detect various biomarkers including sugar, cholesterol, urea during onset or progression of disease.

2.7.4 Affinity biosensors

Affinity biosensors are based on a recognition element derived from biological molecules including antibody, DNA, receptor protein, biomemetic materials combined with a transducer to produce a measurable output signal that is proportional to the concentration of target analyte [17]. The assays based on affinity are usually quite complex and require different components and configuration needs as a multistep process. However, this technique has varying complexity in comparison to a simple assays-based immunosensor to complex ELISA and electrophysiological receptor.

The operational characteristics of biosensors are determined by their design and structural features. The sensor sensitivity, cost, physical limitations and signal processing properties are primarily determined by the signal transducer. The instrument cost is determined by the signal transducer primarily. This also decides the size, portability, data acquisition and signal processing. The sensor interface plays an important role in operational characteristics in many ways owing to binding of an analyte with a bio-affinity-based sensor that is stoichiometric in nature, therefore immobilization of affinity element is crucial.

2.7.5 Immunosensors

Analytical devices which are precisely based on affinity are known as immunosensors. Such type of sensors consists of an antibody or antigen as biorecognition moieties, which are immobilized on the transducer surface, showing immunochemical reactions providing the basis of the analysis. Immunosensors have long been known for their pivotal role in the label-free and non-invasive detection of various biomolecules like cancerous molecules, proteins, lipids, LDLs and microorganisms like bacteria and viruses due to high specificity. Immunosensors are known to be very sensitive and could detect molar concentration of biomolecules up to pico- and femto-range. Immunosensor-based tools are able to detect the changes in various parameters like RI, current, resistance etc, which come from the immunocomplexes formed by the reaction occuring between the antigen and antibody.

Traditionally, an immunoassay employs an antibody (Y) that possesses two sites capable of binding to antigens. The binding between an antigen and its corresponding antibody is characterized by a high degree of specificity, reproducibility, and suitability for detecting a wide range of target biomolecules in biosensing applications. The paratope refers to a specific binding region that is located on the surface of Y and is responsible for recognizing and attaching to the antigen (Ag). However, an antigen possesses an epitope that plays a crucial role in the identification process of the immune system, namely through the assistance of antibodies or T cells. The creation of an Ag–Y complex necessitates a greater level of complementarity between the binding sites of Ag and Y in order to facilitate non-covalent interaction.

2.7.6 Microbial biosensors

Microbial biosensors utilize microorganisms with a transducer to produce rapid, accurate and sensitive detection of target analytes. These biosensors are used in diverse fields such as medicine, monitoring of the environment, food processing, defense and safety. The former microbial biosensors utilized the functions of respiration and metabolism to detect a substance as substrate or inhibitor of these processes. Currently, a microorganism based on a reporter gene fused with an inducible gene promoter is modified genetically and widely used to assay bioavability and toxicity. Microorganisms basically provide improvement of performance to detect a range of chemical substances via genetic modification in the broad range of pH and temperature, making them an ideal biological sensing material [18].

2.7.7 DNA-based biosensors

DNA-based sensors employ nucleic acids as the biorecognition elements on the surfaces of transducers. DNA-based biosensors have recently emerged as a compelling approach due to their quick performance and cost-effectiveness in identifying specific DNA sequences. These techniques are dependent on the immobilization of a DNA probe, which consists of a single-stranded oligonucleotide, onto the surface of a transducer. The transducers under consideration encompass optical, electrochemical, and piezo-electric varieties. The probe DNA exhibits specificity towards the target complementary DNA sequence, which is identified by the process of hybridization, leading to the generation of a detectable signal. The conversion of the specific binding energy between a single stranded DNA probe and its complementary DNA strand results in the generation of relative output signals. Different amplification techniques including electrochemicals such as amperometric, potentiometric and impedimetric and optical such as SPR, absorption, FRET, fluorescence etc, have been employed for fabrication of DNA-based sensors. Various transducing materials such as carbon-based, metal nanoparticles, semiconductor nanomaterials, nanocomposites etc have been utilized due to their large surface-to-volume ratio and biocompatibity with DNA [19].

2.7.8 Phage sensors

In this method a bacteriophage is immobilized at the surface of the sensor to detect pathogens in the sample. Phage-mediated biosensors demonstrate high sensitivity, precision, and dependability in their outcomes. Biosensors utilizing bacteriophages have been employed for the direct identification of pathogens in perishable food items, particularly milk and water [20]. Recently, phages-based optical biosensors have been employed for the diagnosis of food-borne pathogens and several pathogens have been detected using such biosensors.

2.7.9 Optical biosensors

Optical biosensors use an optical transducer for biorecognition of biomolecules that generate a signal directly proportional to the target analyte concentration. Optical biosensors can exploit a range of biological materials as biorecognition elements such as antigens, antibodies, enzymes, nucleic acids, receptors, whole cells and tissues. The change in the optical properties like surface plasmon resonance, evanescent wave fluorescence and optical waveguide interferometery are monitored to measure the interaction of the target analyte with the recognition element [21].

2.7.10 Cantilever-based biosensors

The key element in most of the mechanical biosensors is a cantilever having a specific resonance frequency or amplitude. Cantilever devices measure the quasi-static deflection of the cantilever caused upon binding of biomolecules with a functional group on the device surface. As the biomolecules bind, stress on the surface developed due to electrostatic repulsion or attraction causes the change of frequency/amplitude. The amount of deflection is generally measured by a laser beam incident on the cantilever. This technique has been employed to examine binding proteins and DNA [22].

2.7.11 Bio-MEMS

Biomedical (or biological) microelectromechanical systems (Bio-MEMS) have emerged as a new area for biological and medical applications. It is often referred as lab-on-a-chip or micro total analysis system. This method is more focused on technology of mechanical parts and microfabrication for various applications. Alternatively, lab-on-a-chip is related to miniaturization and incorporation of laboratory processes and experiments on a single chip. Bio-MEMS can be broadly defined as the science of operating at microscale level for biomedical and biological applications such as proteomics, genomics, point-of-care testing etc [23].

2.8 Physical biosensors

2.8.1 Thermometric biosensors

The fundamental properties of biological reactions such as absorption and heat evolution are exploited by thermoelectric biosensors. Calorimetric is an example of thermometric techniques that measure the heat change to calculate degree of reaction or structural dynamics of biomolecules in a solution by measuring the temperature change of circulating fluid due to reaction between substrate and immobilized enzymes. The temperature change evolves both by absorption or radiation of heat during a biochemical reaction which is directly proportional to the molar enthalpy and overall number of products formed in the biochemical reaction.

2.8.2 Acoustic biosensors

Acoustic sensors are basically microelectromechanical systems (MEMS) that use modulation of surface acoustic waves as a function of input parameter. The alterations in amplitude, phase, frequency, or time-delay observed between the input and output electrical signals are utilized for the purpose of quantifying the input characteristics. Piezoelectric materials are used in acoustic sensors to generate waves. Due to excellent mechanical properties and stability, quartz is commonly employed as it is abundant in Nature and allows low-cost manufacturing.

2.8.3 Magnetic biosensors

Magnetic biosensors measure the change in properties of the magnetic field like strength, direction and flux as a function of the input parameter. These sensors are divided in two different groups. The first category of sensor is employed to estimate total magnetic field, whereas the second type is used to estimate vector component of the magnetic field and later is utilized to develop a range of sensors employed.

2.8.4 Wearable skins as biosensors

These sensors are currently being used in various biomedical applications. An important example is smart watches integrated with various health-related issues such as heart rate monitor, pulse oxymeters, gyroscope accelerometer etc. Wearable sensors are user-friendly and do not need having technical expertise [24]. The wearable technology extracts information without involving surgical procedures and implantation that may cause long-term effects.

2.9 Electrochemical biosensors

The electrochemical signal is produced during the exclusive reaction between bio-receptors and target analytes mainly as an enzyme kinetic reaction on a transducer surface with improved signal-to-volume proportion and offering label-free and invasive detection. The target analytes are then quantified depending on the strength of output electrical signal in the form of current, voltage, capacitance and impedance etc. This sensor typically consists of three electrodes; a working electrode, a reference electrode and a counter electrode. The reaction occurs at the surface of the electrode leading either to transfer of electrons across the double layer (give rise to a current) or passing through to double-layer potential (causing a voltage). Therefore, either the current or potential is recorded as a function of input analyte. Electrochemical biosensors are classified on the basis of operating principle such as potentiometric, impedometric, voltammetric, coulometric, conductimetric, amperometric, impedimetric, capacitive etc, which convert the electrochemical reactions into a quantifiable signal.

2.9.1 Potentiometric

This particular chemical biosensor has the capability to ascertain the analytical concentration of a target analyte, whether it is in the form of a gas or a solution. It achieves this by measuring the potential of the electrode, even in the absence of current flow between the working and reference electrodes. The relationship between the value of potential and the concentration of the target analyte in the solution or gas is exactly proportional.

2.9.2 Coulometry methods

This is distinguished from voltammetry and amperometry methods as it does not depend on control of current mass transport to obtain a signal dependent on concentration. This method does not require calibration. In this technique the total current passed is measured directly or indirectly in order to determine the number of passed electrons.

2.9.3 Conductometry methods

The small variation in electrical conductivity of the solution during electrochemical reactions is measured using a sinusoidal signal to avoid the effect of double-layer charging, Faradaic process and concentration polarization by generating an electric field.

2.9.4 Potentiometric titration

This is a chemical analysis technique in which the endpoint is observed using an indicator electrode while changing the concentration during titration and the information is regarding the nature of reaction. These methods are particularly versatile because the indicator electrodes are suitable for examining a wide range of chemical reactions. This technique is reliable, using low cost apparatus and easily available in laboratories.

2.9.4.1 Potentiometric electrochemical cells

The electrochemical cells comprise two half-cells; in each half an electrode is immersed in a solution of ions which play an important role in determining the electrode potential. The two half-cells are connected via a salt bridge which has an inert electrolyte such as KCl. A potentiometric measurement system consists of two electrodes such as reference electrode, anode, cathode and indicator. The potential of a reference electrode is fixed, however, the change of indicators potential depends upon the ion concentration present in the analyte.

2.9.4.1.1 Cyclic voltammetry

Voltammetry electrochemical is a technique in which target analyte information is obtained by measuring the resulting current while varying a potential. Therefore, it is referred as an amperometric tool. Cyclic voltammetry (CV) is valuable to acquire information regarding the electrochemical reaction and redox potential of solutions with target analyte. The voltage is swept in both directions in a range at a fixed rate, as shown in figure 2.4. The enzyme kinetics and progression of the

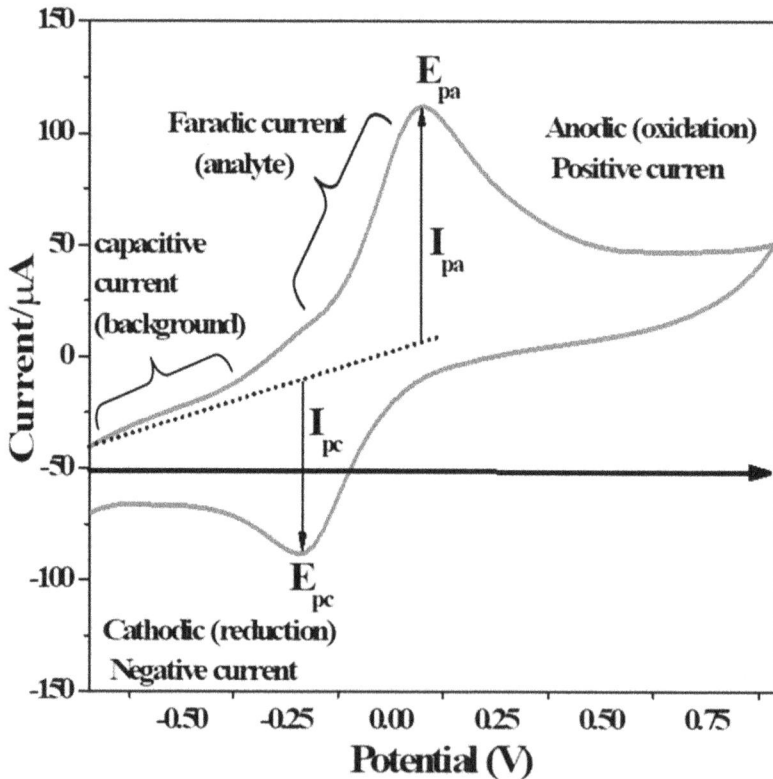

Figure 2.4. Typical voltammogram.

chemical reaction can be monitored by varying the scan rate that offers enough time to permit significant chemical reactions to take place [25]. The current is measured among the working electrode and the counter electrode, while voltage is measured between reference electrode and working electrode. A voltammogram is plotted for different concentrations. The redox peak is obtained and analyzed.

The information regarding the nature of reaction, i.e. reversible, quasi-reversible or non-reversible is estimated from the voltage difference in the oxidation and reduction peaks [26]. The voltammogram shape for a certain compound relies on the scan rate, surface of electrode and concentration of catalyst. For example, increase in concentration of enzymes specific to a reaction at a particular scan rate results in a higher current in comparison to non-catalyzed reactions [27]. CV is not only helpful for sensing but also to understand the processes occurring on the surface of the sensing electrode. The voltammetry methods also measure the current in pulsed mode (current due to charging) upon changing the potential. When potential is applied between working electrode and reference electrode, electron exchange occurs between the working electrode and the electroactive species. The change in the potential difference is due to charging and discharging phenomena by forming an electrical double layer.

2.9.4.1.2 *Impedance spectroscopy*

Electrochemical impedance spectroscopy (EIS) is a powerful analytical tool to estimate the interfacial characteristics of the surface modified electrode. Electrochemical impedance is generally obtained by measuring the current through the cell when AC potential is applied through an electrochemical cell. The angular frequency is varied at a fix applied potential, and the complex impedance is recorded. Therefore, EIS involves the study of both the real and imaginary impedance, referred as electrical resistance and reactance. The information content in EIS is much higher than that obtained using DC techniques. It is also helpful to differentiate between the two electrochemical reactions; to identify diffusion limited reactions and the capacitive behavior of a system.

Impedance spectra are represented by a Nyquist plot which consists of a semicircle region noticed at higher frequencies due to the process of electron transfer at the Z' axis and a linear straight line observed at lower frequencies at an angle of $45°$ to the real axes as shown in figure 2.5. The straight-line segment demonstrates the electron transfer process as diffusion limited. The complex impedance is represented by the sum of real (Z') and imaginary (Z') parts obtained due to resistance and capacitance present in the cell. Charge transfer resistance (R_{ct}) corresponds to the diameter of the semicircle. EIS is capable of studying the intrinsic properties of a material or particular processes that might influence the conductive/resistive or capacitive properties of the electrochemical system. The plot of R_{ct} versus concentration of the analyte is used to extract the information about the system, which makes it the most valuable tool in the development and material analysis for biosensor transduction.

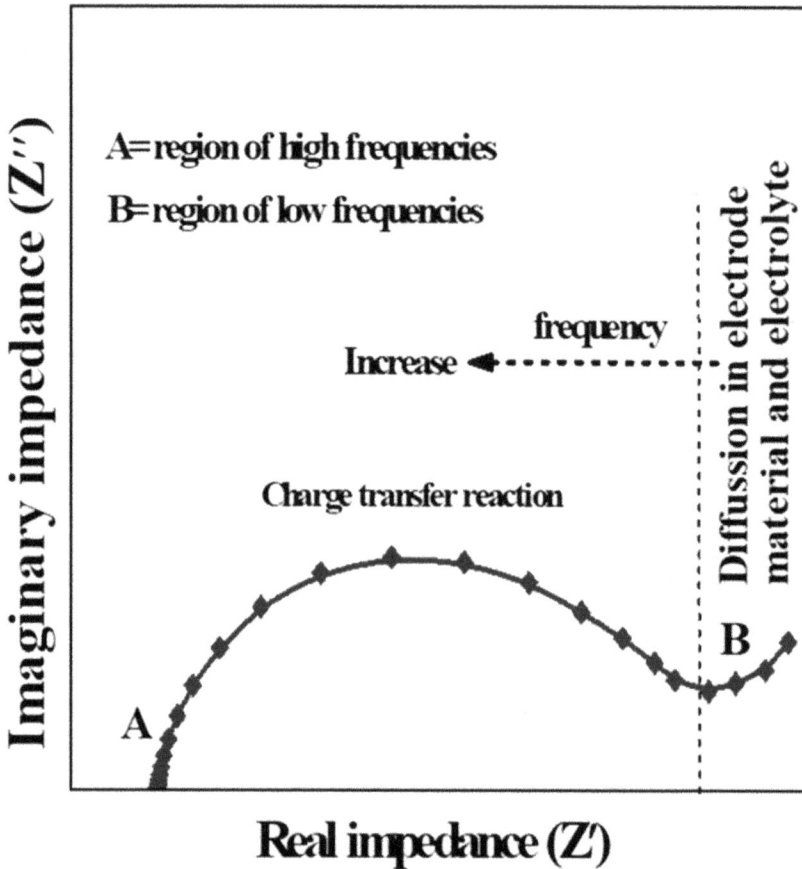

Figure 2.5. Typical EIS curve.

2.10 Materials for biosensors

2.10.1 Nanomaterials for biosensors

Nanomaterials have attracted much interest in the past few years owing to the increasing demand to manage molecules of interest found in the environment. Nanomaterials are grown below 100 nm in all dimensions. Nanotechnology deals with small-sized material, especially below sub-nanometer or a few hundreds of nanometers [3]. Nanomaterials with unique properties have attracted researchers worldwide in different fields including health, food, information technology, security and transport etc. Biosensors have been speculated to realize various needs in the manufacturing of diagnostics with their fast response and portability. Devices for microfluidic biosensors have many advantages, especially in clinical diagnosis. The sensitivity, selectivity and reproducibility of biosensors is still a challenge, and continuous efforts are still being made to improve these parameters and towards the miniaturization of biosensors for quantification of biomolecules together with controlling of microfluids [4]. These miniaturized devices require lowest volume in channels and containers having sizes in microns (10^{-9} to 10^{-18} l), leading to the production of lab-on-a-chip. Nanomaterials have potential for early diagnosis and hence can play a vital role in detecting a disease leading to prognosis and prevention of the disease and improved detection performance with lowest value of limit of detection (LOD). Recently, nanostructured materials having different morphology such as nanowires, nanotubes etc are being explored as transducers in fabrication of biosensors and diagnostic devices. The tailored nanomaterials offer enhanced electrical conductivity, and are biocompatible, therefore, they can be utilized to amplify characteristic output signals [28]. The utilization of nanomaterials has demonstrated to result in improved performance of biosensors such as enhanced sensitivities and lower LOD by magnitude of several orders [29]. Nanostructured materials provide enhanced surface-to-volume ratio, electrocatalytic properties, mechanical strength, chemical activity and diffusivity play a key role in enhanced performance of biosensors.

2.10.2 Gastrointestinal diseases (GIDs) biosensor

The early detection of GIDs plays a significant role in clinical diagnosis and managing of GIDs-related problems or susceptibility to high GI risk, and is important to provide timely therapeutics aid to save lives and reduce healthcare costs. GIDs has become a potential threat to human health and hence rapid, sensitive, accurate, reliable sensing devices are explored for early confirmation of GID [10]. Significant endeavors have been dedicated to the advancement of innovative diagnostic and therapeutic approaches aimed at enhancing patient well-being and extending their lifespan. The enhancement of patient outcomes could be significantly facilitated through advancements in image-based identification, targeted medicine distribution, and metastases ablation. The classical approaches commonly employed in medical practice often fail to meet the expectations of patients as a result of their limited specificity and inadequate patient classification. There is a pressing need for the development of more precise and tailored therapeutic interventions. In pursuit of this objective, researchers have investigated the potential use of nanotechnologies and nano-devices in advancing tailored medicinal techniques. Efforts are also made for early diagnosis of various GI biomarkers for detection of GID such as CRP, anti-neutrophil cytoplasmic antibodies (ANCA), calprotectin etc [30]. Available classical techniques for diagnosis of GID involving classical methods including immunoassays, enzyme-linked immunosorbent assay (ELISA), x-ray, ultrasound, MRI, CT scan, endoscopy etc are performed in central laboratories, which takes a long time to reveal the result after collection of samples from the patient [10].

A number of different methods like electrochemical, capacitor-based biosensors, optical field-effect transistor, piezoelectric or calorimetric biosensors are used for biomarker detection [31, 32]. Nano-biosensors are emerging as a promising substitute to classical methods to detect GIDs biomarkers. These sensors are fast, sensitive, reliable and low concentration level, capable of multi-analyte detection at low-cost, user-friendly and portable [11], and will lead to reduced healthcare expenditure. In addition, nanomaterial-based electrochemicals exhibit better sensor characteristics owing to their unique properties such as conductivity, high surface-to-volume ratio and good biocompatibility with enhanced performance [12, 33].

2.10.2.1 Tailored materials for bio-detection

The identification of physiological and pathological signals within the intestinal system is of utmost importance in order to gain a comprehensive understanding of various disorders. Investigation of the underlying processes inside the GI tract holds promise for advancing the field of oral drug development. This is due to the fact that the absorption of drugs in the intestines is influenced by various factors, including molecular weight, solubility, and others. Overcoming these challenges has long been a key hurdle for numerous pharmaceutical compounds. Given the current focus of numerous contemporary investigations on the conversion of bioactive compounds into oral pharmaceuticals, it becomes imperative to identify and comprehend the receptive signals inside the GI system. While *in vitro* or animal model simulations have successfully discovered physical signals, the number of conclusions drawn from real human body situations remains limited [34]. Currently, the clinical identification of intestinal disorders mostly relies on stool analysis and a limited number of blood-related tests. However, it is important to note that these diagnostic methods do not possess the capability to provide accurate and real-time detection of intestinal diseases. Moreover, the outcomes obtained from the process of detection often lack precision and need a considerable amount of time to be generated.

Moreover, the survival of probes within the digestive system is challenging owing to the unique attributes of the intestinal environment. While the application of conventional molecular probes and antigen–antibody detection methods presents difficulties in real-time detection of the intestine, the signals present in the GI tract still have potential for early intervention in patients to prevent disease progression [35]. The detection and monitoring of intestinal health in contemporary times have proven to be challenging. The primary strategies employed in this circumstance are the utilization of an ingestible device and an *in vitro* customized mechanical analysis.

2.10.2.2 Signals from intestine for detection

Intestinal signals exhibit a significant association with nearly all other organs. While the major activities of the GI tract encompass digestion and absorption, alterations in the physiological composition of the intestine can exert a direct influence on the optimal functioning of several organs such as the kidneys, lungs, brain, liver, and others. One example of potential consequences is the disruption of the intestinal barrier and subsequent translocation of germs, which can lead to illnesses inside the circulatory and respiratory systems [36]. Hence, it is imperative to discern GI symptoms. The assessment and examination of organ functions in the intestine can provide valuable insights into the likelihood of organ damage. This can be achieved by detecting several indicators such as pH, temperature, pressure, gas, and specific compounds.

The most common indicators of abnormal changes in the organs are biomarkers associated with the GI tract. By doing an analysis of the metabolites produced by the gut microbiota, it is possible to explore the correlation between biomarkers and various disorders. The detection of diseases relies on both biological and physical cues. Bowel sounds play a crucial role in the assessment of intestinal obstruction and serve as diagnostic indicators for conditions such as intestinal ischemia and peritonitis. The identification of intestinal contents is a crucial aspect of the study. In order to modify the treatment regimen, it may be necessary to assess the patient's dietary and pharmaceutical consumption through the detection of intestinal contents. Collectively, these characteristics underscore the need of examining gut signals for the purposes of diagnosing illnesses and providing treatment support. Currently, there exists a diverse range of sensors that can be tailored to fulfill specific needs. Electrochemical sensors have the capability to detect many types of waveforms, such as cyclic waves, square waves, and differential pulse, within the GI tract. Voltammetry techniques have the capability to detect bioactive medicinal constituents within the GI tract [37].

2.10.2.3 Sensors for signal detection

Thus far, oral sensors have been employed in various manners for the purpose of detecting microsignals, including alterations in intestinal pH, temperature, and pressure. An example of a commercially available device capable of evaluating the pH levels within the GI tract is the SmartPill capsule endoscope [38]. Furthermore, the biomarkers present in the digestive system, including proteins, DNA, electrolytes, and physiological gases, can be utilized as potential targets for the real-time assessment of both health and disease conditions [39]. For example, the presence of calprotectin and lactoferrin, which are markers of intestinal inflammation, has been found to be correlated with ulcerative colitis. Moreover, the presence of specialized and precise sensing elements enables the identification and analysis of signals within the GI fluid. For instance, the GCN2 molecule in the intestinal region exhibits a robust response to the amino acid signal. Enteritis can be induced by a deficiency of leucine in the intestinal tract. Hence, the presence of intestinal inflammation can be predicted through the monitoring of leucine levels inside the colon [40].

The identification of human diseases can be facilitated by considering not only the small molecules present in the colon, but also the intestinal microbiota, which serves as a significant biomarker. Qin *et al* established a causal relationship between modifications in the human gut microbiota and the occurrence of liver cirrhosis. It is possible to predict the onset of liver disease by monitoring changes in gut flora. Bacterial metabolites are also essential gut signals [41]. According to Yang *et al*'s genome-wide shotgun metagenomic cross-sectional study, significant depression may be triggered by 47 different bacterial species and 50 different metabolites found in feces. Finding these signs may help in figuring out what causes mental illness [42]. Moreover, gut flora has a big impact on how medications are metabolized. Multiple studies have demonstrated that microbes possess the ability to alter medicine molecules subsequent to their oral delivery, resulting in drug activation (as exemplified by sulfasalazine), inactivation (as exemplified by digoxin), and modifications in toxicity (as exemplified by solivudine). A thorough analysis of the connection between microorganisms and drugs was conducted by Zimmermann *et al* in one of these studies, and the results confirmed the existence of 30 different enzyme types involved in the bacterially encoded drug metabolism.

The outcome of medication metabolism in the body could be understood by tracking these enzymes, opening the door to precision medicine and tailored care [43]. These signals have a strong connection to basic medical research. A highly effective approach for the advancement of practical applications in fundamental medicine is the development of tailored sensors that rely on biological signal pathways. The assessment of the patient's systemic organ function and the prediction of disease progression, as well as the evaluation of therapy efficacy, can be achieved through the utilization of intestinal microsignals. Hence, by means of the real-time identification and digital administration of patients' intestinal signals, the potential for individualized treatment and precision medicine becomes boundless. Endoscopy has been effectively implemented in clinical settings.

2.10.2.4 Application of engineered sensors

A specialized sensor designed for the purpose of detecting GI illnesses is sometimes referred to as an ingestible device. The detection of luminal signals is commonly achieved by the utilization of electrochemical, electromagnetic, optical, and auditory measurements, owing to the advantages associated with real-time monitoring and remote control. These devices are currently a crucial component of the evaluation process for many GI diseases [34]. These devices are preferred for GI examinations because they are simple to use, cause little disruption to the patients' daily routines, and result in no trauma, damage, discomfort, or cross-infection. They also increase the inspection's breadth and decrease the low tolerance and inappropriateness of the normal insert endoscopy. They can be used to specifically diagnose diseases of the digestive system, such as abdominal pain, intestinal tumors, etc, that a standard GI endoscopy is unable to detect. As a result of these factors, they are commonly employed, although not universally favored, for the assessment of the GI system in geriatric, debilitated, and critically ill individuals. The initial purpose of these ingestible devices was to gather data pertaining to anatomical abnormalities inside the GI system. Subsequent research has demonstrated the considerable potential of these devices in the detection of internal physiological signals. As a result, a multitude of ingestible devices have been subsequently designed to sense pressure, temperature, and pH levels within the alimentary canal.

2.10.2.5 CRP biosensor

CRP is an annular (ring-shaped) pentameric protein of molecular weight 27.18 kDa, found in the blood plasma where inflammation is being widely utilized as an early diagnostic biomarker of GID. In a healthy individual, CRP in serum is present in low concentrations i.e. less than 0.3 mg dl^{-1} [44]. CRP concentration in blood serum rises by many folds (three times) from the normal range following the appearance of initial symptoms of GID. CRP is mostly created in the liver in response to an acute inflammatory stimulus. However, there is some data suggesting that CRP production may also occur in the kidneys and atherosclerotic tissues [45]. In the acute-phase response of inflammation, there is a sudden and significant increase in CRP concentration in the bloodstream. This increase is observed to rise from approximately

0.8 mg l^{-1} to a range of $600-1000$ mg l^{-1}, with the peak value often occurring around 48 h following the onset of inflammation [46]. The half-life of CRP is around 19 h, and the concentration in the bloodstream promptly reverts to basal levels upon cessation of the stimulus that triggered the heightened production [47]. Within the clinical environment, the prevailing techniques for detecting CRP involve the utilization of immunonephelometric and immunoturbidimetric tests employing a solitary polyclonal antibody. However, it is worth noting that enzyme-linked immunosorbent assays (ELISA) have also gained significant popularity and are widely employed. Nevertheless, the implementation of these techniques requires a significant amount of time and the expertise of qualified individuals [48]. Consequently, CRP is regarded as one of the earliest biomarkers utilized for the identification and confirmation of GID [49]. In recent times, there has been a proliferation of studies focused on the detection of CRP. Liu *et al* presented a study on the development of a microfluidic device that incorporates a capacitive biosensor utilizing three-dimensional (3D) interdigital electrode arrays [50]. In their study, Takaloo *et al* conducted bending experiments to evaluate the performance of flexible biosensors with carbon nanotubes as the deposition material. The biosensor's surface was coated with carbon nanotubes for the purpose of detecting CRP through the utilization of CV and EIS. The LOD achieved for CRP detection ranged from 0.02 to 0.8 nanograms per milliliter (ng ml^{-1}) [51]. In their study, Tu *et al* presented a novel wearable and wireless patch designed for the real-time electrochemical detection of CRP [52].

2.10.2.6 3D sensor materials for GID detection

Sensors are advantageous for developing 3D models for *in vitro* signal detection with more accurate simulation in addition to diagnosis. Researchers could gain a better understanding of diseases by replicating the interactions between cells and their microenvironments, according to Bissell and Radisky's 2001 suggestion [53]. An important tool for studying disease processes and illness detection is 3D culture in sensing materials. For instance, Dhimolea *et al* created organoids models using both tumor cell lines and cancer cell samples from patient samples using the 3D culturing technique. The patient's tumor's status following treatment was evaluated using the organoid model. In the course of their investigation, the researchers proposed an original mechanism of drug resistance in cancer cells that exhibit adaptive survival capabilities, which is linked to the occurrence of diapause in animal embryos. A novel target for tumor-resistant therapy was identified subsequent to its discovery by comprehensive pharmacological screening. To effectively detect illness indicators, it is imperative that both *in vivo* and *in vitro* sensors exhibit a high degree of reliability and accuracy. Nevertheless, *in vivo* application necessitates more stringent safety regulations due to the significantly elevated level of risk associated with it. When designing *in vitro* sensors, it is essential to consider the incorporation of biosafety materials. On the other hand, the development of *in vivo* sensors necessitates careful consideration of their effects on organ function, mitigation of blood toxicity, and various other factors. It is imperative for researchers to thoroughly investigate the challenges associated with the removal and degradation of *in vivo* sensors, as well as the eventual destiny of these sensors.

2.11 Summary and future perspectives

This chapter examines the present advancements in specialized sensors utilized for the detection of intestinal illnesses and explores the potential for further enhancement in the development of such sensors. The investigation of bio-detection, imageable materials, sensors for dynamic detection, and the potential utility of these materials in tailored sensor systems may contribute to personalized diagnosis and healthcare. Despite the significant progress achieved in this field, there persist unresolved obstacles that necessitate attention in order to augment the extensive acceptance and therapeutic effectiveness of tailored sensors. The current state of fundamental research on integrated technology is inadequate, however, there is a growing demand for the integration of diagnostic and treatment methods. The key obstacle to this diagnosis–treatment integration, however, is how to accomplish precise targeting and accumulation in the lesions. When it comes to disease detection, the targeting ability of sensor materials is especially inadequate, which results in issues with analytical errors, a lack of specificity, a vulnerability to interference, and results that are only somewhat dependable. Consequently, forthcoming research endeavors may prioritize the advancement of specialized sensor materials and the development of more intelligent, multifunctional devices that exhibit heightened specificity and enhanced capabilities for precise manipulation within living organisms. According to our opinion, sensor materials can support the coordinated functioning of diagnostic and therapeutic processes via intelligent, adaptable modules that allow for accurate targeting and control. It is strongly anticipated that the development of many industries, such as healthcare, health monitoring, military defense, civilian use, etc, will be accelerated by the employment of sensor materials, and that this will greatly enhance many aspects of human existence.

References

[1] Wang R, Li Z, Liu S and Zhang D 2023 Global, regional, and national burden of 10 digestive diseases in 204 countries and territories from 1990 to 2019 *Front. Public Health* **11** 1061453
[2] Arnold M, Abnet C C, Neale R E, Vignat J, Giovannucci E L, McGlynn K A *et al* 2020 Global burden of 5 major types of gastrointestinal cancer *Gastroenterology* **159** 335–49
[3] McQuaid K R 1998 Gastrointestinal diseases. Risk factors and prevention *Gastroenterology* **114** 1347–8
[4] Greenwood-Van Meerveld B, Johnson A C and Grundy D 2017 Gastrointestinal physiology and function *Gastrointestinal Pharmacology* (Springer) pp 1–16
[5] Ananthakrishnan A N 2013 Environmental risk factors for inflammatory bowel disease *Gastroenterol. Hepatol* **9** 367
[6] Kaneko J J, Harvey J W and Bruss M L 2008 *Clinical Biochemistry of Domestic Animals* (New York: Academic)
[7] Allen T W and Tulchinsky M 2013 Nuclear medicine tests for acute gastrointestinal conditions *Seminars Nucl Med* **43** 88–101

  [8] Ling W, Li Y, Jiang W, Sui Y and Zhao H-L 2015 Common mechanism of pathogenesis in gastrointestinal diseases implied by consistent efficacy of single Chinese medicine formula: a PRISMA-compliant systematic review and meta-analysis *Medicine* **94** e1111
  [9] Ranjbar R, Ghasemian M, Maniati M, Khatami S H, Jamali N and Taheri-Anganeh M 2022 Gastrointestinal disorder biomarkers *Clin. Chim. Acta* **530** 13–26
 [10] Qureshi A, Gurbuz Y and Niazi J H 2012 Biosensors for cardiac biomarkers detection: a review *Sens. Actuators* B **171** 62–76
 [11] de Ávila B E F, Escamilla-Gómez V, Lanzone V, Campuzano S, Pedrero M, Compagnone D *et al* 2014 Multiplexed determination of amino-terminal Pro-B-type natriuretic peptide and C-reactive protein cardiac biomarkers in human serum at a disposable electrochemical magnetoimmunosensor *Electroanalysis* **26** 254–61
 [12] Justino C I, Rocha-Santos T A and Duarte A C 2013 Advances in point-of-care technologies with biosensors based on carbon nanotubes *TrAC, Trends Anal. Chem.* **45** 24–36
 [13] Ronkainen N J and Okon S L 2014 Nanomaterial-based electrochemical immunosensors for clinically significant biomarkers *Materials* **7** 4669–709
 [14] Azeem B, KuShaari K and Man Z 2016 Effect of coating thickness on release characteristics of controlled release urea produced in fluidized bed using waterborne starch biopolymer as coating material *Procedia Eng.* **148** 282–9
 [15] Turner A, Karube I and Wilson G S 1987 *Biosensors: Fundamentals and Applications* (Oxford: Oxford University Press)
 [16] Cavalcanti A, Shirinzadeh B, Zhang M and Kretly L C 2008 Nanorobot hardware architecture for medical defense *Sensors* **8** 2932–58
 [17] Turner A P 1989 Current trends in biosensor research and development *Sens. Actuators* **17** 433–50
 [18] Lei Y, Chen W and Mulchandani A 2006 Microbial biosensors *Anal. Chim. Acta* **568** 200–10
 [19] Rahman M, Li X-B, Lopa N S, Ahn S J and Lee J-J 2015 Electrochemical DNA hybridization sensors based on conducting polymers *Sensors* **15** 3801–29
 [20] Anany H, Brovko L, El Dougdoug N K, Sohar J, Fenn H, Alasiri N *et al* 2018 Print to detect: a rapid and ultrasensitive phage-based dipstick assay for foodborne pathogens *Anal. Bioanal. Chem.* **410** 1217–30
 [21] Damborský P, Švitel J and Katrlík J 2016 Optical biosensors *Essays Biochem.* **60** 91–100
 [22] Wee K W, Kang G Y, Park J, Kang J Y, Yoon D S, Park J H *et al* 2005 Novel electrical detection of label-free disease marker proteins using piezoresistive self-sensing micro-cantilevers *Biosens. Bioelectron.* **20** 1932–8
 [23] Saliterman S 2006 *Fundamentals of BioMEMS and Medical Microdevices* (Bellingham, WA: SPIE Press)
 [24] Elsherif M, Hassan M U, Yetisen A K and Butt H 2018 Wearable contact lens biosensors for continuous glucose monitoring using smartphones *ACS Nano* **12** 5452–62
 [25] Eggins B R 2008 *Chemical Sensors and Biosensors* (New York: Wiley)
 [26] Voltammetry G-J D C 1993 *Simulation and Analysis of Reaction Mechanisms* (New York: Wiley-VCH)
 [27] Liu Y, Yuan R, Chai Y, Tang D, Dai J and Zhong X 2006 Direct electrochemistry of horseradish peroxidase immobilized on gold colloid/cysteine/nafion-modified platinum disk electrode *Sens. Actuators* B **115** 109–15
 [28] Colvin V L 2003 The potential environmental impact of engineered nanomaterials *Nat. Biotechnol.* **21** 1166–70

[29] Haque M, Fouad H, Seo H-K, Othman A Y, Kulkarni A and Ansari Z A 2020 Investigation of Mn doped ZnO nanoparticles towards ascertaining myocardial infarction through an electrochemical detection of myoglobin *IEEE Access* **8** 164678–92

[30] Kehl D W, Iqbal N, Fard A, Kipper B A, Landa A D L P and Maisel A S 2012 Biomarkers in acute myocardial injury *Transl. Res.* **159** 252–64

[31] Salvo P, Dini V, Kirchhain A, Janowska A, Oranges T, Chiricozzi A *et al* 2017 Sensors and biosensors for C-reactive protein, temperature and pH, and their applications for monitoring wound healing: a review *Sensors* **17** 2952

[32] Ozkan S A 2012 *Electroanalytical Methods in Pharmaceutical Analysis and their Validation* (New York: HNB Publishing)

[33] Fenzl C, Hirsch T and Baeumner A J 2016 Nanomaterials as versatile tools for signal amplification in (bio) analytical applications *TrAC, Trends Anal. Chem.* **79** 306–16

[34] Steiger C, Abramson A, Nadeau P, Chandrakasan A P, Langer R and Traverso G 2019 Ingestible electronics for diagnostics and therapy *Nat. Rev. Mater.* **4** 83–98

[35] Fan Y and Pedersen O 2021 Gut microbiota in human metabolic health and disease *Nat. Rev. Microbiol.* **19** 55–71

[36] Pluznick J L 2020 The gut microbiota in kidney disease *Science* **369** 1426–7

[37] Mage P, Ferguson B, Maliniak D, Ploense K, Kippin T and Soh H 2017 Closed-loop control of circulating drug levels in live animals *Nat. Biomed. Eng.* **1** 0070

[38] Camilleri M, Thorne N K, Ringel Y, Hasler W L, Kuo B, Esfandyari T *et al* 2010 Wireless pH-motility capsule for colonic transit: prospective comparison with radiopaque markers in chronic constipation *Neurogastroenterol. Motil.* **22** 874–e233

[39] Kalantar-Zadeh K, Berean K J, Ha N, Chrimes A F, Xu K, Grando D *et al* 2018 A human pilot trial of ingestible electronic capsules capable of sensing different gases in the gut *Nat. Electron.* **1** 79–87

[40] Ravindran R, Loebbermann J, Nakaya H I, Khan N, Ma H, Gama L *et al* 2016 The amino acid sensor GCN2 controls gut inflammation by inhibiting inflammasome activation *Nature* **531** 523–7

[41] Qin N, Yang F, Li A, Prifti E, Chen Y, Shao L *et al* 2014 Alterations of the human gut microbiome in liver cirrhosis *Nature* **513** 59–64

[42] Yang J, Zheng P, Li Y, Wu J, Tan X, Zhou J *et al* 2020 Landscapes of bacterial and metabolic signatures and their interaction in major depressive disorders *Sci. Adv.* **6** eaba8555

[43] Zimmermann M, Zimmermann-Kogadeeva M, Wegmann R and Goodman A L 2019 Separating host and microbiome contributions to drug pharmacokinetics and toxicity *Science* **363** eaat9931

[44] Nehring S M, Goyal A and Patel B C 2017 *C Reactive Protein* (StatPearls)

[45] Du Clos T W and Mold C 2004 C-reactive protein: an activator of innate immunity and a modulator of adaptive immunity *Immunol. Res.* **30** 261–77

[46] Reeves G 2007 C-reactive protein *Aust. Prescr* **30** 74–6

[47] Pepys M B and Hirschfield G M 2003 C-reactive protein: a critical update *J. Clin. Invest.* **111** 1805–12

[48] Hennessey H, Afara N, Omanovic S and Padjen A L 2009 Electrochemical investigations of the interaction of C-reactive protein (CRP) with a CRP antibody chemically immobilized on a gold surface *Anal. Chim. Acta* **643** 45–53

[49] Hart P C, Rajab I M, Alebraheem M and Potempa L A 2020 C-reactive protein and cancer
—diagnostic and therapeutic insights *Front. Immunol.* **11** 595835

[50] Liu D, Zhou L, Huang L, Zuo Z, Ho V, Jin L *et al* 2021 Microfluidic integrated capacitive
biosensor for C-reactive protein label-free and real-time detection *Analyst* **146** 5380–8

[51] Takaloo S, Zand M M, Kalantar M and Rezayan A H 2023 Detection of C-reactive protein
using a flexible biosensor with improved bending life *J. Electrochem. Soc.* **170** 057513

[52] Tu J *et al* 2023 A wireless patch for the monitoring of C-reactive protein in sweat *Nat.
Biomed. Eng.* **7** 1293–306

[53] Bissell M J and Radisky D 2001 Putting tumours in context *Nat. Rev. Cancer* **1** 46–54

IOP Publishing

Nanobiotechnology and Artificial Intelligence in
Gastrointestinal Diseases

Vivek K Chaturvedi, Anurag Kumar Singh, Jay Singh and Dawesh P Yadav

Chapter 3

Nanoscience in controlled drug release in the gastrointestinal tract

Ritu, Bharmjeet, Nida-e-Falak, Asmita Das, Rahul Gupta and Prakash Chandra

The use of nanotechnology in drug delivery has the potential to revolutionize the field by improving the efficacy, safety, and convenience of therapeutic interventions. However, the complexity of the gastrointestinal (GI) tract presents unique challenges that require sophisticated and precise drug release strategies. In recent years, artificial intelligence (AI) has emerged as a powerful tool for optimizing drug delivery systems. Machine learning (ML) algorithms can be used to analyze large amounts of data and predict how drugs will behave in different physiological conditions, allowing for the development of more accurate and personalized drug delivery systems. Moreover, AI can be combined with nanoscience to create intelligent drug delivery systems that respond to the needs of the patient in real time. This chapter will explore the latest advances in the field of nanoscience and AI for controlled drug release in the GI tract and different types of nanomaterials that can be used for drug delivery will be discussed, including liposomes, polymeric nanoparticles, and dendrimers. Also, various methods for controlling drug release will also be covered, including pH-sensitive systems, enzyme-sensitive systems, and stimuli-responsive systems. The use of AI in the development of intelligent drug delivery systems, such as microrobots and smart capsules, will also be discussed. In conclusion, the combination of nanoscience and AI has the potential to revolutionize drug delivery in the GI tract, leading to more effective, personalized, and safe therapies. This chapter will provide an in-depth review of the latest advances in the field and will be of interest to researchers and practitioners in nanoscience, drug delivery, and AI.

3.1 Introduction

Nanoparticles have emerged as highly promising drug delivery vehicles, specifically designed to be less than 100 nm in at least one dimension. Their adaptability enables

doi:10.1088/978-0-7503-6134-7ch3

researchers to create nanoparticles that are specifically suited for therapeutic purposes. These materials include natural or synthetic polymers, lipids, metals, and other biodegradable compounds. One significant advantage of nanoparticles is their superior cellular uptake compared to larger micromolecules, enabling efficient transport and targeted drug delivery within the body. Scientists can precisely control their composition and biological properties, optimizing drug and gene delivery for therapeutic purposes. Whether integrating medications within the nanoparticle's matrix or attaching them to its surface, the flexibility offered by nanoparticles presents diverse strategies for controlled and efficient drug release in the biological environment. With such advancements, nanosystems have undergone extensive investigation as potential tools for precise drug targeting and delivery, holding the potential to revolutionize medical treatments in the future [1].

Despite the many advantages, utilizing nanoparticulate formulations for stomach medication administration has drawbacks. The swift movement of tiny nanoparticles through the stomach and into the intestine is one of these obstacles. However, nanoparticulate formulations offer certain advantages, such as distributing the drug across multiple stomach areas and avoiding the limitations of single-unit forms. Moreover, they may improve mucosal interaction, thereby aiding drug delivery. To address rapid clearance, researchers have incorporated gastroretentive strategies like mucoadhesion and high-density systems into nanoparticulate formulations, showing promising results *in vitro* and *ex vivo*. However, translating these findings to animals and humans proves complex due to physiological factors that impact gastric drug delivery, such as gastric motility, mucus turnover, and high stomach hydration. *In vivo* studies have revealed that nanoparticulate dosage forms can remain in the stomach for up to 3 h in fasted animals, while microparticulate forms remained for over 8 h. Various strategies and animal species influence the retention, with rodents showing mixed results where nanoparticles were found in the forestomach but adhered well to the mucosa in the glandular stomach [2].

The GI tract plays a crucial role in the digestion and absorption of nutrients, but it also possesses mechanisms that can hinder drug absorption. Drugs must navigate through the acidic environment of the stomach, which can degrade some medications and render them less effective. Additionally, the GI tract's enzymes and other elements may break down some medications, further reducing their therapeutic value. In order to protect the body from hazardous chemicals, the GI mucosa poses a formidable barrier to medication absorption. This prevents the passage of larger molecules, especially biologics, which are complex and frequently contain substantial amounts of protein-based pharmaceuticals. Due to these restrictions, many drugs, particularly biologics, are only or mostly available in injectable form.

The enormous molecular size of biologics, which makes it difficult for them to be efficiently absorbed by the GI tract if given orally, is one of their main drawbacks. These fragile biomolecules can be damaged and denatured in the harsh acidic environment of the stomach, becoming less active or even completely inert by the time they reach the site of action. Since many biologics are therefore often provided through injections, patients may find this to be inconvenient and irritating [3].

Innovative strategies are being investigated at the nexus of AI and nanotechnology to address these issues and realize the full potential of biologics for oral delivery. An effective way to improve the oral administration of biologics is by using nanomedicine, which focuses on creating nanoparticles and nanoscale drug delivery devices. It is now possible to safeguard and stabilize biologics as they travel through the GI tract by carefully designing nanoparticles at the nanoscale [4].

To design pharmaceutical delivery systems that are as effective as feasible, AI is required. In order to create nanoparticles that can effectively transport biologics to the target site while minimizing degradation and potential side effects, AI algorithms can analyze a vast amount of data, including pharmacokinetic and pharmacodynamic profiles, biophysical interactions, and patient-specific characteristics. By applying AI-driven medication design, nanoparticles can be tailored to specific biologics and diseases ensuring the best possible drug release and bioavailability [5].

3.2 Challenges in drug delivery to the GI tract

Oral drug delivery offers many advantages but also significant disadvantages because of the intricate architecture of the human GI system. Numerous physiological barriers in the GI system, such as poor drug solubility, instability, and low permeability across mucosal barriers, might make it difficult for medications to be distributed effectively. Furthermore, even in healthy individuals, the physiology of the GI tract can vary significantly [6]. As a result, during the formulation design process, significant thought must be given, taking into account the following factors.

3.2.1 Residence time

To maximize drug delivery, it is essential to know how long the drug formulation stays in various parts of the GI tract. Drug absorption and release might be affected by the unique features of the various GI tract regions. For medications and dosage formulations with region-specific targeting or absorption qualities, GI transit time is an important consideration. A dose form might leave the stomach at a variety of times, from a few minutes to several hours. Age, posture, gender, osmolarity, and food intake are only a few of the variables that affect gastric transit time [7]. Gastric transit can take between 0 and 2 h while fasting, but it can take up to 6 h while fed. The average small intestine transit time is 3 to 4 h, however, in healthy people, it can vary from 2 to 6 h. Colonic transit periods might range from 6 to 70 h, according to reports. Gender and the timing of bowel movements both affect how quickly food moves through the GI tract; females often have longer colonic transit periods [8].

3.2.2 Influence of the GI environment

The GI environment can have a big impact on how well a medication formulation is delivered to the target site of action. Additionally, it may have an impact on the drug's solubility and stability, which may result in diminished effectiveness or unfavorable side effects. Along the GI tract, the pH of the GI environment varies from the stomach, which is very acidic (pH 1.5–2 in the fasted state), to the small intestine, which is more alkaline (pH 6–7.4), and the colon, which is more basic (pH

6.7 at the rectum) [9]. However, dietary choices and microbial metabolism can cause individual pH differences. These pH variations affect drug molecule ionization and absorption and can be used for delayed-release therapy. Effective oral medicine administration is complicated by the GI tract's ongoing secretion of GI mucus. The mucus serves as a lubricant and protective barrier and is made up of water, mucin proteins, and proteoglycans. The thickest mucus layers are found in the colon and stomach, protecting against gastric acid and preserving a stable environment for gut microorganisms. The mucus layer, particularly for hydrophobic compounds, can obstruct drug permeability, which can shorten the period that medicine remains in the body [10].

3.2.3 Intestinal fluid volume

Considering the volume of intestinal fluid is essential as it affects the dissolution and dispersal of the drug formulation. The available fluid volume can influence drug solubility and, consequently, absorption. Luminal fluidity plays a crucial role in GI function as it enables digestion, supports nutrient and drug absorption, and facilitates the smooth transit of intestinal contents without damaging the epithelial lining. In a healthy adult, daily water balance in the GI tract involves various secretions (saliva, gastric juice, pancreatic juice, and others) and absorptions (small and large intestine).

In particular in the lower GI tract, fluid-to-matter ratios have an impact on pH and can impair drug delivery and absorption. Consuming food has a substantial impact on the GI tract's fluid balance, bile salt levels, and digestive enzyme levels. Changes in intestinal fluid volumes can alter intestinal transit periods as well as the medication uptake by cells at the site of action. Additionally, a change in the gut flora and a reduction in reabsorption might impact the digestion and absorption of carbs and polysaccharides by diluting digestive enzymes. These differences may have an impact on how traditional medication formulations are absorbed by the GI tract [11].

3.2.4 Metabolism in the GI tract

It is important to consider how a drug or formulation degrades in the GI tract, whether by microbial or enzymatic means. Such metabolism can change a drug's bioavailability and efficacy, which can affect its therapeutic advantages. Enzymatic and microbiological processes degrade medications and dosage forms in the GI tract. Salivary, gastric, and intestinal fluids include enzymes that digest proteins, lipids, and carbs [12]. Major food-digesting enzymes are found in the stomach and small intestine, which has an impact on the stability of drugs and local drug distribution. With more than 500 bacterial species, the intestinal microbiome promotes intestinal health and aids in digesting. The colon is a target for drug delivery utilizing non-starch polysaccharide coatings because it ferments carbs there. Individuals' microbiomes differ according to genetic and environmental variables, although the leading species (Firmicutes, Bacteroidetes, Proteobacteria, Actinobacteria, and Fusobacteria) stay constant. It is interesting to note that dietary consumption affects the microbiome in the small intestine, which is less dense and changeable. It is a group of genera that includes *Turicibacter*, *Escherichia*, and *Clostridium* and is involved in the control of metabolism. More research is needed to determine how the small intestinal bacteria affects oral dose forms and drug absorption [13].

3.3 Role of nanoscience in drug delivery

3.3.1 Importance of nanotechnology-based techniques in controlled drug release in the GI tract

A controlled delivery system ensures that an optimum concentration of a drug is maintained in the blood so as to protect the body from adverse effects [14]. Drugs can be built into nanoparticles for controlled release in order to maintain a sustained response. By altering nanoparticle properties including size, surface charge, and composition, the rate of drug release can be precisely controlled to achieve the desired therapeutic effects [15]. Nanotechnology-based approaches have drawn a lot of interest and demonstrated considerable promise as a significant therapeutic option for GI diseases as nanotechnology provides protection of sensitive drugs and enhanced drug stability [16]. Certain drugs are susceptible to deterioration, but by being enclosed within a nanoparticle, these drugs can withstand the tough GI environment which includes bile salts, enzymes, and HCl exposure. This extends the biological half-life of the drug [3] and enhances its stability [15, 17].

3.3.2 Targeted drug delivery

By adding site-specific ligands or antibodies to the surface of the nanoparticles, which enable them to recognize and bind to particular receptors, one can target particular parts of the GI tract, such as the colon, small intestine, or stomach [15, 18].

3.3.3 Increased bioavailability

By enhancing the solubility as well as the rate of dissolution of less-soluble drugs, nanoparticles can increase their oral bioavailability. The drug can hence be distributed and absorbed more effectively throughout the GI tract, improving [3] the effectiveness of therapy [15, 17].

3.3.4 Reduced toxicity and side effects

Excessive amounts of drug in normal tissues can have adverse consequences which can be decreased by controlled nanotechnology-based drug release systems. These delivery systems improve the therapeutic index by confining drug release at the target site while minimizing exposure to normal cells [15, 17].

3.3.5 Imaging and diagnostic capabilities

Imaging agents or contrast agents can be incorporated into nanoparticles to provide non-invasive imaging of the GI tract. As a result, personalized medicine and treatment optimization are made possible by the real-time monitoring of drug release, biodistribution, and therapeutic response [15].

3.3.6 Drug designing

While designing a nano drug delivery system, the surface charge is a crucial factor to be taken into account since all the interactions with the cells, receptors, or other biomolecules are significantly dependent on the surface charge. A suitable surface charge aids the nanoparticles to maintain colloidal stability by preventing their aggregation or sedimentation leading to increased shelf life of nanomedicines during storage and retention of therapeutic properties of nanomedicine during administration [14].

3.3.7 Delivery system

Another significant factor to be taken into account is surface hydrophobicity as it also influences the behaviour of a nanoparticle in a biological environment by affecting the cellular uptake, protein adsorption, and stability of the nanomedicine. Hydrophobic nanoparticles possess enhanced cellular uptake as they can favorably interact with lipids by a layer of cell membrane that facilitates the endocytosis process. Hydrophobic surfaces have a higher tendency to adsorb proteins that can decide the distribution, immune response, and biological journey of the nanoparticles (figure 3.1) [19].

The third factor to consider is the optimization of the drug release profile which directly impacts the performance and efficacy of a nanomedicine. The surface properties of the shell in which the drug is contained greatly influence the rate at which the drug is released. For example, hydrophobic nanoparticles interact strongly with hydrophobic drugs, leading to drug release, whereas the hydrophilic drug in the same shell will be released faster since it has weaker interactions with the

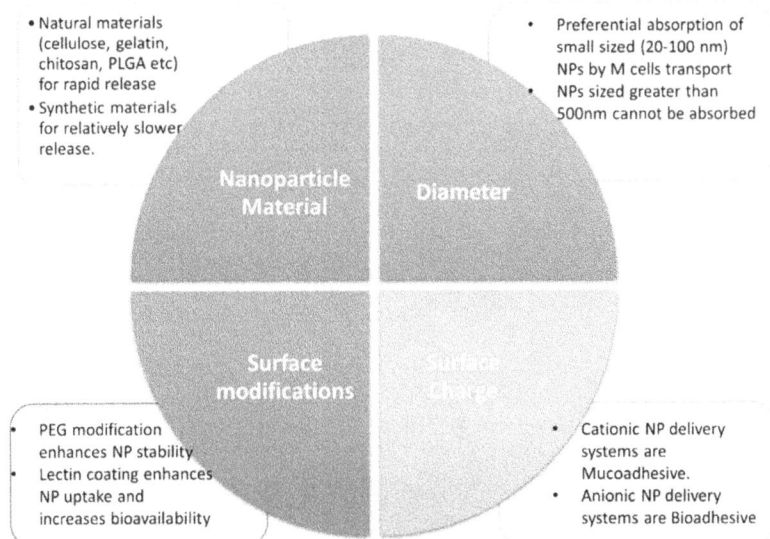

Figure 3.1. Significant elements to be considered while designing a nanoparticle drug.

shell. The controlled drug release strategies should also be selected according to the nature of the disease, the location of the target site, and the surface properties of the encapsulated drug (figure 3.1) [19, 20].

3.4 Methods of nanomedicine formulation

Conventional techniques used for nanomedicine formulation are the solvent evaporation method (figure 3.2) and ionic gelation method. In the solvent evaporation method, a polymer and a drug are dissolved in a volatile solvent which is then allowed to evaporate to precipitate out the nanoparticles. Ionic gelation on the other hand depends on the interaction of ions with opposite charges to form crosslinked mesh-like networks (figure 3.3) [20].

Supercritical fluid technology is one of the recent and widely utilized approaches in nanomedicine design. Supercritical fluids are employed as solvents for dissolution of polymers. Owing to its inflammability, less toxicity and ability to exist as both liquid and gas above mild critical conditions, carbon dioxide is a widely used supercritical solvent. A supercritical fluid can either aid in nanoparticle formation while it rapidly expands via a small pointed tube causing separation of solutes (rapid expansion of supercritical solutions) or when a drug is first dissolved quickly in supercritical fluid and then precipitated out by antisolvent addition. Supercritical fluids are reported to be used for coating nanoparticles making them more porous and facilitating effective drug penetration. They can also extract contaminants or unwanted remanent solvents from nanoformulations supporting the purification process [15, 21].

Uniform particle size and consistent shape are critical to the effectiveness of a drug delivery process and the particle replication technique provides precisely

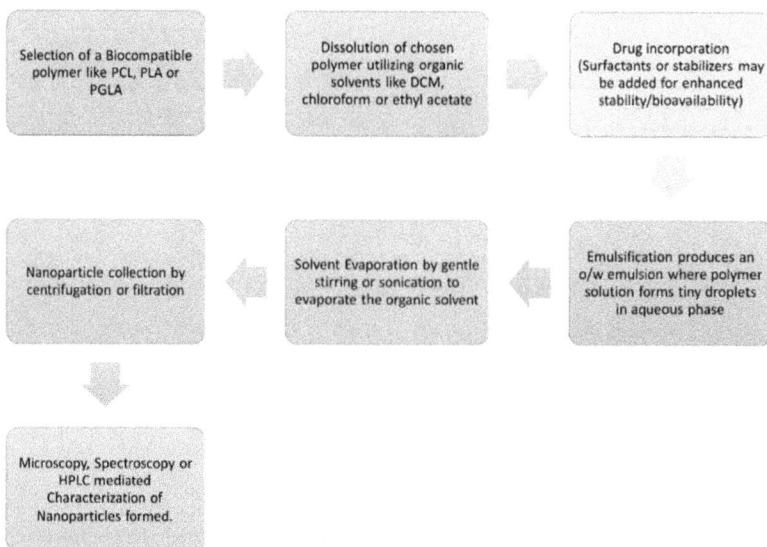

Figure 3.2. Steps explaining solvent evaporation method for nanomedicine formulation.

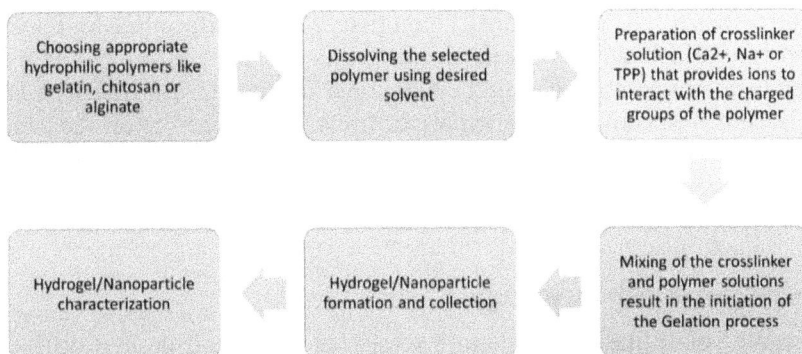

Figure 3.3. Flowchart explaining ionic gelation method for nanomedicine formulation.

controlled nanoparticle synthesis assuring homogeneity and batch-to-batch reproducibility. In this technique, numerous copies of nanoparticles are prepared by using a master replica or mold. Techniques like soft lithography in which a soft elastomeric mold is created by using PDMS to be further used as a template for nanoparticle production or nanoimprint lithography that exploits a stiff mold to imprint the required pattern onto a precursor material for nanoparticle synthesis, also come into play [15, 20, 21].

3.5 Drug release strategies

3.5.1 Active targeting strategies

In order to optimize therapeutic outcomes and minimize harm to healthy cells, active targeting strategies in nanoparticle-based drug delivery utilize the modification of nanoparticle surfaces with targeted ligands. Nanoparticles can specifically bind to receptors or biomarkers that are overexpressed specifically on the diseased cells differentiating them from normal cells, by interacting with targeted ligands. This enhances the accuracy of the therapy by promoting the attaching and absorption of nanoparticles by the target cells [22]. Active targeting methods involve targeting via cell membranes, targeting via antibodies, and targeting via receptors. Active targeting frequently employs receptor-mediated targeting. If the target cells have unique receptors that are either absent or barely expressed in normal cells, this strategy is especially helpful. Another successful strategy is antibody-mediated targeting, in which antibodies designed for disease-associated antigens are coupled to the surface of the nanoparticle. This strategy is widely used in cancer therapy because it allows for precision tumor targeting by creating antibodies that specifically target tumor antigens. While in a cell membrane-mediated strategy, nanoparticles can successfully migrate to the appropriate target tissues or cells by utilizing the cell membranes of cells that have specific targeting capabilities, such as immune cells or cancer cells [8].

Precise and better therapeutic results for conditions affecting the colon such as IBD and colon cancer have been achieved by active targeting. In an inflamed colon, drug delivery to macrophages by aiming at receptors like mannose receptors or macrophage galactose-type lectin enhances site-specific drug deposition and therapeutic efficacy [23, 24]. Inflamed colon tissues show surface ICAM-1 and CD98 overexpression which aids in the selective targeting and aggregation of nanoparticles at desired locations by conjugating these nanoparticles to ICAM-1[25] or CD98 [26] specific ligands, respectively. Overexpressed transferrin receptors on the cancer cell surface aid in selective nanoparticle binding and uptake of these nanoparticles by receptor-mediated endocytosis when they have ligands customized to transferrin receptors attached to them, in the treatment of colon cancer [8, 23, 26].

3.5.2 Stimuli-based delivery strategy

To overcome issues like the premature release of drugs and desired drug concentration not reaching the target location, the focus is shifting toward stimulus-responsive delivery strategies. Stimuli-based drugs are capable of reacting to a particular stimulus at the desired location by changing their physiochemical characteristics and disassembling or breaking down specific linkers. To enable precise and regulated drug release, these stimuli frequently depend on variations between the surrounding conditions of healthy and diseased tissues or cells.

Major alterations in the GI tract can be observed during a chronic disease like Crohn's disease or ulcerative colitis (UC), including penetration by macrophages and lymphocytes, enhanced production of mucus, compromised intestinal barrier as a consequence of inflammation, ulcers, and crypt distortion that causes altered GI motility affecting the pH, intestinal volume as well as epithelial permeability [8]. In another instance, the tumor microenvironment differs from normal tissues in a number of ways, and these variations can be used as activation-inducing endogenous cues. Acidic pH, elevated ROS levels, overexpressed enzymes, increased ATP concentrations, high redox potential and are some of the prevalent triggers present in the tumor microenvironment (table 3.1) [23].

3.5.3 pH-dependent drug release

The difference in the pH of diseased tissue as well as normal tissues can be utilized to design a pH-responsive drug delivery system that can undergo changes like swelling

Table 3.1. Polymeric nanoparticle coatings along with their optimum pH [15, 8].

pH range	5.0	5.5	6.0	7.0
Polymer coatings	Polyvinyl acetate phthalate	Hydroxypropyl methylcellulose phthalate 55	Cellulose acetate phthalate	Eudragit® S-100
	Hydroxypropyl methylcellulose phthalate 50	Eudragit® L 30D-55		
		Eudragit® L 100 55	Eudragit® L-100	Eudragit® FS 30D
		Cellulose acetate trimellitate		

or degradation at a specific pH leading to the release of the encapsulated drug under regulated conditions, releasing at the precise moment and location. Polymers that are pH sensitive might show an altered solubility or structure as a consequence of fluctuations in pH. One can either employ pH sensitive matrix or coatings while designing nanoparticles that allow them to swell and rupture at a specific pH, leading to site-specific regulated drug release or pH-responsive linkers can be employed, which can be made stable at neutral pH but cleave or degrade at acidic pH levels leading to release of the medicine (table 3.1) [27, 28].

3.5.4 ROS-dependent drug release

These methods provide specific therapy for GI diseases by exploiting the reactive oxygen species (ROS) gradient as a drug release trigger. In contrast to healthy tissues, enhanced ROS production, including superoxide radicals and H_2O_2, has been reported in diseased or inflamed GI tissues. ROS-sensitive linkers, moieties, and matrix materials are employed which cleave or undergo structural alterations in the presence of an oxidizing environment, i.e., when ROS are present. The drug is hence released due to the disassembly of the encapsulating nanoparticle at the desired release site lowering systemic toxicity and off-target effects to the bare minimum [15, 8].

Studies reveal that the biopsies collected from inflamed mucosa of UC patients show 10–100-fold greater ROS levels than normal conditions. These increased amounts are often restricted to the diseased area and keep on increasing with the development of the disease. Activated ROS generation by phagocytes is a significant factor contributing to inflammation during UC that can in turn directly harm the biological constituents of the cells [29, 30].

Additionally, specific ligands or surface alterations can be added to ROS-dependent delivery systems to ensure target delivery by increased specificity, i.e., coupling of active targeting and ROS responsiveness methods. Ligands that show specific binding toward overexpressed biomarkers on diseased GI tissues might be functionalized onto the surface of ROS-dependent drug-delivering nanoparticles so that the drug can be released at the intended place.

3.5.5 Time-dependent dosage forms

The objective of time-dependent dosage forms is to create a delivery system that releases the drug into the colon after a certain amount of time in the stomach and small intestine. Ethyl cellulose and hydroxypropyl methylcellulose (HPMC), two hydrophilic polymers, are frequently used in time-dependent formulations. These polymers can gradually enlarge over a period of time and are integrated into the coating or matrix of the dosage form. The hydrophilic polymers expand and swell up as they gradually take in the water while traveling through the stomach and small intestine, causing a lag phase that delays the drug's release until it arrives at the appropriate site in the colon. The enlarged hydrophilic polymers start to further hydrate and disintegrate in the colon, where the transit time is greater and the environment is better suited to drug absorption. Ultimately, this procedure results in the drug being released in a continuous and regulated manner, maximizing drug

Table 3.2. Functional groups that can be employed as linkers for different stimuli-responsive strategies [32].

pH responsive	Redox responsive	Light responsive
Silyl ether	Thioketal	Anthracene
Orthoester	Disulphide	Arylmethyl
Cis-aconityl	PBA/PBE	O-nitrobenzyl
Acetal	Oxalate ester	Azobenzene
Hydrazone	Diselenium	Coumarinyl ester
Imine	Vinyldithioether	Spiropyan

delivery to the colon and other specified areas of the GI tract and reducing drug wastage (table 3.2) [15, 31].

3.5.6 Gastro retentive strategies

Another challenge faced during drug delivery in GI diseases is the rapid elimination of drugs from the stomach, so to retain the drug in the stomach for longer durations, researchers have been exploring gastroretentive strategies that prevent drug loss and ensure localized drug action [33]. Mucoadhesive systems and high-density systems are two frequently used techniques. Utilizing certain polymeric materials or coats with adhesive capabilities, mucoadhesive methods enable the adhesion of nano-particles to the mucus membrane covering the stomach wall. These adhesive interactions tend to increase the residence period of the nanoparticles in the stomach and slow down their quick evacuation ensuring controlled drug release and improved drug absorption, whereas the goal of high-density systems is to make the nanoformulation denser than gastric fluids in order to avoid buoyant character-istics and promote retention. Substances like chitosan, Carbopol, polycarbophil, and lectins are the extensively used coatings in these drug delivery systems [33, 34].

Mucoadhesive systems are generally cationic since they have to interact with the negative charges on the inflamed mucus. Colonic mucus is rich in negative charge due to highly substituted sialic acid and sulfate carbohydrate residues making cationic mucoadhesive nanoparticle delivery systems, a colon-specific delivery strategy. On the other hand, anionic delivery methods are bioadhesive as they interact and stick to the inflamed tissue rich in positively charged proteins, by electrostatic interactions. High-density polymers or heavy metals can be added so that the nanoformulations become denser and the longer the nanoparticles stay in the stomach, the longer the drug is released ensuring better bioavailability and less toxicity [33, 34].

The development and optimization of these gastroretentive systems necessitate a thorough evaluation of a number of elements including choice of a suitable biocompatible polymer, size of nanoparticle, modifications or alterations to be made onto the surface of nanoparticle and formulation techniques. These elements in turn affect how well the gastroretentive nanoparticulate composition works including its density and adhesive tendencies. [8, 35]. These strategies have proven to be quite beneficial against local digestive disorders like bacterial infections, gastric ulcers and even gastritis.

3.5.7 Photothermal and photodynamic approach

Nanoparticles with photothermal characteristics including gold nanorods or carbon nanotubes, are employed in photothermal therapy (PTT). To promote their preferential deposition in the diseased or cancer cells within the GI tract, the nanoparticles might be functionalized with certain ligands or targeting moieties. These nanoparticles can take in certain light wavelengths and transform this absorbed light into heat energy. Near infrared has the ability to activate these nanoparticles once they have reached the intended location. The light energy is subsequently transformed into heat which specifically kills cancer cells providing therapeutic consequences. This photothermal reaction can also aid in speeding up the drug release from the nanoparticles [15]. When used in photodynamic treatment (PDT), photosensitizers that are very often organic compounds, can produce ROS when activated by light. These photosensitizers deposit within the cancer cells or diseased areas and upon exposure to a particular light wavelength, high ROS production is initiated which can cause cell death or slow down the tumor growth. Different photosensitizers can be employed for the PDT like first-generation photosensitizers which include hematoporphyrins. Under this category, performer sodium is widely used as a therapeutic agent against esophageal cancer but first-generation photosensitizers are generally non-specific and absorb less light which leads to less ROS generation resulting in poor therapeutic efficacy. To eradicate these shortcomings, second-generation photosensitizers came into existence, including chlorins and phthalocyanine which show high tumour specificity and penetration, fewer side effects and light absorption at a particular wavelength (table 3.3) [36].

3.6 Types of nanoparticles in drug delivery

3.6.1 Liposomes

Dr Alec D Bangham made their discovery in 1964 at the Babraham Institute at the University of Cambridge [41]. The Greek words 'Lipos' (fat) and 'Soma' (body) are where the name 'liposome' originates [42]. Aqueous artificial vesicles with a spherical form and a diameter of 30 nm to several micrometers called liposomes have one or more circumferential lipid bilayers around them [43]. Numerous factors, such as magnitude, lipid composition, production technique, and surface charge have an impact on liposome properties. Liposomes are superior drug delivery devices because they protect the constituents they contain from physiological deterioration [44], increasing the drug's half-life, limiting the release of therapeutic molecules [45], and offering enhanced safety and safety. Cholesterol, sphingomyelin, and glycerolphospholipid are the main ingredients utilized in commercially available products. Furthermore, by passively or actively directing their payload to the location, the maximum tolerated dose, systemic side effects, and therapeutic outcomes can all be improved using liposomes [46].

Based on compartment structure and lamellarity, liposomes can be classified as unilamellar vesicles (ULVs), oligolamellar vesicles (OLVs), multilamellar vesicles

Table 3.3. This table depicts the different nanoformulation utilized in the treatment different GI diseases along with the underlying mechanism involved.

Disease	Drug delivery approach	Nanoformulation	Mechanism of action	References
Esophageal cancer	Photothermal ablation therapy	Chitosan-coated gold-gold sulphide nanoparticles	Cancer cells coated with nanoparticles are subjected to x-ray irradiation that destroys them leaving healthy cells unharmed.	[37]
	Photodynamic therapy	• Porfimer sodium • Aminolevulinic acid • Foscan • Phthalocyanine	Application of a photosensitizer on the cancer cells that can be activated at a certain wavelength to produce ROS that damages the cells.	[36]
Gastric cancer	Stimuli-responsive strategy	Paclitaxel loaded nanoparticles incorporated with tentradine	Tentradine is used to boost up the stability of Paclitaxel nanoparticles and produces ROS while paclitaxel simultaneously eliminates antioxidants leading to cell death.	[37]
Crohon's disease and ulcerative colitis	Active targeting	Hyaluronic acid loaded polymeric nanoparticles with tripeptide coating	Accurately bind to amplified CD44 receptors expressed on inflamed epithelial cells.	[26]
		Mesalazine incorporated pectin-silica-based nanoparticles	Pectin is dissolved in the colon by enzyme pectinase assuring controlled release of Mesalazine in the colon.	
		Mannosylated PGLA-PEG nanoparticles	Target amplified Folate receptors expressed at the inflammatory sites.	
	pH-dependent dosage	Resveratrol incorporated into poly (N, N-dimethylamino ethyl methylacrylate) nanoparticles Eudragit-coated budesonide-loaded PLGA nanoparticles	Polymer layers protect the drug from upper GI degradation and trigger release only at a specific pH creating a delayed as well as extended drug release profile.	[15, 8]
	Charge-mediated Targeting	Positively charged chitosan nanoparticles	The mucus released by inflamed colon is abundant in negatively charged carbohydrates which results in stronger and specific binding.	

(Continued)

Table 3.3. (*Continued*)

Disease	Drug delivery approach	Nanoformulation	Mechanism of action	References
Colon cancer	pH-responsive dosage forms	Quercetin dihydrate loaded Eudragit® S100 coated nanoparticles	The pH-dependent polymer covering dissolves at an ideal pH of 7, ensuring regulated medication release in the colon.	[38]
	Active targeting and photodynamic therapy	EGFR conjugated Fucoidan/ alginate loaded hydrogel utilizing chlorin e6 photosensitizer	The nanoparticles target amplified EGFR on cancer cells and deliver the apoptotic agent fucoidan while the photosensitizer coats the cells and can produce ROS when stimulated.	[39]
	Photothermal therapy	IR780 loaded chitosan nanoparticles	Destruction of cancer cells using irradiations without sabotaging the healthy cells.	[40]
	Colon-specific drug delivery	Resistant starch film coated incorporated with fluorescein microparticles	Drugs delivered to colon specifically by providing resistance to drug release in the upper GI tract withstanding the gastric pH and enzymatic degradation.	[40]
		Pectin-Aminothiophenol coated Metronidazole loaded microparticles	The environment of colon is rich in pectinolytic enzymes that ensure the specific drug release in colon.	[40]
Colorectal cancer	Target delivery	IL-12 incorporated chitosan nanoparticles (utilizing TPP as crosslinking agent)	Reduction of tumor metastasis once IL-12 is provided to the cancer cells.	[37]
	Active targeting	Methotrexate incorporated folic acid conjugated guar gum nanoparticles	Specific delivery of drug to the folate receptors overexpressed on the colon cancer cells ensuring no drug pre-release in the upper GI tract.	[37]

(MLVs), and multivesicular liposomes (MVLs). OLVs and MLVs both have structures resembling onions, but OLVs also have two to five or more concentric lipid bilayers. Unlike MLVs, MVLs have a structure resembling a honeycomb and include a single-bilayer lipid membrane enclosing hundreds of non-concentric water chambers. Small unilamellar vesicles (SUVs, 30–100 nm), large unilamellar vesicles (LUVs, >100 nm), and giant unilamellar vesicles (GUVs, >1000 nm) are the three categories into which ULVs can be further subdivided based on particle size. Because of their prolonged circulation times and capacity to passively target the sick region, the majority of currently available commercial products—such as Doxil— are SUVs. Owing to its multiple chambers, the MVL structure may store a considerable amount of drug-aqueous solution and offer prolonged release due to the dispersion of drug molecules and the erosion/degradation of liposomes [47].

Different liposome preparation techniques have been created. The ethanol injection, double emulsion, and thin-film hydration techniques are among the frequently employed production procedures. The development of the drug solution(s) and drug loading; in the case of passive drug loading, this step is combined with step 1; the preparation of MLVs or ULVs; the reduction in size, if necessary; the aseptic processing; the buffer exchange and concentration; the aseptic processing; the lyophilization, if necessary; and the packaging.

The two primary strategies for medication loading are active and passive drug loading. Drug molecules may interact with lipids in ionic, covalent, non-covalent, electrostatic, or steric ways that cause the drug to be confined inside the inner aqueous space or included in the bilayer of liposomes. AmBisome, Arikayce, Visudyne, DepoDur, DepoCyte, and Expel are examples of commercialized liposomal products that use the passive drug loading strategy. Vyxeos, the first approved liposome containing daunorubicin and cytarabine in the same vesicle, employs a combination of active and passive loading (figure 3.4) [48].

When compared to other nanocarriers, liposomes are known for having minimal intrinsic toxicity; this is mostly because of the natural phospholipids that make up most of them [49]. The most often employed phospholipids in the creation of liposomes are sphingomyelins and lecithin, which may be found in soy and eggs [50]. The ability of liposomes to specifically target diseased tissues by functionalizing them with targeting moieties has been recognized, and they are valued for these positive qualities. For their vast therapeutic pharmaceutical uses as drug delivery systems, they provide a plethora of potential.

3.6.2 Polymeric nanoparticles

Macromolecules known as polymers are created by joining monomers to form straight or branching strands. As long as they have at least two functional groups where they may interact with another monomer, these monomers can have any structure. A polymer might be created to have certain qualities by using the right monomer(s). Due to their excellent synthetic adaptability, polymers may be tailored to specific needs by researchers. Chemical derivatization might be used to directly customize polymers for use in biopolymers [51], or from artificial monomers, which

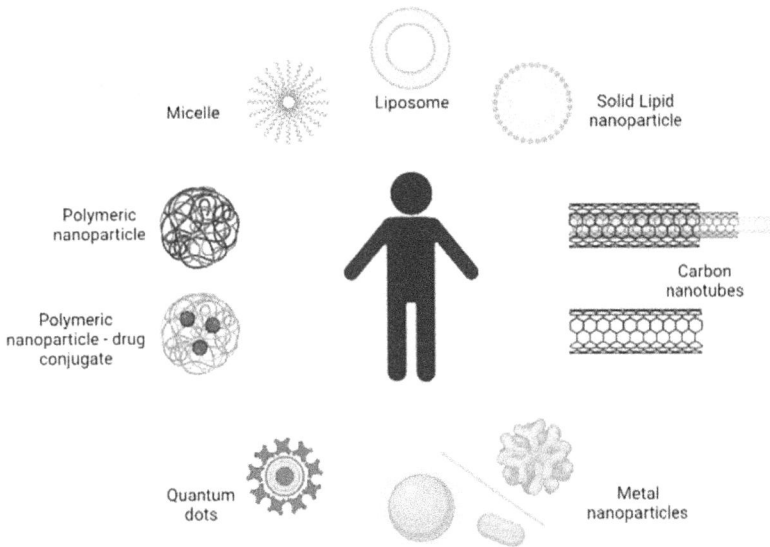

Figure 3.4. Nanoparticle-based drug delivery systems.

can result in a wide variety of forms and uses. As stabilizing agents, surfactants are necessary for the creation of polymeric nanoparticles. The majority of commonly used surfactants consist of an ionic functional group that can be cationic (like sodium laurate), anionic (like benzalkonium chloride), or non-ionic (like ethoxylated amines) attached to a hydrocarbon chain (hydrophobic portion) [52]. Low molecular weight polymers such as block copolymers (e.g., Pluronic P123) can also act as surfactants [53]. Reduced nanoparticle surface tension and increased affinity for lipidic structures are two benefits of the stabilizers [54]. When surfactant surface-modified nanoparticle systems are utilized, studies of pharmacokinetics and biodistribution demonstrate enhanced retention of the medication in the body and lower toxicity [55].

Due to their increased surface area, polymeric nanoparticles show many different surface functional groups, making them ideal for targeted drug delivery [56]. In addition, they are simple to operate and modify. With no chemical reaction, the medication loading capacity is likewise large and simple. Polymeric nanoparticles have a lot of benefits, but they also have some drawbacks, such as toxicity from certain surfactants used during preparation and the complexity of scaling up production.

Pharmaceuticals made of polymers work as inert carriers to deliver therapeutic molecules to certain locations. Polymers can be organic and synthetic. For instance, PAMAM dendrimers are biocompatible and may encapsulate different therapeutic compounds, but their main disadvantage is toxicity [57]. PEGylated PAMAM dendrimers have been created to address this, lowering cytotoxicity and liver damage [58]. PEGylation of polymers improves biodistribution and pharmacokinetics, as seen in PEGylated surfers with HPMA double bonds. Gelatin and albumin, two proteins with intriguing properties that make them useful building blocks for the production of nanoparticles, are also very stable and non-antigenic [59].

Numerous polymers, such as chitosan, alginate, PLGA (poly (lactic-co-glycolic acid), and PLA (polylactic acid), as well as collagen, are used to make nanoparticles because they are biocompatible and biodegradable [60]. Each contains special qualities including controlled release, pH sensitivity, and the capacity to transport drugs. A non-ionic hydrophilic polyester called PEG (Poly (ethylene glycol)) is used to stabilize nanoparticles, stop them from aggregating, and lessen immune recognition [61]. Ovomucin, which is obtained from egg whites, is a naturally occurring polymer with certain biological roles, although some people may experience allergic responses to it (figure 3.4).

The advantages of PEG and PLGA are combined in PEG-PLGA, a block copolymer that makes it simple to self-assemble into micelles that can contain and release pharmaceuticals under regulated conditions [62]. Even for hydrophilic pharmaceuticals, it is biodegradable and provides good drug encapsulation. Overall, polymeric nanoparticles show considerable promise for applications in targeted drug delivery and nanomedicine, but a comprehensive analysis of their characteristics and possible limitations is necessary before they can be developed and used.

3.6.3 Metallic nanoparticles

A significant avenue for the creation of novel medical technology is metal nanomaterials. Metal nanoparticles' long-term safety in medicine is still mostly unknown [63]. Several biological applications, such as site-specific *in vivo* imaging, cancer detection, and cancer therapy, have already made use of these particles, treatment for neurological diseases, treatment for HIV/AIDS, treatment for eye and respiratory diseases, and cancer therapy [64]. One of the many uses for metal nanoparticles is drug delivery [65]. Nanomaterial surface modification is essential to maintain nanoparticle stability and avoid aggregation. Surface modifications of noble metals, such as thiol groups, amines, and carboxylic acids, are common [66]. To decrease non-specific protein absorption and increase therapeutic effectiveness, nanoparticle surfaces are modified using long-chain polymers like PEG [67].

The exceptional physicochemical features of silver nanoparticles (AgNPs) and a variety of biological activities, such as antibacterial, antiviral, anti-fungal, and antioxidant capabilities, have made them well known [68]. When AgNPs contact with bacteria, silver ions are released, delaying membrane penetration and inhibiting cellular enzymes. Gold nanoparticles (AuNPs) can deliver pharmacological compounds, proteins, and chemotherapeutic drugs into their targets and are efficient radiosensitizers [69]. AuNPs are adaptable nanocarriers that exhibit beneficial properties in the biomedical industry, such as surface functionalization [70]. Palladium nanoparticles (PdNPs) have demonstrated antibacterial and cytotoxic effects as self-therapeutics and have significant mechanical and catalytic properties [71]. Owing to their expansive surface and capacity to combat cancer, germs, and free radicals, platinum nanoparticles (PtNPs) are now being studied in a number of biotechnological and pharmaceutical disciplines [72]. Due to their distinctive qualities, low toxicity, and potent antibacterial properties, copper nanoparticles

(CuNPs) have grown in popularity [73]. Other metal nanoparticles, such as those made of zinc oxide (ZnO), titanium dioxide (TiO$_2$), and metal sulfide nanoparticles, have intriguing possibilities for anti-cancer, anti-diabetic, and anti-inflammatory drug delivery systems (figure 3.4).

3.6.4 Quantum dots

Researchers have been more interested in quantum dots (QDs) because of their extraordinary electromagnetic, luminescent, and adaptable surface chemistry, which allows for real-time monitoring of QDs vehicle transit and drug release at both systemic and cellular levels. Inorganic nanomaterials known as QDs have large luminous excitation spectra and narrow symmetrical excitation spectra that suffer significant Stokes shifts [74]. Typically, QDs are made of a covering substance to prevent photobleaching and leakage and a metallic core material that may transmit fluorescence. The core material is chosen to provide the highest quantum yield. Researchers are interested in the outstanding electromagnetic, luminous, and controllable surface chemistry of QDs, which allows for real-time monitoring of QDs vehicle transit and drug release at both systemic and cellular levels. The inorganic nanomaterials known as QDs possess broad, symmetrical excitation spectra with weak Stokes shifts and broad, brilliant excitation spectral. Carbon dots (CDs), a type of commonly used graphene QD, have cemented their position as nanostructures due to their high cost-effectiveness, good solubility, simple function-alization, pleasant fluorescence emission, appealing chemical composition, simplic-ity of large-scale synthesis, and photochemical stability. Surface passivation enhances fluorescence while surface functionalization increases solubility in both aqueous and non-aqueous fluids [75]. Synthetic fluorescent CDs, according to reports, emit light in the deep blue (430 nm) to near-infrared (730 nm) ranges [76]. Due to these characteristics, CDs are well positioned to give unmatched performance for a variety of applications, including photodynamic treatment, biosensing, bioimaging, drug administration, and electrocatalysis [75]. Natural carbon dots (NCDs) are fluorescent, which provides real-time monitoring and sensing capabilities to enhance medication distribution. NCDs are biocompatible contrast agents that are both safe and effective for directing the course of drug release, particularly for medications that are not water-soluble. Sensing and tracking probe, photoactivated antibacterial agents, antioxidants, and neurodegenerative agents are the special uses of NCDs in drug administration (figure 3.4).

3.7 Approved nanomedicines

A large portion of the nanomedicines that are now being researched are improved release mechanisms for active ingredients that are already being utilized to treat patients. [77]. They are assessed for this sort of strategy if the pharmacokinetic profile and biodistribution of these active ingredients are altered by the prolonged release. If the active component is applied to the target tissue and demonstrates improved cell uptake/absorption and has a lower organism toxicity profile, it can be concluded that the nanoformulation is superior to the present formulation in this situation [78].

Some of the most often researched nanocarriers for drug delivery include dendrimers, micelles, liposomes, solid lipid nanoparticles, polymeric nanoparticles, and superparamagnetic iron oxide nanoparticles [79]. Tables 3.4–3.8 include details on nanotechnology-based products that have already been given FDA clearance. Notably, these nanomedicines are commonly able to improve the pharmacokinetic characteristics of the medication in issue while reducing its toxicity. They are often created for medications with severe toxicity and poor water solubility.

3.8 Application of AI in GI disease

In recent years, the application of AI in therapeutics for GI diseases has witnessed significant expansion. Advanced diagnostic technologies, such as capsule endoscopy, have benefited greatly from the incorporation of AI analysis, leading to improved patient outcomes and more targeted treatment approaches [86]. One area where AI has demonstrated great potential is in the classification of patients with biliary strictures and the identification of potential biomarkers in human bile. AI provides accurate patient categorization through the use of neural network models, assisting in early identification and intervention [87]. Additionally, the development of colorectal cancer prevention strategies has benefited greatly from the use of ML algorithms to medical examination records. Through retrospective and prospective clinical studies, AI assists in the diagnosis and prognosis prediction of a variety of GI diseases, including gastroesophageal reflux disease, atrophic corpus gastritis, acute pancreatitis, acute lower GI bleeding, esophageal cancer, nonvariceal upper GI bleeding, UC, and IBD [88]. Clinicians may make better judgments and give patients individualized care by utilizing these AI-powered technologies. AI has also demonstrated impressive promise for assisting in the identification and categorization of colorectal polyps, which may boost the use of colonoscopy for effective colorectal cancer therapies. With the use of this technology, which was created utilizing convolutional neural network (CNN) models, medical personnel may identify and characterize polyps with more precision [89]. Additionally, AI-guided tissue analysis has become a useful tool for forecasting outcomes in patients with stage III colon cancer, ultimately resulting in improved patient treatment with the help of pathologists. Doctors can develop customized treatment strategies by utilizing AI to analyze tissue samples and obtain important information on the behavior of the malignancy. Furthermore, AI utilization has proven effective in classifying Barrett's esophagus cancer, providing a more efficient and accurate diagnosis for this condition. An AI-based clinical decision-support system has been created for celiac disease, allowing for more accurate and quick diagnoses [90]. The identification of significant genes linked to the pathogenesis and prognosis of esophageal squamous cell carcinoma has also been greatly aided by bioinformatics analyses. These discoveries might aid in the creation of specific molecular treatments for the illness [91]. For locally advanced rectal adenocarcinoma, AI-driven identification of long non-coding RNA signatures has offered the ability to predict patient responses to

Table 3.4. FDA-approved polymer nanoparticles coupled with pharmaceuticals or biologicals.

Name	Loaded drug/biologics	Advantage	Indication	Approved year	References
Adagen®/pegademase bovine	PEGylated ADA enzyme	Decrease immunogenicity and improve circulation time	SCID	1990	[77, 80]
Oncaspar®/pegaspargase	PEGylated L-asparaginase	Improve stability	Acute lymphoblastic leukemia	1994	[77, 81, 82]
Copaxone®/Glatopa	Random copolymer of L-alanine, L-glutamine, L-tyrosine and L-lysine	Controlled molecular weight and clearance characteristics	Multiple sclerosis	1996	[77, 81]
Renagel®[sevelamer hydrochloride/Renagel®[sevelamer carbonate]	Poly (allylamine hydrochloride)	improve circulation time	Chronic kidney disease	2000	[83]
PegIntron®	PEGylated IFN alpha-2a	Improve stability	Hepatitis C	2001	[77, 81]
Eligard®	PLGH and leuprolide	Improve circulation time and controlled drug release	Prostate cancer	2002	[77, 80]
Neulasta®/pegfilgrastim	PEGylated GCSF protein	Improve stability	Neutropenia	2002	[77, 81]
Pegasys®	PEGylated IFN alpha-2a	Improve stability	Hepatitis B and C	2002	[77, 80, 81]
Rebinyn	GlycoPEGylated Coagulation factor IX	Effective control in bleeding	Haemophilia B	2017	[77]
Cimzia®/certolizumab pegol	PEGylated Certolizumab fragment	Improve stability and circulation time	Crohn's disease; Rheumatoid arthritis; Psoriatic Arthritis; Ankylosing Spondylitis	2008 2009 2013 2013	[77]

Krystexxa®/pegloticase	PEGylated porcine-like uricase	Improve stability	Chronic gout	2010	[77, 80]
Plegridy®	PEGylated IFN beta-1a	Improve stability	Multiple Sclerosis	2014	[77, 80]
ADYNOVATE	PEGylated factor VIII	Improve stability	Hemophilia	2015	[77]
Zilretta	Triamcinolone acetonide with a PLGA matrix microspheres	Extended pain relief over 12 weeks	Osteoarthritis	2017	[77]
Mircera®/Methoxy polyethylene glycol-epoetin beta	Synthetic ESA	Improve stability	Anemia associated with chronic kidney disease	2007	[77]
Somavert®/pegvisomant	PEGylated HGH receptor antagonist	Improve stability	Acromegaly	2003	[77]

ADA—Adenosine deaminase, IFN-Interferon, PLGH—poly DL-lactide-coglycolide, GCSF—Glycine cleavage system H, HGH—Human growth hormone, VEGF—Vascular endothelial growth factor, ESA - Erythropoiesis stimulating agent, SCID—Severe combined immunodeficiency disease.

Table 3.5. FDA-approved liposome formulations coupled with drugs or biologics.

Name	Loaded drug/biologics	Advantage	Indication	Approved year	References
Doxil®/Caelyx™	Doxorubicin	Improve on-site delivery, decrease systematic toxicity	Karposi's sarcoma; Ovarian cancer; multiple myeloma	1995 2005 2008	[77, 80–82, 84]
DaunoXome®	Daunorubicin	Improve on-site delivery, decrease systematic toxicity	Karposi's sarcoma	1995	[80, 82, 84]
Abelcet®	Amphotericin B	Reduce toxicity	Fungal infections	1995	[77, 80, 81]
DepoCyt©	Cytarabine	Improve on-site delivery, decrease systematic toxicity	Lymphomatous meningitis	1996	[77, 80–82]
AmBisome®	Amphotericin B	Reduce nephrotoxicity	Fungal/protozoal infections	1997	[77, 80, 81, 84]
Curosurf®/Poractant alpha	SP-8 and SP-C proteins	Reduce toxicity and improve controlled release	Pulmonary surfactant for respiratory distress syndrome	1999	[77]
Visudyne®	Verteporfin	Improve on-site delivery, photosensitive release	Macular degeneration, wet age-related; myopia; ocular histoplasmosis	2000	[77, 80, 84]
DepoDur®	Morphine sulphate	Improve controlled release	Analgesia	2004	[77, 80]
Marqibo®	Vincristine	Improve on-site delivery, decrease systematic toxicity	Acute lymphoblastic leukemia	2012	[77, 80–82, 84]
Onivyde®	Irinotecan	Improve on-site delivery, decrease systematic toxicity	Pancreatic cancer	2015	[77, 80, 82, 84]
Vyxeos	Daunorubicin and cytarabine	Improve controlled release	AML or AML-MRC	2017	[77]

AML—Acute myeloid leukemia, AML-MRC—Acute myeloid leukemia with myelodysplasia-related changes.

Table 3.6. FDA approved micellar nanoparticles coupled with drugs or biologics.

Name	Loaded drug/ biologics	Advantage	Indication	Approved year	References
Estrasorb™	Estradiol	Improve controlled release	Menopausal therapy	2003	[77, 80]

Table 3.7. FDA approved protein nanoparticles coupled with drugs or biologics.

Name	Description	Advantage	Indication	Approved year	References
Ontak®	Combination of IL-2 and diphtheria toxin with engineered protein	Improve stability	Cutaneous T-cell lymphoma	1999	[77]
Abraxane®/ ABI-007	Paclitaxel nanoparticles bound with albumin	Decrease immunogenicity and improve circulation time	Breast cancer; NSCLC; Pancreatic cancer	2005 2012 2013	[77, 80–82, 84]

NSCLC—Non small cell lung cancer

neoadjuvant chemoradiotherapy. This personalized approach can optimize treatment plans and improve patient outcomes [92]. Additionally, predictive biomarkers have been found in the entire blood of IBD patients thanks to ML, facilitating the use of customized treatments. By analyzing vast amounts of patient data, AI aids in tailoring treatment strategies to individual needs.

3.9 Future perspectives and challenges

In today's rapidly advancing technological landscape, achieving interoperability among various technologies is essential due to the immense amount of data available at the big data level. Nanoscience and nanotechnology offer vast possibilities, dealing with objects as small as molecules and atoms. However, at such a minute scale, a wealth of information is contained in collective data, necessitating data analytics and mining. AI and its subsets, ML and deep learning, play crucial roles in this endeavor [88]. AI has made significant strides across various industries, particularly in medicine, and the convergence of AI with nanoscience holds immense potential for nanomedicine, including fields like cancer cell research, biomedicine, and nanobiology. Integrating AI with nanotechnology becomes indispensable when dealing with nanomedicine and nanoscale drug delivery systems.

In order to establish effective therapeutic strategies, AI has been employed in identifying cancer subtypes, especially concerning cancer cell phenotypes like

Table 3.8. FDA approved nanocrystals coupled with drugs or biologics.

Name	Description	Advantage	Indication	Approved year	References
INFeD®	Iron dextran	Increases the dosage	Iron deficiency in chronic kidney disease	1957	[77]
DexIron®/Dexferrum®	Iron dextran	Increases the dosage	Iron deficiency in chronic kidney disease	1957	[77, 84]
Feridex®/Endorem®	SPION coated with dextran	Supermagnetic effects	Imaging agent	1996	[84]
Ferrlecit®	Sodium ferric gluconate	Increases the dosage	Iron deficiency in chronic kidney disease	1999	[77, 84]
Venofer®	Iron sucrose	Increases the dosage	Iron deficiency in chronic kidney disease	2000	[77, 84]
Rapamune®	Sirolimus	Increase bioavailability	Immunosuppressant	2000	[77, 80]
Megace ES®	Megestrol acetate	Reduce dose	Anti-anorexic	2001	[77, 80]
GastroMARK™; umirem®	SPION coated with silicone	Supermagnetic effects	Imaging agent	2001	[85]
Avinza®	Morphine sulphate	Increase bioavailability, release and drug loading	Psychostimulant	2002	[77]
Ritalin LA®	Methylphenidate HCl	Increase bioavailability, and drug loading	Psychostimulant	2002	[77]
Zanaflex®	Tizanidine HCl	Increase bioavailability, and drug loading	Muscle relaxant	2002	[77]
Vitoss®	Calcium phosphate	Allow cell adhesion and growth	Bone substitute	2003	[77]
OsSatura®	Hydroxyapatite	Allow cell adhesion and growth	Bone substitute	2003	[77]
Emend®	Aprepitant	Increase bioavailability and allow faster absorption	Antiemetic	2003	[77, 80]

Product	Composition	Function	Indication	Year	References
Tricor®	Fenofibrate	Increase bioavailability	Hyperlipidemia	2004	[77, 80]
Ostim®	Hydroxyapatite	Allow cell adhesion and growth	Bone substitute	2004	[77]
Focalin XR®	Dexmethylphenidate HCl	Increase bioavailability, and drug loading	Psychostimulant	2005	[77]
NanOss®	Hydroxyapatite	Allow cell adhesion and growth	Bone substitute	2005	[77]
EquivaBone®	Hydroxyapatite	Allow cell adhesion and growth	Bone substitute	2009	[77]
Invega® Sustenna®	Paliperidone palmitate	Controlled drug release	Schizophrenia	2009	[77]
			Schizoaffective disorder	2014	[77]
Feraheme™/ferumoxytol	Ferumoxytol SPION with polyglucose sorbitol carboxymethylether	Reduced dosages and sustained steady release are made possible by magnetite suspension.	Iron deficiency in chronic kidney disease	2009	[77, 80, 81, 84]
Inorganic and metallic nanoparticles Nanotherm®	Iron oxide	Supermagnetic effects and allow cell uptake	Glioblastoma	2010	[82]
Ryanodex®	Paliperidone palmitate	Faster administration	Malignant hypothermia	2014	[77]

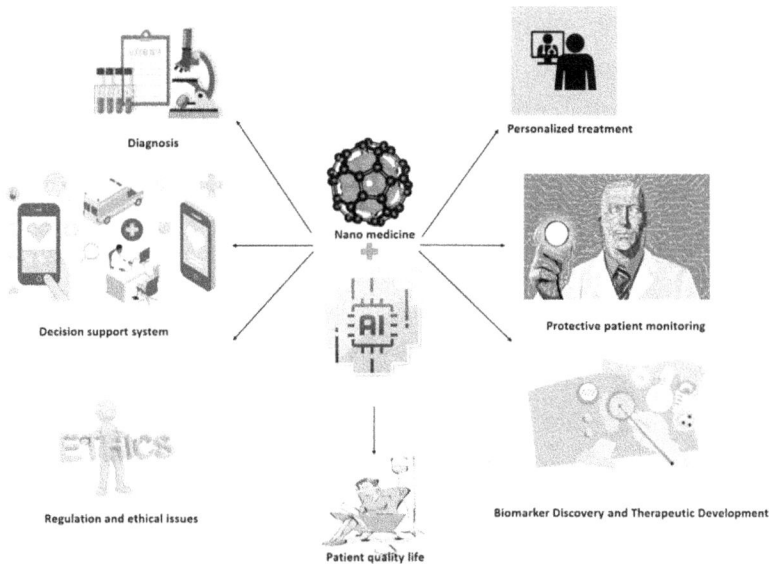

Figure 3.5. Application of AI and nanomedicine in different fields.

epithelial–mesenchymal transition in diffuse-type gastric cancer. This approach allows for more targeted treatments based on specific cancer characteristics. Finally, the gut–brain axis represents another crucial area where ML algorithms can be applied to GID therapy. AI can help unravel the complex interactions between the GI system and the brain, providing valuable insights for the development of innovative therapeutic approaches. The various aspects of AI's integration with nanoscience and nanotechnology in nanomedicine, particularly in the field of gastroenterology are shown in figure 3.5.

3.9.1 Diagnostics

AI systems have proven to be remarkably accurate in analyzing images from medical procedures like colonoscopies and endoscopies. These clever computers can spot irregularities, GI disease early warning indicators, and even potentially malignant tumors that could be hard for human experts to find. Early disease detection and diagnosis can result in quicker interventions and improved patient outcomes [93].

3.9.2 Individualized treatment

The development of individualized treatment regimens is made possible by AI's ability to assess substantial volumes of patient-specific data, such as genetic data, medical history, lifestyle factors, and reactions to prior therapies. These individualized treatments are created to meet the unique aspects of each patient's disease, resulting in more focused, efficient treatments with fewer side effects [94].

3.9.3 Proactive patient monitoring

AI-powered systems can keep track of patients constantly by evaluating data in real-time through sensors, wearable technology, and other sources. Healthcare workers can respond early and avert any emergencies by quickly identifying any symptoms of disease complications or exacerbation. This in-the-moment observation improves patient care and guarantees improved illness control [95].

3.9.4 Decision support systems

The creation of decision-support systems for medical practitioners is made possible by AI's capacity to process and evaluate enormous volumes of clinical and medical data. These tools can offer recommendations for treatments that are supported by the available data, assisting physicians in making well-informed choices regarding patient care. A healthcare system that is more effective and efficient is one that combines human competence and AI [96].

3.9.5 Biomarker discovery and therapeutic development

AI can assist in the discovery of novel biomarkers connected to GI illnesses, offering important insights into the pathophysiology of the condition and possible therapeutic targets. This knowledge could hasten medication development procedures and result in the identification of brand new GI disease treatment modalities [97, 98].

3.9.6 Patient outcomes and quality of life

By combining AI with nanomedicine and gastroenterology, we want to improve patient outcomes and raise the general standard of living for those with GI illnesses. AI-driven solutions have a substantial influence on patient care and management by offering early and accurate diagnoses, individualized treatment regimens, and real-time monitoring.

3.9.7 Regulation and ethical issues

While AI presents exciting breakthroughs, it is crucial to address issues like data privacy, ethics, and the need for strong regulatory frameworks. To maintain patient safety and confidence, it is essential to integrate AI in healthcare responsibly [99].

3.10 Conclusion

In particular, cancer cell research, biomedicine, and nanobiology have benefited from the integration of AI with nanoscience and nanotechnology in nanomedicine, which has shown promising results in the field of gastroenterology. The extraordinary precision in diagnosing GI disorders from medical imaging made possible by AI's capacity to evaluate massive volumes of data has enabled early therapies and improved patient outcomes. The treatment of GI diseases has also been transformed by AI-generated individualized treatment regimens based on patient-specific data, which optimize medicines and reduce side effects. AI-powered technologies enable ongoing patient monitoring and quickly identify symptoms of illness escalation. The use of decision-support technologies improves physician decision-making by offering evidence-based treatment suggestions. For ethical AI applications in healthcare, regulatory frameworks and ethical issues must be taken into account. AI and human expertise working together have the potential to significantly advance GI medicines, helping patients all around the world.

References

[1] Lombardo D, Kiselev M A and Caccamo M T 2019 Smart nanoparticles for drug delivery application: development of versatile nanocarrier platforms in biotechnology and nano-medicine *J. Nanomater.* **2019** 3702518

[2] Patra J K, Das G, Fraceto L F, Campos E V R, Rodriguez-Torres M D P, Acosta-Torres L S *et al* 2018 Nano based drug delivery systems: recent developments and future prospects *J. Nanobiotechnol.* **16** 1–33

[3] Alqahtani M S, Kazi M, Alsenaidy M A and Ahmad M Z 2021 Advances in oral drug delivery *Front. Pharmacol.* **12** 618411

[4] Soltani M, Kashkooli F M, Souri M, Harofte S Z, Harati T, Khadem A *et al* 2021 Enhancing clinical translation of cancer using nanoinformatics *Cancers (Basel)* **13** 2481

[5] Paul D, Sanap G, Shenoy S, Kalyane D, Kalia K and Tekade R K 2021 Artificial intelligence in drug discovery and development *Drug Discov. Today* **26** 80

[6] Lou J, Duan H, Qin Q, Teng Z, Gan F, Zhou X *et al* 2023 Advances in oral drug delivery systems: challenges and opportunities *Pharmaceutics* **15** 484

[7] Stillhart C, Vučićević K, Augustijns P, Basit A W, Batchelor H, Flanagan T R *et al* 2020 Impact of gastrointestinal physiology on drug absorption in special populations—an UNGAP review *Eur. J. Pharm. Sci.* **147** 105280

[8] Hua S 2020 Advances in oral drug delivery for regional targeting in the gastrointestinal tract—influence of physiological, pathophysiological and pharmaceutical factors *Front. Pharmacol.* **11** 524

[9] Van Den Abeele J, Rubbens J, Brouwers J and Augustjns P 2017 The dynamic gastric environment and its impact on drug and formulation behaviour *Eur. J. Pharm. Sci.* **96** 207–31

[10] Abuhelwa A Y, Foster D J R and Upton R N 2016 A quantitative review and meta-models of the variability and factors affecting oral drug absorption—part I: gastrointestinal pH *AAPS J.* **18** 1309–21

[11] Azman M, Sabri A H, Anjani Q K, Mustaffa M F and Hamid K A 2022 Intestinal absorption study: challenges and absorption enhancement strategies in improving oral drug delivery *Pharmaceuticals* **15** 975

[12] Choonara B F, Choonara Y E, Kumar P, Bijukumar D, du Toit L C and Pillay V 2014 A review of advanced oral drug delivery technologies facilitating the protection and absorption of protein and peptide molecules *Biotechnol. Adv.* **32** 1269–82

[13] Bakshi H A, Quinn G A, Aljabali A A A, Hakkim F L, Farzand R, Nasef M M *et al* 2021 Exploiting the metabolism of the gut microbiome as a vehicle for targeted drug delivery to the colon *Pharmaceuticals* **14** 1211

[14] Permanadewi I, Kumoro A C, Wardhani D H and Aryanti N 2019 Modelling of controlled drug release in gastrointestinal tract simulation *J. Phys.: Conf. Ser.* **1295** 012063

[15] Chavda V P 2018 Nanobased nano drug delivery: a comprehensive review *Applications of Targeted Nano Drugs and Delivery Systems: Nanoscience and Nanotechnology in Drug Delivery* (Amsterdam: Elsevier) pp 69–92

[16] Umapathy V R, Natarajan P M and Swamikannu B 2023 Review of the role of nanotechnology in overcoming the challenges faced in oral cancer diagnosis and treatment *Molecules* **28** 5395

[17] Krishna R, Rizk M L, Larson P J, Schulz V, Friedman E, Gupta P *et al* 2016 Novel gastroretentive controlled release formulations for once-daily administration: assessment of clinical feasibility and formulation concept for raltegravir *Ther. Innov. Regul. Sci.* **50** 777–90

[18] Liu R, Luo C, Pang Z, Zhang J, Ruan S, Wu M *et al* 2023 Advances of nanoparticles as drug delivery systems for disease diagnosis and treatment *Chin. Chem. Lett.* **34** 107518

[19] Liu J, Leng P and Liu Y 2021 Oral drug delivery with nanoparticles into the gastrointestinal mucosa *Fundam. Clin. Pharmacol.* **35:** 86–96

[20] Macedo A S, Castro P M, Roque L, Thomé N G, Reis C P, Pintado M E *et al* 2020 Novel and revisited approaches in nanoparticle systems for buccal drug delivery *J. Control. Release* **320** 125–41

[21] Mamidi N and Delgadillo R M V 2021 Design, fabrication and drug release potential of dual stimuli-responsive composite hydrogel nanoparticle interfaces *Colloids Surf. B Biointerfaces* **204** 111819

[22] Chen W, Sun Z and Lu L 2021 Targeted engineering of medicinal chemistry for cancer therapy: recent advances and perspectives *Angew. Chem.-Int. Ed.* **60** 5626–43

[23] Coco R, Plapied L, Pourcelle V, Jérôme C, Brayden D J, Schneider Y J *et al* 2013 Drug delivery to inflamed colon by nanoparticles: comparison of different strategies *Int. J. Pharm.* **440** 3–12

[24] Xiao B, Laroui H, Viennois E, Ayyadurai S, Charania M A, Zhang Y *et al* 2014 Nanoparticles with surface antibody against CD98 and carrying CD98 small interfering RNA reduce colitis in mice *Gastroenterology* **146** 1289–300

[25] Mane V and Muro S 2012 Biodistribution and endocytosis of ICAM-1-targeting antibodies versus nanocarriers in the gastrointestinal tract in mice *Int. J. Nanomed.* **7** 4223–37

[26] Chen F, Liu Q, Xiong Y and Xu L 2021 Current strategies and potential prospects of nanomedicine-mediated therapy in inflammatory bowel disease *Int. J. Nanomed.* **16** 4225–37

[27] Thakral S, Thakral N K and Majumdar D K 2013 Eudragit®: a technology evaluation *Expert Opin. Drug Deliv.* **10** 131–49

[28] Liu J, Zhu D, Ling T, Vasileff A and Qiao S Z 2017 S-NiFe$_2$O$_4$ ultra-small nanoparticle built nanosheets for efficient water splitting in alkaline and neutral pH *Nano Energy* **40** 264–73

[29] Simmonds N J, Allen R E, Stevens T R J, Niall R, Van Someren M, Blake D R *et al* 1992 Chemiluminescence assay of mucosal reactive oxygen metabolites in inflammatory bowel disease *Gastroenterology* **103** 186–96

[30] Lih-Brody L, Powell S R, Collier K P, Reddy G M, Cerchia R, Kahn E *et al* 1996 Increased oxidative stress and decreased antioxidant defenses in mucosa of inflammatory bowel disease *Digest. Dis. Sci.* **41** 2078–86

[31] Gareb B, Eissens A C, Kosterink J G W and Frijlink H W 2016 Development of a zero-order sustained-release tablet containing mesalazine and budesonide intended to treat the distal gastrointestinal tract in inflammatory bowel disease *Eur. J. Pharm. Biopharm.* **103** 32–42

[32] Liu G, Lovell J F, Zhang L and Zhang Y 2020 Stimulus-responsive nanomedicines for disease diagnosis and treatment *Int. J. Mol. Sci.* **21** 1–44

[33] Das S, Kaur S and Kumar Rai V 2021 Gastro-retentive drug delivery systems: a recent update on clinical pertinence and drug delivery *Drug Deliv. and Transl. Res.* **11** 1849–77

[34] Kumar M and Kaushik D 2018 An overview on various approaches and recent patents on gastroretentive drug delivery systems *Recent Pat. Drug Deliv. Formul* **12** 84–92

[35] Hua S, Marks E, Schneider J J and Keely S 2015 Advances in oral nano-delivery systems for colon targeted drug delivery in inflammatory bowel disease: selective targeting to diseased versus healthy tissue *Nanomed. Nanotechnol. Biol. Med.* **11** 1117–32

[36] Didamson O C and Abrahamse H 2021 Targeted photodynamic diagnosis and therapy for esophageal cancer: potential role of functionalized nanomedicine *Pharmaceutics* **13** 1943

[37] Riasat R and Guangjun N 2016 Effects of nanoparticles on gastrointestinal disorders and therapy *J. Clin. Toxicol.* **6** 1000313

[38] Sunoqrot S and Abujamous L 2019 pH-sensitive polymeric nanoparticles of quercetin as a potential colon cancer-targeted nanomedicine *J. Drug Deliv. Sci. Technol.* **52** 670–6

[39] Shanmugapriya K, Kim H and Kang H W 2020 Epidermal growth factor receptor conjugated fucoidan/alginates loaded hydrogel for activating EGFR/AKT signaling pathways in colon cancer cells during targeted photodynamic therapy *Int. J. Biol. Macromol.* **158** 1163–74

[40] Wahab S, Alshahrani M Y, Ahmad M F and Abbas H 2021 Current trends and future perspectives of nanomedicine for the management of colon cancer *Eur. J. Pharmacol.* **910** 174464

[41] Daraee H, Etemadi A, Kouhi M, Alimirzalu S and Akbarzadeh A 2016 Application of liposomes in medicine and drug delivery *Artif. Cells Nanomed. Biotechnol.* **44** 381–91

[42] Kumar A, Badde S, Kamble R and Pokharkar V B 2010 Development and characterization of liposomal drug delivery system for nimesulide *Int. J. Pharm. Pharmaceut. Sci.* **2** 87–9

[43] Mazur F, Bally M, Städler B and Chandrawati R 2017 Liposomes and lipid bilayers in biosensors *Adv. Colloid Interface Sci.* **249** 88–99

[44] Niu M, Lu Y, Hovgaard L, Guan P, Tan Y, Lian R *et al* 2012 Hypoglycemic activity and oral bioavailability of insulin-loaded liposomes containing bile salts in rats: the effect of cholate type, particle size and administered dose *Eur. J. Pharm. Biopharm.* **81** 265–72

[45] Wang N, Wang T, Li T and Deng Y 2009 Modulation of the physicochemical state of interior agents to prepare controlled release liposomes *Colloids Surf. B Biointerfaces* **69** 232–8

[46] Zeng H, Qi Y, Zhang Z, Liu C, Peng W and Zhang Y 2021 Nanomaterials toward the treatment of Alzheimer's disease: recent advances and future trends *Chin. Chem. Lett.* **32** 1857–68

[47] Guimarães D, Cavaco-Paulo A and Nogueira E 2021 Design of liposomes as drug delivery system for therapeutic applications *Int. J. Pharm.* **601** 120571

[48] Mayer L, Janoff A, Swenson C and Louie A 2008 Fixed drug ratios for treatment of hematopoietic cancers and proliferative disorders *US Patent* US20070901772P 20070216 http://v3.espacenet.com/textdoc?DB=EPODOC&IDX=CN101657098

[49] Li C, Zhang Y, Wan Y, Wang J, Lin J, Li Z *et al* 2021 STING-activating drug delivery systems: design strategies and biomedical applications *Chin. Chem. Lett.* **32** 1615–25

[50] Gadekar V, Borade Y, Kannaujia S, Rajpoot K, Anup N, Tambe V *et al* 2021 Nanomedicines accessible in the market for clinical interventions *J. Control. Release* **330** 372–97

[51] Liu R, Zhao J, Han Q, Hu X, Wang D, Zhang X *et al* 2018 One-step assembly of a biomimetic biopolymer coating for particle surface engineering *Adv. Mater.* **30** e1802851

[52] Cortés H, Hernández-Parra H, Bernal-Chávez S A, Prado-Audelo M L D, Caballero-Florán I H, Borbolla-Jiménez F V *et al* 2021 Non-ionic surfactants for stabilization of polymeric nanoparticles for biomedical uses *Materials* **14** 3197

[53] Zhao T, Elzatahry A, Li X and Zhao D 2019 Single-micelle-directed synthesis of mesoporous materials *Nat. Rev. Mater.* **4** 775–91

[54] Belletti D, Grabrucker A M, Pederzoli F, Menrath I, Cappello V, Vandelli M A *et al* 2016 Exploiting the versatility of cholesterol in nanoparticles formulation *Int. J. Pharm.* **511** 331–40

[55] Joseph E and Saha R N 2017 Investigations on pharmacokinetics and biodistribution of polymeric and solid lipid nanoparticulate systems of atypical antipsychotic drug: effect of material used and surface modification *Drug Dev. Ind. Pharm.* **43** 678–86

[56] Dey A, Koli U, Dandekar P and Jain R 2016 Investigating behaviour of polymers in nanoparticles of chitosan oligosaccharides coated with hyaluronic acid *Polymer (Guildf)* **93** 44–52

[57] Taghavi Pourianazar N, Mutlu P and Gunduz U 2014 Bioapplications of poly(amidoamine) (PAMAM) dendrimers in nanomedicine *J. Nanopart. Res.* **16** 2342

[58] Luong D, Kesharwani P, Deshmukh R, Mohd Amin M C I, Gupta U, Greish K *et al* 2016 PEGylated PAMAM dendrimers: enhancing efficacy and mitigating toxicity for effective anticancer drug and gene delivery *Acta Biomater.* **43** 14–29

[59] Elzoghby A O, Samy W M and Elgindy N A 2012 Albumin-based nanoparticles as potential controlled release drug delivery systems *J. Control. Release* **157** 168–82

[60] Pandey P, Patel J and Kumar S 2022 Toward eco-friendly nanotechnology-based polymers for drug delivery applications *Sustainable Nanotechnology* (New York: Wiley) pp 89–116

[61] Sur S, Rathore A, Dave V, Reddy K R, Chouhan R S and Sadhu V 2019 Recent developments in functionalized polymer nanoparticles for efficient drug delivery system *Nano-Struct. Nano-Objects* **20** 100397

[62] Shi J, Yu L and Ding J 2021 PEG-based thermosensitive and biodegradable hydrogels *Acta Biomater.* **128** 42–59

[63] Hofmann-Amtenbrink M, Grainger D W and Hofmann H 2015 Nanoparticles in medicine: current challenges facing inorganic nanoparticle toxicity assessments and standardizations *Nanomedicine* **11** 1689–94

[64] Åkerman M E, Chan W C W, Laakkonen P, Bhatia S N and Ruoslahti E 2002 Nanocrystal targeting *in vivo Proc. Natl. Acad. Sci.* **99** 12617–21

[65] Faraji A H and Wipf P 2009 Nanoparticles in cellular drug delivery *Bioorg. Med. Chem.* **17** 2950–62

[66] Patzke G R, Zhou Y, Kontic R and Conrad F 2011 Oxide nanomaterials: synthetic developments, mechanistic studies, and technological innovations *Angew. Chem. Int. Ed.* **50** 826–59

[67] Suk J S, Xu Q, Kim N, Hanes J and Ensign L M 2016 PEGylation as a strategy for improving nanoparticle-based drug and gene delivery *Adv. Drug Deliv. Rev.* **99** 28–51

[68] Le Ouay B and Stellacci F 2015 Antibacterial activity of silver nanoparticles: a surface science insight *Nano Today* **10** 339–54

[69] Jain S, Hirst D G and O'Sullivan J M 2012 Gold nanoparticles as novel agents for cancer therapy *Br. J. Radiol.* **85** 101–13

[70] Alkilany A M and Murphy C J 2010 Toxicity and cellular uptake of gold nanoparticles: what we have learned so far? *J. Nanopart. Res.* **12** 2313–33

[71] Yaqoob S B, Adnan R, Rameez Khan R M and Rashid M 2020 Gold, silver, and palladium nanoparticles: a chemical tool for biomedical applications *Front. Chem.* **8** 376

[72] Johnstone T C, Suntharalingam K and Lippard S J 2016 The next generation of platinum drugs: targeted pt(ii) agents, nanoparticle delivery, and Pt(IV) prodrugs *Chem. Rev.* **116** 3436–86

[73] Gawande M B, Goswami A, Felpin F X, Asefa T, Huang X, Silva R *et al* 2016 Cu and Cu-based nanoparticles: synthesis and applications in catalysis *Chem. Rev.* **116** 3722–811

[74] Yao J, Li P, Li L and Yang M 2018 Biochemistry and biomedicine of quantum dots: from biodetection to bioimaging, drug discovery, diagnostics, and therapy *Acta Biomater.* **74** 36–55

[75] Lim S Y, Shen W and Gao Z 2015 Carbon quantum dots and their applications *Chem. Soc. Rev.* **44** 362–81

[76] Yuan T, Meng T, He P, Shi Y, Li Y, Li X *et al* 2019 Carbon quantum dots: an emerging material for optoelectronic applications *J. Mater. Chem. C Mater.* **7** 6820–35

[77] Ventola C L 2017 Progress in nanomedicine: approved and investigational nanodrugs *P T* **42** 742–55

[78] Havel H, Finch G, Strode P, Wolfgang M, Zale S, Bobe I *et al* 2016 Nanomedicines: from bench to bedside and beyond *AAPS J.* **18** 1373–8

[79] Zhu Z, Li Y, Yang X, Pan W and Pan H 2017 The reversion of anti-cancer drug antagonism of tamoxifen and docetaxel by the hyaluronic acid-decorated polymeric nanoparticles *Pharmacol. Res.* **126** 84–96

[80] Grumezescu A M 2017 *Nanoscale Fabrication, Optimization, Scale-up and Biological Aspects of Pharmaceutical Nanotechnology* (Elsevier)

[81] Caster J M, Patel A N, Zhang T and Wang A 2017 Investigational nanomedicines in 2016: a review of nanotherapeutics currently undergoing clinical trials *WIREs Nanomed. Nanobiotechnol.* **9** e1416

[82] Tran S, DeGiovanni P, Piel B and Rai P 2017 Cancer nanomedicine: a review of recent success in drug delivery *Clin Transl Med.* **6** e44

[83] Slatopolsky E A, Burke S K and Dillon M A 1999 RenaGel®, a nonabsorbed calcium- and aluminum-free phosphate binder, lowers serum phosphorus and parathyroid hormone *Kidney Int.* **55** 299–307

[84] Anselmo A C and Mitragotri S 2016 Nanoparticles in the clinic *Bioeng. Transl. Med.* **1** 10–29

[85] Sharma S, Parveen R and Chatterji B P 2021 Toxicology of nanoparticles in drug delivery *Curr. Pathobiol. Rep.* **9** 133–44

[86] Tziortziotis I, Laskaratos F M and Coda S 2021 Role of artificial intelligence in video capsule endoscopy *Diagnostics* **11** 1192

[87] Urman J M, Herranz J M, Uriarte I, Rullán M, Oyón D, González B *et al* 2020 Pilot multi-omic analysis of human bile from benign and malignant biliary strictures: a machine-learning approach *Cancers (Basel)* **12** 1–30

[88] Yang Y J and Bang C S 2019 Application of artificial intelligence in gastroenterology *World J. Gastroenterol.* **25** 1666

[89] Taghiakbari M, Mori Y and von Renteln D 2021 Artificial intelligence-assisted colonoscopy: a review of current state of practice and research *World J. Gastroenterol.* **27** 8103

[90] Hamade N and Sharma P 2021 Artificial intelligence in Barrett's esophagus *Ther. Adv. Gastrointest. Endosc.* **14**

[91] Zhou W, Wu J, Liu X, Ni M, Meng Z, Liu S *et al* 2020 Identification of crucial genes correlated with esophageal cancer by integrated high-throughput data analysis *Medicine* **99** e20340

[92] Machado Carvalho J V, Dutoit V, Corrò C and Koessler T 2023 Promises and challenges of predictive blood biomarkers for locally advanced rectal cancer treated with neoadjuvant chemoradiotherapy *Cells* **12** 413

[93] Goyal H, Mann R, Gandhi Z, Perisetti A, Ali A, Ali K A *et al* 2020 Scope of artificial intelligence in screening and diagnosis of colorectal cancer *J. Clin. Med.* **9** 1–22

[94] Johnson K B, Wei W Q, Weeraratne D, Frisse M E, Misulis K, Rhee K *et al* 2021 Precision medicine, AI, and the future of personalized health care *Clin. Transl. Sci.* **14** 86

[95] Bohr A and Memarzadeh K 2020 The rise of artificial intelligence in healthcare applications *Artif. Intell. Healthc.* **2020** 25–60

[96] Giordano C, Brennan M, Mohamed B, Rashidi P, Modave F and Tighe P 2021 Accessing artificial intelligence for clinical decision-making *Front. Digit. Health* **3** 645232

[97] Vatansever S, Schlessinger A, Wacker D, Kaniskan HÜ, Jin J, Zhou M M *et al* 2021 Artificial intelligence and machine learning-aided drug discovery in central nervous system diseases: state-of-the-arts and future directions *Med. Res. Rev.* **41** 1427

[98] Alqahtani A 2022 Application of artificial intelligence in discovery and development of anticancer and antidiabetic therapeutic agents *Evid. Based Complement Alternat. Med.* **2022** 6201067

[99] Murdoch B 2021 Privacy and artificial intelligence: challenges for protecting health information in a new era *BMC Med. Ethics* **22** 1–5

IOP Publishing

Nanobiotechnology and Artificial Intelligence in
Gastrointestinal Diseases

Vivek K Chaturvedi, Anurag Kumar Singh, Jay Singh and Dawesh P Yadav

Chapter 4

Novel drug delivery systems for inflammatory bowel disease

Ashutosh Kumar, Pratistha Singh, Rajesh Kumar and Sunil Dutt

Crohn's disease (CD) and ulcerative colitis constitute the majority of the chronic and recurrent inflammatory disorder known as inflammatory bowel disease (IBD). These are incurable and complex disease states. The treatment of IBD is complex because of gastrointestinal (GI) tract inflammation and epithelium damage. Several approaches have been used to treat this chronic illness. To treat the inflamed region of the GI tract, selective and site-specific drug delivery methods continue to be important. Antibiotics, steroids, immunosuppressive and high nonsteroidal anti-inflammatory drugs have been used for the treatment of IBD. Targeted drug delivery to the specific inflammatory area of the bowl increases therapeutic efficacy and allows for localized treatment, which lowers systemic toxicity. Some drug formulations have been formulated as targeted delivery to reduce the early signs of inflammation. Drugs made from nanoparticles (NPs) have recently received a lot of attention due to their potential to address these issues. There are various types of nanodrug delivery systems, which can deliver the drug into the inflamed or targeted area of the gut for the prolonged and desired action. Some novel drug delivery systems have been developed for targeting the inflamed area of the gut. These are now frequently employed to deliver medications, proteins, DNA, RNA, genes, polypeptides, medicines, and even vaccinations. Enteric coated pills, prodrugs and hybrid drug delivery systems are examples of some novel drug delivery systems. A stable and functionally developed novel drug delivery system is required in order to deliver the drugs specifically to the disease site, increase the duration of the drug's residence time, and reduce systemic effects. This chapter will discuss the type and the role of novel drug delivery systems in the treatment of IBD along with challenges and future aspects in the treatment of IBD.

4.1 Introduction

IBDs are mostly characterized by ulcerative colitis and CD but also include non-infectious intestinal inflammations. Pathogenesis of the disease is not clear, however, strong new investigative tools are steadily increasing our understanding of the major pathophysiologic processes underlying these disorders, allowing for the creation of potent new medicines [1]. The disease's pathogenesis is likely to involve interactions between genetic factors, environmental conditions (e.g., bacterial pathogens), and abnormal immune system activity. CD is a recurrent systemic inflammatory illness that primarily impacts the GI tract, with extra-intestinal symptoms related with immunological illnesses. Ulcerative colitis is marked by diffuse mucosal inflammation that spreads proximally from the rectum to variable degrees. Although CD mostly impacts the colon, it can spread to other areas of the GI tract, causing transmural inflammation [2]. In contrast, ulcerative colitis is limited to the colon, and the inflammation is primarily involved in the mucosal layer. IBD treatment seeks to minimize symptom severity and extent, as well as to limit disease progression. These disorders are the result of three interdependent cofactors: host vulnerability, intestinal microbiota, and mucosal immunity. CD is related with increased IL-12/IL-23 and IFN-/IL-17 generation, which impacts the small intestine and colon, causing irregular ulcers and full thickness intestinal wall inflammation, often with granulomas. The primary organ affected by ulcerative colitis is the colon, and excessive IL-13 production is linked to it. A continuous mucosal inflammation almost invariably involves the rectum and extends proximally [3]. Conventional immunosuppressive and anti-inflammatory medications, such as corticosteroids, mesalamine compounds, azathioprine, and its derivatives, are used in medical treatment. Our capacity to manage IBD has dramatically improved with the development of newer, targeted medications like anti-TNF-α-antibodies that target the inflammatory cytokine TNF-α. The effects of IL-12 and IL-23 on CD can be prevented by using an anti-IL-12p40 antibody. Classical medications have variable tolerability and high toxicities, and even newer therapies are limited by lower efficacy and related toxicities [4].

The conventional modes of drug administration are parenteral, oral, and rectal, with oral administration being the most extensively used. However, with these regular methods of distribution, difficulties of drug responses and lack of accuracy in delivering medications to affected locations have occurred. Because the physiological environment differs through the GI tract, traditional targeted medication delivery techniques are unable to provide satisfactory outcomes [5]. Furthermore, many regions of inflammation exist in the targeted area of the intestine and the pattern of inflammation is often uneven. As a result, only a little amount of the medication gets to the inflamed regions, whereas the remaining amount might get absorbed into the circulatory system through healthier regions of the digestive tract, causing considerable adverse effects. Novel methods of drug delivery have been developed to address many curative challenges and to provide localized delivery of drugs to target tissues [6].

4.2 Challenges and barriers in drug delivery

The oral route of drug delivery, is the most preferred way of treating GI tract inflammation in patients. However, the oral route of medication delivery is also the most difficult to execute because several obstacles and environmental factors may impede the drug's reach at the site of action [6].

The stomach possesses a high acidic condition, having a pH between 1.0 and 2.5, making it the obstruction to drug absorption. Extrinsic epithelial cells and a mucin-bicarbonate barrier combine to reduce drugs absorption. Pepsins in the stomach may degrade protein drugs. The small intestine, with its large surface area and diverse transport routes, is a prime site for oral drug delivery. However, challenges like the acidic gastric environment, pancreatic enzymes, and the mucosal barrier may hinder drug absorption [7].

The pH level in the colon is higher, with longer residence time, and low enzyme activity compared to the upper GI tract. Gut microbiota can metabolize drugs, affecting release characteristics. The colon needs to be targeted in order to treat bowel illnesses with fewer side effects and smaller dosages.

Normally, the pH in the area that lies connecting the colon and the rectum is 7.0 ± 0.7. However, in people with ulcerative colitis, the pH ranges from 2.7 to 5.5, with an average of 5.3 in those with CD. pH environments and digestive enzymes are biochemical hurdles for oral delivery of drugs. Acidic to alkaline, impacting drug action, absorption and bioavailability. pH variation also influences oral drug delivery design and targeting [8].

4.3 Drugs used in IBD

The use of general strategies to therapy in IBD treatments are generally determined by the extent of the illness and the affected location. Aminosalicylates, cortico-steroids, and immunosuppressive medications are just a few of the typical treatment drugs. Aminosalicylates, particularly 5-amino salicylic acid, are the primary drugs for patients with mild-to-moderate conditions of CD or ulcerative colitis because they work by modulating inflammatory mediators and exhibiting an antioxidant effect [9]. However, using 5-ASA has been associated with a number of side effects, including headaches, fever, flatulence, rashes, nausea, diarrhoea, cramps, and sometimes pancreatitis, nephritis, pancytopenia, and hair loss. Corticosteroids are another class of medications used to treat IBD signs and symptoms, reduce inflammatory conditions, and suppress immunological responses, but their use in long-term therapy is constrained by their adverse drug reaction, which includes infections, Cushing's syndrome, adrenal dysfunction, insomnia, osteoporosis, and impaired kidney function. Immunosuppressive drugs are frequently used as a third-line treatment for IBD patients who are in the chronic active stage and have not shown a meaningful response to 5-ASA and steroids [10].

IBD and other immunological disorders like psoriasis, ankylosing spondylitis, and rheumatoid arthritis are all affected by the cytokine TNF, which is also crucial in their progression. As a new therapy option, TNF-specific monoclonal antibodies were developed and need to be employed in the event that the other drugs are ineffective or have side effects. Despite TNF-targeting biological deliveries have demonstrated remarkable efficiency, particularly in cases when conventional approaches have failed, and use of such medicines may result in undesired adverse effects and hypersensitivity [11]. It is crucial to emphasize the potential for the development of antibodies against anti-TNF agents, the sudden immune response (itching, burning, prolonged hypersensitive response, erythema), infections (specifically when used in association with immunomodulatory drugs like corticosteroids), autoimmunity, and to a lower degree, cancers such as lymphoma. Ustekinumab, a human monoclonal antibody that binds the prevalent p40 component found in IL-12 and IL-23, inhibits the biological function of Th1 and Th17 pathogenic cells [12]. When used as a single therapy, stekinumab was effective in treating persons with moderate to serious IBD who had become resistant to anti-TNF, and it increased their rate of remission. Natalizumab, a recombinant humanized monoclonal antibody directed against α4-integrin from leukocytes, is a crucial biological therapeutic created for inflammatory illnesses. Natalizumab works by blocking T-cell migration to inflamed regions such as the gut. Natalizumab appears to be a potential alternative option for those with IBD who have not responded to conventional medications [13].

4.4 Novel drug delivery system for inflammatory bowel disease

There are negative aspects of conventional drug delivery systems, such as a higher probability of systemic adverse drug reactions and the difficulty in delivering ingredients mainly to the inflamed or diseased portions of GI tracts [14]. For utilization in patients having IBD, drug carriers having dimensions in micro- and nano, such as NPs, microparticles and liposomes, and many more variations, have been created and rigorously evaluated (figure 4.1).

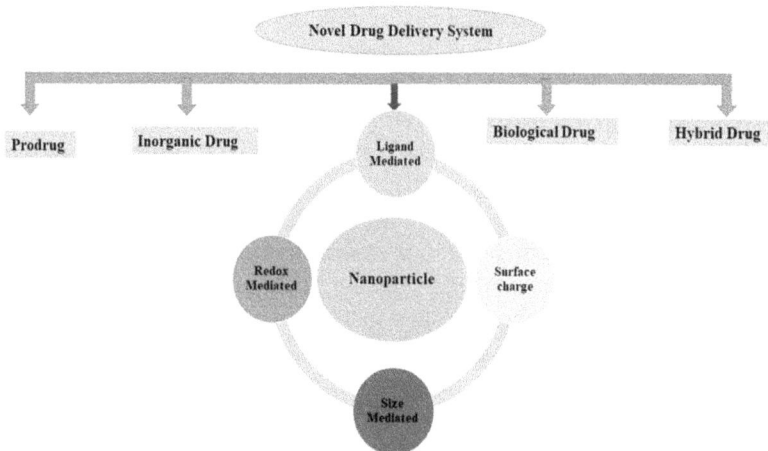

Figure 4.1. Novel drug delivery systems.

4.4.1 Vesicular delivery system

The most recommended method for treating localized illnesses of the colon in the GI tract is oral administration. Inflammation occurs at the ascending portion of the colon, where site-specific medication delivery methods like enemas and suppositories are ineffective. In comparison to the GI tract's proximal locations, the colon has a higher affinity for absorbing water. The limited volume of colonic fluid makes it difficult for drugs to dissolve at the colon site and makes them less bioavailable. If a drug administered at the colon location has a low solubility in water, the vesicular-based route of administration is preferred in order to get over the colonic delivery system's dissolving and penetration problems and achieve the necessary effectiveness [15]. These vesicular delivery devices have the significant benefit of maintaining drug molecules in dissolved state or need very little water to create *in situ* micro- or nanoemulsions. Micro- and nanoemulsions, which are lipid-based vesicular delivery vehicles, are usually selected for active compounds like cyclosporine, tacrolimus, and curcumin that have unpredictable bioavailability and limited water solubility. In GI tract mediums, the appropriate micro- and nanoemulsions improve solubility [16]. These delivery devices' tiny size allows for relatively high interfacial surface contact, which further encourages drug uptake by cells and systemic absorption. The high doses of medication are reduced by all these characteristics of micro- and nanoemulsions. The most often used delivery systems for improving solubility and desired pharmacokinetic profiles with higher patient compliance are lipid vesicular systems [17].

4.4.2 Nanoparticle drug delivery system

4.4.2.1 Target depends on the surface charge

By changing the external charge of the NPs, it is possible to control how they interact with the intestinal mucosa and increase the efficacy of the system used to deliver drugs. Colonic mucins, sulfates, sialic acid, and negatively charged carbohydrate molecules make up the colonic mucosa. Through electrostatic contact, these components allow NPs having positive charge to stick to the intestinal mucosa [18]. In a study, animals who had colitis brought on by 2,4,6-TNBS and oxazolone received both free clodronate and NPs having clodronate loaded on them (Eudragit RL). In animal models of colitis, there was a considerable decrease in myeloperoxidase activity, whereas free clodronate had no such beneficial effects [19]. NPs having negative charge, in contrast, specifically bind to particular proteins with positive charge and more effectively enter the membrane of the intestinal mucosa. Colonic mucosal inflammation damages the epithelium and causes an accumulation of proteins having positive charge, including eosinophil and transferrin (positive charge) proteins [20].

4.4.2.2 Target depends on size

The most typical method used by NPs drug delivery systems to target the inflamed colon is size-dependent targeting. NP penetration into inflamed areas is increased by enhanced permeability and retention (EPR), which is seen during inflammation.

Mucosal fiber networks range in size from 10 to 200 nm, and changing the particle size to nanoformulations facilitates mobility within the network. PLGA NPs (size 200 nm) packed with budesonide gathered at the inflamed gut, according to a different study on mice with oxazolone-induced colitis. Comparing rats with an inflammatory colon to rats with a healthy colon, the 100 nm formulation showed the strongest bio attachment. One study developed an NP sized 40 nm, that reduced inflammation by consuming the excessive reactive oxygen species (ROS) that are present in the inflamed colonic mucosa [21].

4.4.2.3 Target depends on redox
Increased ROS generation, which is restricted to the area of inflammation and associated with disease development, is seen in patients with IBD. ROS accumulated at the site of inflammation and were linked to the disease development. In a study of three mouse colitis models, the drug delivery system could successfully absorb ROS and reduce symptoms. The NPs accrue in the inflammation regions in the intestine. NPs that have been developed that are made of nitroxide radicals (RNPo) alleviate inflammation by exhausting the ROS in the inflamed digestive areas [22].

4.4.2.4 Target depends on ligands
It has been shown that ligand-dependent NPs are an efficient method of drug localization with few adverse effects and higher efficacy in therapy in a localized area of inflammation. NPs targeting inflammatory markers on cell surfaces are used to treat colitis in animals. Colonic mucosal cells overexpress CD98 glycoprotein when there is inflammation and CD98 antibodies are used for targeted action [23]. In a study, NPs (ligand modified) of chitosan/polyethyleneimine loaded with CD98 antibody target inflammation-expressed CD98 glycoprotein. Furthermore, during colitis, it is seen that macrophages and inflamed epithelial cells express CD44 more than usual. In macrophages and inflammatory epithelial cells, CD44 expression tends to rise in colitis. Along with the overexpression of receptors and ligands on intestinal epithelial cells, endothelial adhesion molecules (ECAMs) are also increased. ECAMs designated as vascular adhesion molecules-1 were developed to be resistant to polylactic acid particles modified with monoclonal antibodies. Ligand-modified NPs show potential as an alternative replacement for targeted drug administration in IBD patients [24].

4.5 pH-dependent nano-delivery systems
This drug delivery technique takes advantage of the pH changes found in the GI tract. The pH values in the last portion of the ileum and colon are the highest in the GI tract. The use of pH-sensitive polymers that are biocompatible is one of the simplest ways of developing formulations for pH-dependent administration of drugs. Methacrylic acid copolymers are the most often used pH-dependent coating polymers for oral delivery. The pH at which Eudragits are soluble can be altered by altering the side-group composition. The different ratios of Eudragit S100 and Eudragit L100 are generally used for drug release at pH 6–7 because they dissolve at pH between 6 and 7 [25].

4.6 Inorganic nanoparticles

Because of their ideal physicochemical properties, inorganic NPs have emerged as a promising targeted drug delivery strategy. In a study, histopathology and inflammatory cytokine levels demonstrate that nanocrystalline silver has positive therapeutic benefits on IBD. The anti-inflammatory impact is on a par with or even better than the group receiving sulfasalazine. Mesoporous silica microparticles that contain budesonide can release the medication when the colon microbiota interacts with them [26]. In various biological contexts, inorganic NPs are linked to issues such agglutination, cytotoxicity, free radical production, and instability, which limits their usefulness. Due to the potential harmful effects of systemic exposure, it is necessary to address the biodistribution of inorganic NPs [27].

4.7 Prodrugs based

Another method for delivering drugs to the colon is by the use of prodrugs. In this method, the prodrug is formulated as an in-active ingredient by the combining a pharmacologically active ingredient covalently to a carrier. Due to enzymatic action, the active component is released *in vivo* in a non-specific manner. Gut microbiomes have enzymatic activities (e.g. glycosidase, azoreductase, nitroreductase, galactosidase, deaminase, and xylosidase) which has been used to release the drug from prodrug at the colon specifically. Few medicines contain the right functional groups to conjugate, hence the prodrug-based strategy is not highly adaptable. Prodrugs having colon specificity can be greatly improved by using azo conjugates [28]. The thermal, chemical, and photochemical stability of azo linkages is often very high. Prodrug can be delivered in different forms, some of which are summarized in figure 4.2.

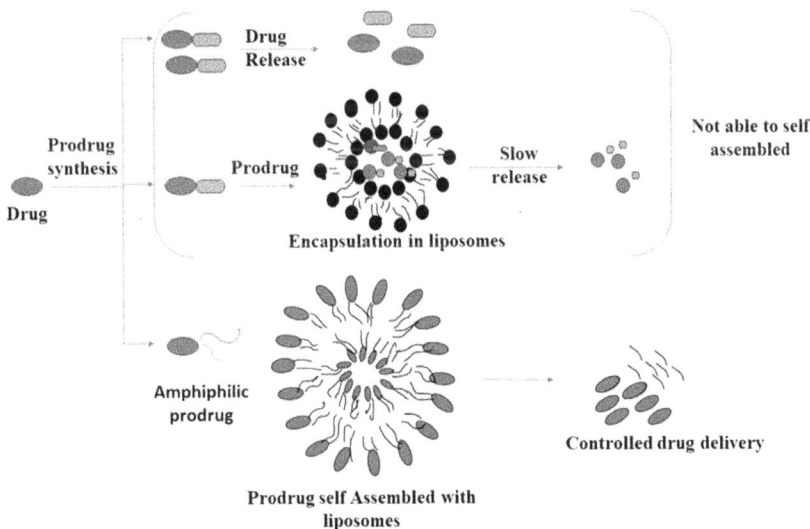

Figure 4.2. Prodrug and prodrug encapsulated in liposomes which cannot be self-assembled, release the drug in uncontrolled or slow release. Self-assembled liposome drug delivery shows controlled drug delivery and having higher drug loading capacity.

4.8 Hybrid drug delivery systems

Hybrid drug delivery systems combine the benefits of various carriers into a single design. The vehicles carrying the drugs are encased in an additional external protective carrier. The site of inflamed colon where the exterior compartment of hybrid drug delivery system dissolved and internal NPs were designed released at the site of action. Orally ingested NPs can be further encapsulated in microparticles to overcome the challenges of orally administered NPs for localized colonic drugs delivery [29]. This innovative method, which consists of NPs in a microparticle-system for drug delivery and incorporates the benefits of both NPs and micro-particles, has been engineered to result in a combined drug delivery system as a better option than single NP- or microparticle-based systems, each of which has unique properties. Microparticles can provide a larger reservoir for drug-loaded NPs that may be manipulated to react to stimuli in the targeted site. At pH 7.4 Eudragit FS30D disolves and in colon and teminal illeum it releases the drug at a specific pH. This pH-sensitive polymer controls the release of drug-loaded NPs in the stomach and initial part of the small intestine. Other studies have proposed the use of oil-in-oil emulsions for the manufacture of NPs encased in enteric microparticle-based systems. However, the oil-in-oil emulsion approach necessitates an extensive, complicated, and multistep process [30].

Hybrid drug delivery systems have a lot of potential for the treatment of IBD, despite the fact that their preparation can often be difficult. The primary purpose of the protective exterior compartment in hybrid drug delivery systems is to shield medicines from denaturation and gastric breakdown at lower pH levels. In order to carry drugs and target inflammatory cells, the internal part of NPs was designed. These investigations frequently make use of changes in conformation in the outer chamber when subjected to the pH range of the GI tract in order to achieve controlled release of the embedded NPs [31].

4.9 Enteric coated formulations

The first reports of smart pills with gastric pH monitoring date back to 1965. Enteric coated, especially microneedle, formulations are pills with microneedles that have been loaded with drugs. Through oral administration, intestine targeted capsule can effectively deliver microneedles into the intestine, where they can be utilized to load drugs, particularly biological agents. Biocompatible polymers are used in the preparation of the microneedles. They release from the capsule and adhere to the areas of the intestine that are swollen and inflammatory, where they slowly deliver the drug ingredient [32]. When the mucosal lining of the GI tract is breached, the biologics held in the reservoir of microneedles, which are either solid or hollow, are released. Microneedles are made of biodegradable polymers and covered with a pH-resistant layer which delivers a very low amount of drug at the acidic pH in the gut. In the treatment of IBDs, the microneedles with the enteric coated system have greater advantages in the future advancement of drug delivery. One important consideration of these drug delivery systems must be noted: due to peristaltic movements these capsules may be degraded in the GI, which could impact the kinetics of drug release. The result of delivery may therefore vary depending on the individual, requiring additional evaluation [33].

4.10 RNA interference-based novel drug delivery

In contrast to traditional oral drug delivery formulations that often take benefit of pH variations, food passages passing time through the GI tract, and gut micro-bacteria differences throughout the GI tract, siRNA-loaded drug delivery systems face significant challenges with inflamed tissue/cell-specific delivery due to tough digestive tract circumstances, mucus and injured epithelial intestinal barrier, absorption issues, local targeting capacity, and intracellular drug absorption [34].

Besides the above-mentioned facts, therapeutic benefits mucosal repair and immuno-logical equilibrium restoration at the sites of disease are brought on by the RNA interference (RNAi) technology, which modifies gene expression linked to susceptibility and the release of cytokines that are pro-inflammatory related to IBD. In general, microRNA (miRNA), and short interfering RNA (siRNA) are the two types of RNAi molecules typically employed in the treatment of IBD. Unlike conventional medicines, which decrease immune system function throughout the body, RNAi therapy exclusively exerts its therapeutic effects in intestinal tissues [35]. Due to its ability to cure inflammation in the GI tract by repressing cytokines that are pro-inflammatory, small interfering RNAs (siRNAs) have drawn a lot of interest from investigators. However, endogenous ribonucleases and pH changes cause naked RNA to decay *in vivo*. Additionally, RNAi therapy could result in immunostimulation and unwanted off-target consequences. To get over these challenges, siRNA and miRNA nanovectors were developed [36].

As an external double-stranded RNA, siRNA was created to target mRNA breakdown through the RNAi cascade. SiRNA is a chemosynthetic RNA duplex that has a 2 nt 3′ overhang and a length of 19–23 nucleotides. As an alternative, siRNA can also be produced through the cytosolic breakdown of RNA that is double-stranded by a dicer. The net negative charge of RNA impedes

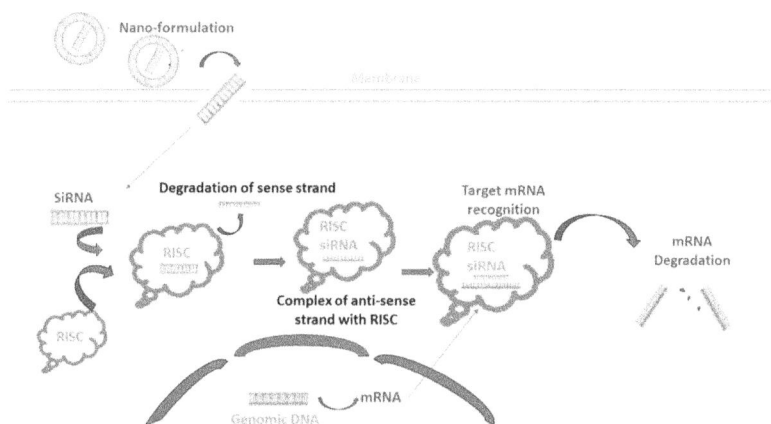

Figure 4.3. siRNA nanodrug delivery system. RISC: RNA-induced silencing complex, siRNA: small interfering RNA.

cytomembrane penetration due to electrostatic resistance from the anionic cell membrane. Therefore, chemical medication of RNA vector is necessary to reach the inflammation site. The majority of viral vectors have a high transfection effectiveness. Immune toxicity and the possibility of gene inclusion into recipient DNA, have prompted scientists to look for safer carriers in gene delivery techniques [37]. The low repeatability of viral vectors must also be taken into account in substantial commercial manufacturing. As a result, non-viral NPs have received a lot of attention. The siRNA delivery mechanism is shown in figure 4.3.

Present-day approaches for treating IBD with siRNA and miRNA NPs include NPs based on polysaccharide, liposomes, NPs based on polylactide (PLA), calcium phosphate, poly(d,l-lactide-co-glycolide acid) (PLGA)-based NPs, thioketal and NPs-in-microsphere oral system.

4.11 Toxicity profiling of IBD

IBD, which includes conditions such as CD and ulcerative colitis, can have various effects on the body, including potential toxicities associated with both the disease itself and the medications used for treatment. Here's a brief overview of the toxicity profile associated with IBD [38] (figure 4.4).

4.11.1 Corticosteroids

Steroids have been used for many years to get IBD into remission. Chronic use, characterized by therapy for more than three months, has been associated with several issues, including higher length of stay, infections, higher risk of infection, adrenal suppression, worsening of IBD, and even death. Numerous studies have assessed the risk of infectious complications in patients with IBD receiving corticosteroid medication, as it predisposes them to infections [39]. A comparison of the safety of infliximab

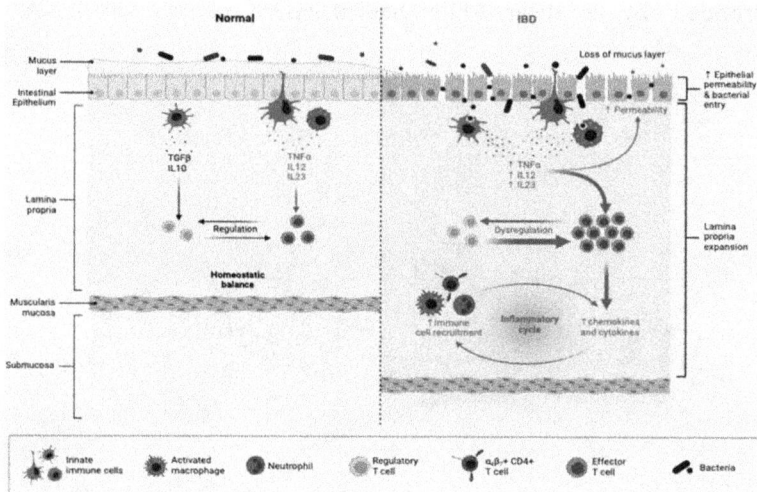

Figure 4.4. Normal intestinal epithelium or IBD showing abnormalities of the immune system.

with nonbiological drug therapy was conducted using the TREAT registry (Crohn's Therapy Resource, Evaluation, and Assessment Tool registry), and the results showed that prednisone therapy was independently linked to both an increased risk of mortality (HR 2.14; 95% CI 1.55–2.95) and serious infections (HR 1.57; 95% CI 1.17–2.10). [23]. After multivariate analysis, glucocorticosteroids alone produced an OR of 2.2 (95% CI 1.0–4.9) in a case-control study including 100 IBD patients with opportunistic infections. However, the number of immunosuppressive medications increased the risk of infection (OR 14.5; 95% CI 4.9–43.0 for two or three medicines) [40]. A retrospective cohort research found that the use of glucocorticosteroid treatment greatly increased the risk of postoperative infection in IBD patients undergoing elective bowel surgery (OR 3.69, 95% CI 1.24–10.97 for all infectious complications). Another case-control analysis found that in patients receiving infliximab, Glucocorticosteroids were the sole independent risk factor for infections (OR 2.69; 95% CI 1.18–6.12). Where CIs represent confidence intervals, ORs represent odds ratios [14].

Many adverse effects affecting the musculoskeletal system, endocrine balance, metabolic system, neuropsychiatric wellbeing, GI system, skin, eyes, infectious risk, cardiovascular system, and hematological system have been linked to the widespread use of corticosteroids [41].

Corticosteroids can have different harmful consequences based on a variety of criteria, such as the individual's susceptibility to them, gender, dose and length of therapy, and mode of administration. Moon face, mood swings, sleeplessness, GI intolerance, weakness, fluid retention, weight gain, increased hunger, raised blood glucose, amenorrhea, sluggish wound healing, striae, and acneiform rash are typical side effects of short-term medication. More severe side effects may arise from long-term supraphysiological dosages of corticosteroids, which are often used to treat CD (i.e., equivalent to more than 7.5 mg of prednisone daily). Corticosteroid medication administered on alternate days can help reduce the suppression of the hypothalamic-pituitary-adrenal axis as well as a number of other negative effects [42].

4.11.2 Immuno modulators

Drugs like azathioprine, 6-mercaptopurine, and methotrexate are used for maintenance therapy. They can cause bone marrow suppression, liver toxicity, and an increased risk of infections or malignancies. Concomitant administration of MTX with adalimumab has been shown to decrease the clearance and increase the concentration of adalimumab. Considering the available PK and immunogenicity data for both adalimumab and infliximab, it is reasonable to expect a decrease in antibody formation, an increase in serum drug concentrations and a related improvement in efficacy with concomitant IMM use. Based on the results of our analysis, these effects may not translate into clinical benefit when adding adalimumab therapy in patients with inadequate disease control on immunomodulator therapy [43].

4.11.3 Biologic therapies

TNF-alpha inhibitors (e.g., infliximab, adalimumab) and other biologics (e.g., vedolizumab) are commonly used for moderate to severe IBD. They may increase the risk of infections, infusion reactions, development of antibodies, and, rarely, paradoxical worsening of symptoms or malignancies. A few instances include the severe cytokine release syndrome that was seen in healthy volunteers receiving treatment with a monoclonal antibody directed against CD28; the decline in heart failure and reactivation of mycobacterial infections with anti-tumour necrosis factor (TNF) agents; and the extremely rare occurrence of fatal viral encephalitis with natalizumab, an anti-integrin antibody. Thankfully, strict post-marketing surveillance programs and registries have made it possible to identify the majority of these issues early on, and suitable policies and procedures have been created to both avoid and treat them [44].

It is critical that the balance between efficacy and safety is carefully considered for each patient, given the following facts: most patients treated with biologics require induction and maintenance therapy; most are immunogenic and may lose their effect over time; the optimal role of biologics in the management of CD and ulcerative colitis is still poorly defined; and the cost of these agents is likely to remain high [36].

4.11.4 JAK inhibitors

For moderate to severe ulcerative colitis, these comparatively recent drugs are licensed. Infections, elevated liver enzymes, and GI perforations are possible side effects. There is a need for new alternatives for treating IBD because the current medications have some drawbacks. Treatment trials are underway for IBD and other immune-mediated disorders involving inflammation. With tofacitinib's regulatory approval for the treatment of rheumatoid arthritis in 2012 and its positive risk-benefit ratio in phase 3 studies for ulcerative colitis, both in patients with no prior experience with TNF and in those with experience, Janus kinase (JAK) inhibitors appear to be leading the field among them. Tests on other substances that have JAK inhibitory action are showing encouraging outcomes [45].

The possibility of Janus kinase inhibitors, also known as AK inhibitors, to treat IBD, which encompasses ailments such as ulcerative colitis and CD, has been studied. The digestive system is chronically inflamed in certain disorders.

JAK inhibitors have the potential to be harmful, even though they have demonstrated promise in the management of IBD symptoms by modifying the immune response. Since JAK inhibitors disrupt cytokine signaling pathways involved in the inflammatory response, some of these toxicities may be connected to the wider immunosuppressive effects of these drugs.

The risks associated with infection, GI side effects, hepatotoxicity, dermatological effects, hematologic toxicities, immunogenicity, and cancer risk [3].

4.11.5 Immune dysregulation in IBD

IBD is a group of diseases that includes abnormalities of the immune system in the GI tract and includes CD and ulcerative colitis. Chronic inflammation is caused by this imbalance, which includes an overreaction of the immune system to the gut microbiota and other luminal antigens. Numerous cytokines, including interleukins (IL), tumor necrosis factor-alpha (TNF-α), and interferons (IFNs), are important participants in this process [46].

4.11.6 Gastrointestinal effects

JAK inhibitors have the ability to modify cytokine signaling, which may upset the delicate balance of immune responses in the gut and cause GI side effects include diarrhea, stomach discomfort, or worsening of pre-existing GI symptoms [47].

4.11.7 Antibiotics

Certain antibiotics, such as ciprofloxacin and metronidazole, are occasionally used to address side effects or in addition to other treatments. They may result in allergic responses, disturbances in the microbiota, or unsettled stomachs.

Numerous antibiotics are associated with pseudomembranous colitis; ampicillin is associated with hemorrhagic colitis; chemotherapy is associated with neutropenic colitis; and deferoxamine is associated with Yersinia enterocolitis. Mechanisms of these toxicities include altering normal bowel flora, weakening immunologic defenses, promoting microorganism virulence, and mucosal injury [48].

4.11.8 Cyclosporine

Used in many severe cases of ulcerative colitis, it can cause nephrotoxicity, hypertension, and increased susceptibility to infections. Cytotoxic agents were first used to treat neoplastic diseases because of their capacity to interfere with the synthesis of proteins and nucleic acids. But it was discovered that these substances also weaken the immune system while being used. Subsequent research on this often undesirable impact led to helpful therapy recommendations for non-neoplastic disorders where autoimmune processes were thought to play a significant role in the etiology [49]. The studies have led to the development of cytotoxic drugs and, more recently, cyclosporine as crucial components of treatment plans for a variety of autoimmune disorders. However, these drugs may still result in side effects from the treatment or even death. Therefore, while treating a non-neoplastic condition, it is especially crucial to consider the advantages and disadvantages of cytotoxic treatment [50].

4.11.9 Nutritional deficiencies

Deficiencies in vitamins (including B12 and D), minerals (such iron and calcium), and other vital nutrients can result from malabsorption, reduced appetite, and altered nutrient absorption caused by inflammation. Every patient with IBD should have access to a dietitian since nutritional evaluations and dietary recommendations are essential to the treatment of this condition. Patients who have just been diagnosed frequently believe that their pre-illness diet played a role in the onset of their IBD. Nevertheless, there is little epidemiological data to substantiate nutrition as a risk factor. Though its precise role in the food chain is unknown, it is interesting to see how the meal interacts with the gut flora. With IBD, nutritional issues are frequent. Up to 85% of patients have malnutrition, while 18%–62% of patients with ulcerative colitis and up to 80% of patients with CD experience weight loss [51].

4.11.10 Surgery-related complications

Surgery could be required for certain people in order to treat severe instances or complications from IBD. Risks associated with surgery include bleeding, infection, intestinal blockage, and the requirement for a permanent ostomy. Patients underwent an open colectomy with ileostomy formation, according to research. After the colon was removed, 64 individuals had ulcerative colitis, and 16 had indeterminate colitis, according to the histopathological analysis. T2 N0 cancer and significant dysplasia were seen in two of the patients. An appendix-related carcinoid tumor was found in two individuals [52]. During follow-up, the diagnosis of two patients was changed to CD; both had indeterminate colitis in the colectomy material and later had progressive perianal illness that was compatible with CD. The hospital stay following surgery was nine (range 4–171) days on average. Seven individuals stayed in hospital for more than 21 days after colectomy [53].

4.11.11 Increased risk of colorectal cancer

People who have have severe ulcerative colitis for a long time may be more likely to have colorectal cancer. It is advised to have surveillance colonoscopies on a regular basis to check for dysplasia or early cancer symptoms. To manage IBD and minimize toxicities while maximizing the patient's overall health, a multidisciplinary strategy comprising gastroenterologists, nutritionists, mental health specialists, and other specialists is necessary. To reduce dangers and optimize benefits, personalized treatment programs and close monitoring are necessary [54].

4.12 Current prospective of IBD

A person with IBD may be born with genetic risk factors or may be exposed to environmental variables such as nutrition, drugs, smoking, and intestinal flora after birth. The prognosis of IBD is still influenced by some environmental variables and IBD therapy even after the illness has started. The prognosis is also influenced by other genetic variables, such as pharmacogenetic genes, which interact with environmental factors and the therapy of IBD [55]. Despite being predetermined at birth, these genetic variables are linked to the course of the disease once it has begun. Consequently, variations in nucleotide sequences derived from germlines have been the main focus of research looking into the genetic components linked to IBD. A case of VEO-IBD was recently described, and it appears that the disease's pathophysiology may have been influenced by the mosaicism of the CYBB mutation. In the realm of IBD [56] (figure 4.5).

4.12.1 Personalized medicine and immunological therapies

In IBD, there is an increasing focus on individualized treatment plans. This entails customizing therapy regimens according to the unique attributes of each patient, such as

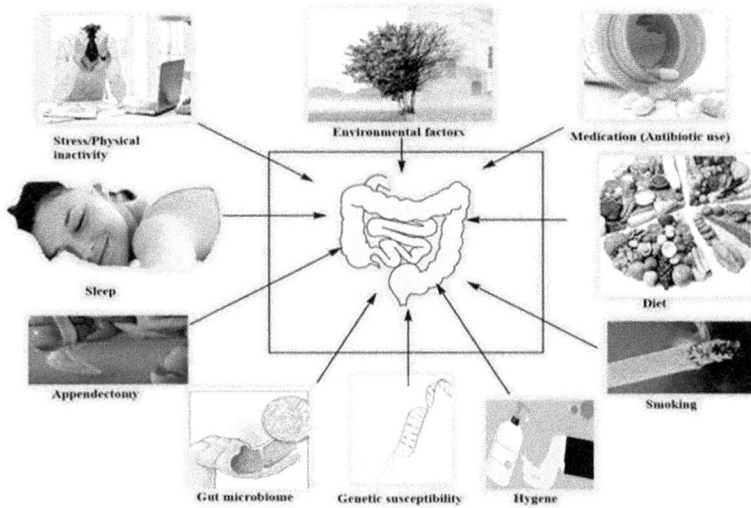

Figure 4.5. Toxicities and some variables influencing inflammatory bowel syndrome.

the illness phenotype, genetic composition, composition of the microbiome, and reaction to prior treatments. This individualized strategy to maximize treatment outcomes and reduce adverse effects is being driven by advancements in precision medicine, genetic testing, and biomarker discovery [57]. When it comes to the pathophysiology of IBD, the gut microbiota is paramount. The goal of ongoing study is to get a deeper understanding of the intricate relationships that exist between the immune system, intestinal barrier function, and gut microbiota in people with IBD. This involves looking into microbial metabolites, microbial dysbiosis, and the possible medical benefit of probiotics, prebiotics, fecal microbiota transplantation (FMT), and other microbiome-targeted therapeutics [7]. The development of innovative immuno-logical therapeutics for IBD that specifically target immune system components implicated in disease pathogenesis is still of interest. This comprises immuno-modulating treatments meant to restore immune tolerance and balance, as well as biologic drugs that target cytokines like interleukin-23 (IL-23) and JAK inhibitors [58].

4.12.2 Disease monitoring and surgical advances

One of the main objectives of treatment for IBD patients is to achieve mucosal healing, which is characterized as the cessation of inflammation and the restoration of normal mucosal architecture. The use of non-invasive imaging methods for tracking illness progression and evaluating treatment outcomes is growing, such as fecal biomarkers and magnetic resonance enterography. These techniques provide information on the state of mucosal healing, disease activity, and the necessity of therapy optimization. IBD is managed in part by nutritional therapies, which can be used as an adjuvant or main therapy [59]. Research on the effectiveness of specified formula meals, exclusive enteral nutrition, and certain food components in bringing IBD patients into and maintaining remission, modifying their gut flora, and enhancing their nutritional status and quality of life is still underway. An essential component of IBD therapy is still surgical surgery, especially for those with problems such as strictures, fistulas, or dysplasia. For patients needing surgery for IBD, advancements in less invasive surgical procedures, such as laparoscopic and robotic-assisted surgery, have resulted in lower morbidity, shorter hospital stays, and better postoperative results [60].

4.12.3 Development of IL-6 signaling inhibitors

Studies on IL-6-deficient animals have demonstrated the involvement of IL-6 in the pathogenesis of several inflammatory diseases, including viral and bacterial infections, arthritis, experimental colitis, and multiple sclerosis. Consequently, IL-6 inhibition emerged as a viable therapeutic strategy that was prepared for clinical use. In principle, IL-6 signalling may be suppressed by using antibodies against any component of the receptor signalling complex; however, gp130, IL-6R, or IL-6 blockage alone is sufficient to completely silence IL-6-mediated signalling. In the West, IBD178 affects at least 0.5% of the population [61]. With the advent of many biologics, anti-TNF medications remain the cornerstone of the IBD treatment plan. Therefore, it could seem obvious to select IBD for the first phase II clinical trial of olamkicept. This was indeed a risky decision because phase II clinical trials using IL-6 and IL-6R antibodies for IBD were stopped due to undesirable side effects, such as intestinal perforation [62].

4.12.4 Genome-wide association studies (GWAS)

GWAS have identified over 240 genetic loci associated with susceptibility to IBD. These loci encompass genes involved in various biological pathways, including innate and adaptive immunity, epithelial barrier function, autophagy, and microbial recognition. Despite these discoveries, the majority of the heritability of IBD remains unexplained, suggesting that additional genetic variants and mechanisms contribute to disease risk. CD has benefited greatly from this technology, with the IL-17/IL-23 axis, autophagy, and innate lymphoid cells being identified as important components in CD pathogenesis. Our growing comprehension of the genetic make-up of CD has also brought to light the possibility that the development of the illness may be aided by an inability to regulate aberrant immune responses [63].

4.12.5 Rare variant analysis

In addition to common genetic variants identified through GWAS, rare and low-frequency variants with larger effect sizes are being investigated using next-generation sequencing approaches. Studies have identified rare variants in genes such as IL36RL, NOD2, IL23R, and ATG16L1 that confer increased risk of IBD. Rare variant analysis provides insights into the genetic architecture of IBD and may help elucidate disease mechanisms in subsets of patients. SNPs rs150582502 and rs149199982 are identified by experts as potential private, uncommon, high effect variations for CD based on recent studies. Through modulating the Wnt/β-Catenin pathway, PYGB (glycogen phosphorylase B) has been demonstrated to stimulate cellular proliferation in a variety of tumor forms. $5'$–$3'$ exoribonuclease 2, which is involved in transcription termination, is encoded by XRN2. Research on XRN2 has shown that it plays a role in DNA repair, and mutations in the gene have been linked to a number of cancer types [64].

Another study examined genetic variants from the perspective of the patient rather than the genes. For each paediatric case a profile of deleterious variations is determined across a comprehensive panel of known IBD genes. Paediatric IBD patients carry a wide spectrum of low-frequency variants within candidate IBD genes. *In silico* analyses indicate a substantial proportion of these mutations are potentially deleterious. Consistent with complex inheritance, this small subset of patients with severe IBD exhibit a varied profile of mutation with limited sharing of specific variants across the set of eight exomes. The main objective is to identify the spectrum of rare and novel variation in known IBD susceptibility genes using exome sequencing analysis in eight individual cases of childhood onset severe disease [65].

4.12.6 Functional genomics and gene expression studies

Integrating genetic data with functional genomics approaches, such as epigenomics, transcriptomics, and proteomics, enables the characterization of disease-relevant pathways and cell types involved in IBD pathogenesis. These studies help prioritize candidate genes, identify potential drug targets, and elucidate the molecular mechanisms underlying IBD susceptibility and progression. The host–microbiota interactions and DNA methylation control the OS genes that cause CD, according to the multiomics integration research. This furnishes proof for subsequent focused functional study with the objective of formulating appropriate therapeutic strategies and averting sickness.

Polygenic risk scores combine information from multiple genetic variants to calculate an individual's genetic risk for developing IBD. Polygenic risk scores (PRS) have shown utility in predicting disease risk, stratifying patients based on genetic susceptibility, and identifying individuals at higher risk of disease complications or poor treatment outcomes. As larger cohorts and more comprehensive genetic data become available, the predictive accuracy of PRS is expected to improve [66].

Scientists have developed Exfoliome sequencing (Exfo-seq), an innovative non-invasive method to measure the GI transcriptome directly from stool. The approach makes use of the trace amounts of human RNA molecules (i.e., the exfoliome) that are present within stool due to natural turnover of intestinal cells. Exfo-seq has great potential as a non-invasive method to guide IBD diagnosis, treatment, long-term care, and future pharmaceutical development [67].

4.12.7 Therapeutic targets

Genetic discoveries in IBD have facilitated the development of targeted therapies directed at specific pathways implicated in disease pathogenesis. For example, biologic agents targeting cytokines such as tumor necrosis factor (TNF), interleukin-12/23 (IL-12/23), and integrins have revolutionized IBD treatment. As our understanding of the genetic basis of IBD advances, there is growing interest in developing personalized treatment approaches based on an individual's genetic profile, with the aim of optimizing therapeutic response and minimizing adverse effects [68].

The key to managing IBD has been to use precision medicine to personalize patient care. Using the present arsenal of biologics and small molecules in a one-size-fits-all manner results in much higher non-response rates and worse than optimal clinical outcomes. Breaking through this therapeutic ceiling will still require overcoming a number of obstacles, including accurately predicting the course of the disease, obtaining an early diagnosis of IBD, ideally even in the pre-clinical stage, and adjusting a patient's therapy regimen to suit their unique pharmacokinetic and pharmacodynamic profiles [69].

4.12.8 Gene-environment interactions

Genetic susceptibility to IBD interacts with environmental factors, such as diet, gut microbiota, and lifestyle, to influence disease risk and phenotype. Understanding gene–environment (GxE) interactions is critical for unraveling the complex etiology of IBD and developing targeted interventions aimed at modulating environmental factors to prevent or mitigate disease development. Recent discoveries about the pathophysiology of IBD have brought to light the intricate interactions among the environment, the genome, and the epigenome. Even with the remarkable progress in genomics that has allowed for the discovery of more than 200 susceptibility loci, the estimated heritability and illness variance in IBD are primarily explained by these loci. 'Missing heritability' is most likely caused by GxE interactions, which may operate via epigenetic pathways. Children's and adults' epigenomes are altered by a number of environmental variables, including diet, tobacco use, and the microbiome. These changes may have an effect on an individual's susceptibility to certain diseases. In early life, other GxE interaction pathways are also directly relevant. [70].

In the future, advances in genomic technologies, multiomics integration, large-scale collaborative efforts, and data sharing initiatives will continue to drive progress in IBD genetics research. These efforts hold promise for elucidating disease mechanisms, identifying novel therapeutic targets, and ultimately improving outcomes for individuals affected by IBD.

Overall, ongoing research in these areas holds promise for advancing our understanding of IBD pathogenesis, improving treatment strategies, and ultimately enhancing outcomes and quality of life for individuals living with these chronic inflammatory disorders [71].

4.13 Future prospective of IBD

IBD is a long-term inflammatory illness of the GI system that mostly affects people with CD and ulcerative colitis. Because drug delivery systems can increase patient compliance, reduce side effects, and improve treatment efficacy, they are highly promising for the therapy of IBD in the future. In light of IBD, the following are potential future thoughts on medication delivery systems [2].

4.13.1 Targeted drug delivery and site-specific release

Patients with IBD may have their advanced medication delivery systems tailored to target particular GI tract areas that are inflamed. By doing so, therapeutic efficacy can be maximized while minimizing systemic exposure to the medicine and minimizing adverse effects. Drugs can be developed into controlled-release formulations to release at certain places where inflammation is concentrated inside the GI system. This can reduce exposure to healthy tissues while maintaining appropriate medication concentrations at the target location [72].

4.13.2 Microparticles-based delivery systems

For the treatment of IBD, drug delivery methods based on NPs and microparticles provide several benefits, such as increased mucosal penetration, prolonged release kinetics, and better drug stability. These systems are capable of encasing and delivering to the site of inflammation a wide range of therapeutic agents, such as biologics, immunomodulators, and anti-inflammatory medications. Drug delivery methods for IBD are being developed to increase the oral bioavailability and targeted distribution of medications. These methods include enteric coated formulations, NPs, and mucoadhesive hydrogels. These mechanisms can help deliver medication into the intestine, where inflammation originates, and shield medication from breaking down in the stomach's acidic environment [63].

4.13.3 Biological therapies

For the treatment of IBD, drug delivery methods for biological therapies—such as cytokine inhibitors and monoclonal antibodies—are being investigated. These systems have the potential to increase the therapeutic efficacy of biologics, decrease dosage frequency, and lengthen their duration in circulation. Novel approaches to medication administration for IBD are being made possible by developments in pharmacogenomics and biomarker research [73]. Clinicians may tailor treatment plans and choose the best medication delivery method for each patient by identifying genetic markers and illness biomarkers. Oral, nasal, and transdermal drug administration are examples of non-invasive drug delivery methods that are being researched as substitutes for injecting medications to treat IBD. Convenience, less discomfort for the patient, and better patient compliance are benefits of these methods [74].

4.13.4 Combination therapies

In order to treat IBD, drug delivery systems can help co-deliver many therapeutic drugs with complimentary modes of action. Combination treatments have the potential to improve treatment results and slow the emergence of drug resistance by addressing many facets of inflammation and disease progression [75]. All things considered, there is a bright future ahead for drug delivery systems in the treatment of IBD, as research continues to be carried out on new and creative ways to improve medication targeting, effectiveness, and patient outcomes. In the years to come, new medication delivery approaches for IBD are anticipated to be fueled by ongoing developments in nanotechnology, biomaterials, and personalized medicine [76].

4.14 Conclusion

By targeting active drug to specific regions of inflammation, novel delivery technologies have improved the treatment of IBD. It increases safety and efficacy and decreases systemic adverse effects. The development of novel drug delivery that can regulate the release of a drug in the GI tract when it is activated by environmental factors like pH, bacteria, or enzymatic degradation can be attributed to methods based on the simplest polymeric NPs. For drug administration in IBD, a variety of encapsulated systems have been developed including liposomes, NPs, prodrugs, inorganic particles, hybrid systems, enteric coated microneedle tablets, and biological delivery systems. Due to the benefits of oral delivery over parenteral routes, oral nanomedicines delivering siRNA are among the latest generation of such treatments and are a very appealing approach to treat disorders, particularly IBD. However, more study is required to prove the effectiveness and safety of the various innovative drugs delivery systems.

References

[1] Stidham R W and Takenaka K 2022 Artificial intelligence for disease assessment in inflammatory bowel disease: how will it change our practice? *Gastroenterology* **162** 1493–506

[2] Vasilakakis M D, Koulaouzidis A, Marlicz W and Iakovidis D K 2020 The future of capsule endoscopy in clinical practice: from diagnostic to therapeutic experimental prototype capsules *Prz. Gastroenterol.* **15** 179–93

[3] Malone J C and Thavamani A Physiology, Gastrocolic Reflex. StatPearls [Internet]. https://ncbi.nlm.nih.gov/books/NBK549888/ (accessed 6 August 2023)

[4] Pau A K and George J M 2014 Antiretroviral therapy: current drugs *Infect. Dis. Clin. North Am.* **28** 371

[5] Kim J and Jesus O D 2023 Medication routes of administration *StatPearls [Internet].* https://ncbi.nlm.nih.gov/books/NBK568677/ (accessed 1 March 2024)

[6] Singh H and Sharma G 2023 Recent development of novel drug delivery of herbal drugs *RPS Pharm. Pharmacol. Rep.* **2** 1–8

[7] Thomas T J, Tajmir-Riahi H-A and Pillai C K S 2019 Biodegradable polymers for gene delivery *Molecules* **24** 3744

[8] Yamazaki I 1987 Free radical mechanisms in enzyme reactions *Free Radic. Biol. Med.* **3** 397–404

[9] Lüering N, Kucharzik T, Stoll R and Domschke W 1998 Das system der unspezifischen abwehr bei chronisch-entzundlichen darmerkrankungen (CED)—Pathophysiologische und therapeutische aspekte *Z. Gastroenterol* **36** 173–87

[10] Groß V, Andus T, Leser H G, Roth M and Schölmerich J 1991 Inflammatory mediators in chronic inflammatory bowel diseases *Klin. Wochenschr.* **69** 981–7

[11] Nguyen V X, li Nguyen V T and Nguyen C C 2010 Appropriate use of endoscopy in the diagnosis and treatment of gastrointestinal diseases: up-to-date indications for primary care providers *Int. J. Gen. Med.* **3** 345

[12] Frøkjaer J B, Drewes A M, Gregersen H, Brøndum Frøkjaer J and Duvnjak M 2009 Imaging of the gastrointestinal tract-novel technologies guidelines clinical practice *World J. Gastroenterol.* **15** 160–8

[13] Cohen J and Greenwald D A 2022 Overview of upper gastrointestinal endoscopy (esophagogastroduodenoscopy)—UpToDate [Internet]. https://uptodate.com/contents/overview-of-upper-gastrointestinal-endoscopy-esophagogastroduodenoscopy (accessed 6 August 2023)

[14] Lambert R 2012 Endoscopy in screening for digestive cancer *World J. Gastrointest. Endosc.* **4** 518

[15] Qaseem A, Mustafa R A, Hicks L A, Wilt T J, Crandall C J, Fitterman N *et al* 2019 Screening for colorectal cancer in asymptomatic average-risk adults: a guidance statement from the american college of physicians HHS public access *Ann. Intern. Med.* **3002:** 643–54

[16] Nassani N, Alsheikh M, Carroll B, Nguyen D and Carroll R E 2020 Theranostic gastrointestinal endoscopy: bringing healing light to the Lumen *Clin. Transl. Gastroenterol* **11** e00119

[17] Smolsky J, Kaur S, Hayashi C, Batra S K and Krasnoslobodtsev A V 2017 Surface-enhanced raman scattering-based immunoassay technologies for detection of disease biomarkers *Biosensors* **7** 7

[18] Monika P, Chandraprabha M N, Rangarajan A, Waiker P V and Chidambara Murthy K N 2021 Challenges in healing wound: role of complementary and alternative medicine *Front. Nutr.* **8** 791899

[19] Laurano R, Boffito M, Ciardelli G and Chiono V 2022 Wound dressing products: a translational investigation from the bench to the market *Eng. Regen.* **3** 182–200

[20] Ma W, Zhan Y, Zhang Y, Mao C, Xie X and Lin Y 2021 The biological applications of DNA nanomaterials: current challenges and future directions *Signal Transduct. Target Ther.* **6** 1–28

[21] Cardoza C, Nagtode V, Pratap A and Mali S N 2022 Emerging applications of nanotechnology in cosmeceutical health science: latest updates *Heal. Sci. Rev.* **4** 100051

[22] Yildirimer L, Thanh N T K, Loizidou M and Seifalian A M 2011 Toxicology and clinical potential of nanoparticles *Nano Today* **6** 585–607

[23] Habeeb Rahuman H B, Dhandapani R, Narayanan S, Palanivel V, Paramasivam R, Subbarayalu R *et al* 2022 Medicinal plants mediated the green synthesis of silver nanoparticles and their biomedical applications *IET Nanobiotechnol.* **16** 115

[24] Missaoui W N, Arnold R D and Cummings B S 2018 Toxicological status of nanoparticles: what we know and what we don't know *Chem. Biol. Interact.* **295** 1

[25] Krishnan P D, Banas D, Durai R D, Kabanov D, Hosnedlova B, Kepinska M *et al* 2020 Silver nanomaterials for wound dressing applications *Pharmaceutics* **12** 1–27

[26] Sieber S, Grossen P, Detampel P, Siegfried S, Witzigmann D and Huwyler J 2017 Zebrafish as an early stage screening tool to study the systemic circulation of nanoparticulate drug delivery systems in vivo *J. Control Rel.* **264** 180–91

[27] Maiti D, Tong X, Mou X and Yang K 2018 Carbon-based nanomaterials for biomedical applications: a recent study *Front. Pharmacol.* **9** 1401

[28] Monteiro N, Martins A, Reis R L and Neves N M 2014 Liposomes in tissue engineering and regenerative medicine *J. R. Soc. Interface* **11** 20140459

[29] Jain S, Jain V and Mahajan S C 2014 Lipid based vesicular drug delivery systems *Adv. Pharm* **2014** 1–12

[30] Silva A C, Moreira J N, Manuel J, Lobo S, Subhan A, Filipczak N *et al* 2023 Advances with lipid-based nanosystems for siRNA delivery to breast cancers *Pharmaceuticals (Basel)* **16** 970

[31] Attama A A, Agbo C P, Onokala O B, Kenechukwu F C, Ugwueze M E, Mbah C C *et al* 2023 Applications of nanoemulsions as drug delivery vehicle for phytoconstituents *Nanotechnology in Herbal Medicine: Applications and Innovations* (Elsevier) pp 119–94

[32] Yu B, Tai H C, Xue W, Lee L J and Lee R J 2010 Receptor-targeted nanocarriers for therapeutic delivery to cancer *Mol. Membr. Biol.* **27** 286

[33] Yao Y, Zhou Y, Liu L, Xu Y, Chen Q, Wang Y *et al* 2020 Nanoparticle-based drug delivery in cancer therapy and its role in overcoming drug resistance *Front. Mol. Biosci.* **7** 558493

[34] Luo M, Lee L K C, Peng B, Choi C H J, Tong W Y and Voelcker N H 2022 Delivering the promise of gene therapy with nanomedicines in treating central nervous system diseases *Adv. Sci.* **9** 2201740

[35] Khan I, Saeed K and Khan I 2019 Nanoparticles: properties, applications and toxicities *Arab J Chem.* **12** 908–31

[36] Sukhanova A, Bozrova S, Sokolov P, Berestovoy M, Karaulov A and Nabiev I 2018 Dependence of nanoparticle toxicity on their physical and chemical properties *Nanoscale Res. Lett.* **13** 1–21

[37] Park H J and Moon D E 2010 Pharmacologic management of chronic pain *Korean J. Pain* **23** 99

[38] Jain A K and Thareja S 2019 *In vitro* and *in vivo* characterization of pharmaceutical nanocarriers used for drug delivery *Artific. Cells Nanomed. Biotechnol.* **47** 524–39

[39] Roobol S J, Hartjes T A, Slotman J A, De Kruijff R M, Torrelo G, Abraham T E *et al* 2020 Uptake and subcellular distribution of radiolabeled polymersomes for radiotherapy *Nanotheranostics* **2020** 14–25

[40] Mandal S, Zhou Y, Shibata A and Destache C J 2015 View online-export citation crossmark confocal fluorescence microscopy: an ultra-sensitive tool used to evaluate intracellular antiretroviral nano-drug delivery in HeLa cells confocal fluorescence microscopy: an ultra-sensitive tool used to evaluate intracellular antiretroviral nano-drug delivery in HeLa cells *AIP Adv.* **5** 84803

[41] Ro T H, Mathew M A and Misra S 2015 Value of screening endoscopy in evaluation of esophageal, gastric and colon cancers *World J. Gastroenterol.* **21** 9693

[42] Mcguigan A, Kelly P, Turkington R C, Jones C, Coleman H G and Mccain S 2023 Pancreatic cancer: a review of clinical diagnosis, epidemiology, treatment and outcomes *World J. Gastroenterol.* **24** 4846–61

[43] Mosleh-Shirazi S, Abbasi M, Moaddeli M R, Vaez A, Shafiee M, Kasaee S R *et al* 2022 Nanotechnology advances in the detection and treatment of cancer: an overview *Nanotheranostics* **6** 400–23

[44] Haleem A, Javaid M, Singh R P, Rab S and Suman R 2023 Applications of nanotechnology in medical field: a brief review *Glob. Heal. J. Homepage* **7** 70–7

[45] Ding Y-N, Xue M, Tang Q-S, Wang L-J, Ding H-Y, Li H *et al* 2023 Immunotherapy-based novel nanoparticles in the treatment of gastrointestinal cancer: trends and challenges *World J. Gastroenterol.* **28** 5403–19

[46] Gullo I, Grillo F, Mastracci L, Vanoli A, Carneiro F, Saragoni L *et al* 2020 Precancerous lesions of the stomach, gastric cancer and hereditary gastric cancer syndromes *Pathologica* **112** 166–85

[47] Dessale M, Mengistu G and Mengist H M 2022 Nanotechnology: a promising approach for cancer diagnosis, therapeutics and theragnosis *Int. J. Nanomed.* **17** 3735–49

[48] Cheng Z, Li M, Dey R and Chen Y 2020 Proteolysis-targeting chimera (PROTAC) for targeted protein degradation and cancer therapy *J. Hematol. Oncol.* **14** 85

[49] Cheng Z, Li M, Dey R and Chen Y 2021 Nanomaterials for cancer therapy: current progress and perspectives *J. Hematol. Oncol.* **14** 1–27

[50] Nabil G, Bhise K, Sau S, Atef M, El-Banna H A and Iyer A K 2019 Nano-engineered delivery systems for cancer imaging and therapy: recent advances, future direction and patent evaluation *Drug Discov. Today* **24** 462

[51] Udenni Gunathilake T M S, Ching Y C, Ching K Y, Chuah C H and Abdullah L C 2017 Biomedical and microbiological applications of bio-based porous materials: a review *Polymers (Basel)* **9** 160

[52] Wang L, Hu C and Shao L 2017 The antimicrobial activity of nanoparticles: present situation and prospects for the future *Int. J. Nanomed.* **12** 1227

[53] Bera D, Qian L, Tseng T K and Holloway P H 2010 Quantum dots and their multimodal applications: a review *Mater* **3** 2260–345

[54] Singh A, Prasad L B, Shiv K, Kumar R and Garai S 2023 Synthesis, characterization, and *in vitro* antibacterial and cytotoxic study of Co(II), Ni(II), Cu(II), and Zn(II) complexes of N-(4-methoxybenzyl) N-(phenylethyl) dithiocarbamate ligand *J. Mol. Struct.* **1288** 135835

[55] Kumar A, Kumar B, Kumar R, Kumar A, Singh M, Tiwari V *et al* 2022 Acute and subacute toxicity study of ethanolic extract of *Calotropis procera* (Aiton) dryand flower in *Swiss albino* mice *Phytomed. Plus* **2** 100224

[56] Naso M F, Tomkowicz B, Perry W L and Strohl W R 2017 Adeno-Associated Virus (AAV) as a vector for gene therapy *Biodrugs* **31** 317

[57] Lee C S *et al* 2017 Adenovirus-mediated gene delivery: potential applications for gene and cell-based therapies in the new era of personalized medicine *Int. J. Nanomed.* **12** 2373–84

[58] Seyedian S S, Nokhostin F and Dargahi Malamir M 2019 A review of the diagnosis, prevention, and treatment methods of inflammatory bowel disease *J. Med. Life* **12** 113–22

[59] Thakur A and Foged C 2020 Nanoparticles for mucosal vaccine delivery *Nanoengineered Biomaterials for Advanced Drug Delivery* **2020** (Woodhead) pp 603–46

[60] Cojocaru M, Inimioara, Cojocaru M, Silosi I and Doina Vrabie C 2011 Gastrointestinal manifestations in systemic autoimmune diseases *Maedica A J. Clin. Med.* **6** 45–51

[61] Cederbaum A I 2001 Introduction—serial review: alcohol, oxidative stress and cell injury *Free Radic. Biol. Med.* **31** 1524–6

[62] Patra J K, Das G, Fraceto L F, Campos E V R, Rodriguez-Torres M D P, Acosta-Torres L S *et al* 2018 Nano based drug delivery systems: recent developments and future prospects *J. Nanobiotechnol.* **16** 1–33

[63] Din F U, Aman W, Ullah I, Qureshi O S, Mustapha O, Shafique S *et al* 2017 Effective use of nanocarriers as drug delivery systems for the treatment of selected tumors *Int. J. Nanomedicine* **12** 7291–309

[64] Riley R S, June C H, Langer R and Mitchell M J 2019 Delivery technologies for cancer immunotherapy HHS public access *Na.t Rev. Drug Discov* **18** 175–96

[65] Cells E, Brzuszkiewicz E, Gottschalk G, Buchrieser C, Dobrindt U and Oswald E 2006 The mucus and mucins of the goblet cells and enterocytes provide the first defense line of the gastrointestinal tract and interact with the immune system *Immunol. Rev.* **260** 87–107

[66] Johansson M E V, Sjövall H and Hansson G C 2013 The gastrointestinal mucus system in health and disease *Nat. Rev. Gastroenterol. Hepatol.* **10** 352

[67] Baracat F, Moura E, Bernardo W, Pu L Z, Mendonça E, Moura D *et al* 2016 Endoscopic hemostasis for peptic ulcer bleeding: systematic review and meta-analyses of randomized controlled trials *Surg. Endosc.* **30** 2155–68

[68] Ibrahim M, El-Mikkawy A, Hamid M A, Abdalla H, Mostafa I and Devière J 2019 Early application of haemostatic powder added to standard management for oesophagogastric variceal bleeding: a randomised trial *Gut* **68** 844–53

[69] Mangiavillano B, Pagano N, Baron T H and Luigiano C 2015 Outcome of stenting in biliary and pancreatic benign and malignant diseases: a comprehensive review *World J. Gastroenterol.* **21** 9038

[70] Bokov D, Jalil A T, Chupradit S, Suksatan W, Ansari M J, Shewael I H *et al* 2021 Nanomaterial by sol–gel method: synthesis and application

[71] Kopylov U and Seidman E G 2014 Role of capsule endoscopy in inflammatory bowel disease *World J. Gastroenterol.* **20** 1155–64

[72] Bahadar H, Maqbool F, Niaz K and Abdollahi M 2016 Toxicity of nanoparticles and an overview of current experimental models *Iran Biomed. J.* **20** 1–11

[73] Nazari P M, Reza Talebi P A, Hosseini Sharifabad P M, Abbasi P A, Khoradmehr P A, Hossein Danafar P A *et al* 2016 Acute and chronic effects of gold nanoparticles on sperm parameters and chromatin structure in mice *Int. J. Reprod. BioMed.* **14** 637–42

[74] Kher C and Kumar S 2022 The application of nanotechnology and nanomaterials in cancer diagnosis and treatment: a review *Cureus* **14** e29059

[75] Ricciotti E and FitzGerald G A 2011 Prostaglandins and inflammation *Arterioscler. Thromb. Vasc. Biol.* **31** 986

[76] Parasher G, Wong M and Rawat M 2020 Evolving role of artificial intelligence in gastrointestinal endoscopy conflict-of-interest statement: specialty type: gastroenterology and hepatology *World J. Gastroenterol.* **26** 7287–98

IOP Publishing

Nanobiotechnology and Artificial Intelligence in
Gastrointestinal Diseases

Vivek K Chaturvedi, Anurag Kumar Singh, Jay Singh and Dawesh P Yadav

Chapter 5

Nanotechnology in gastrointestinal endoscopy

Rajesh Kumar, Sunil Dutt, Ankush Goyal,
Ashutosh Kumar and Brijesh Kumar

Nanotechnology is a field which deals with the development of intentional design and characterizations of nanoscale particles (1–100 nm) for the diagnosis, treatment, mitigation of illnesses as well as other desirable uses. These engineered devices are controlled by their size and shape through physical characteristics to produce the intended impact at subcellular and molecular level with unique attributes. These nanoparticles (NPs), which can cross the blood–brain barrier and have the capacity to avoid immune system interception, have a longer half-life than microparticles, making them suitable for use as drug delivery vehicles. Quantum dot and cadmium selenide semiconductor NPs are two diagnostic techniques that may simultaneously scan a blood sample for various proteins, viruses, and other desirable compounds. Environmental NPs can reach the human body through several pathways, including the gastrointestinal (GI) tract. As soon as anything is consumed, it easily passes through the mucus layer and interacts with the enterocytes. Nanopowder as hemostatic agent in gastric ulcer bleed, prevention of clogging of plastic stents, nano-based capsule endoscopy, molecular imaging and optical biopsy, biosensing and maneuvering technology, nanorobots are some tools used in the diagnostic and therapeutic endoscopy such as the endoscopic hemostasis of peptic ulcer bleeding, prevention of clogging of plastic stent and advance capsule endoscopy. These NPs, which are either approved for clinical use or are undergoing clinical trials, have technical challenges and potential adverse reactions like back pain, vasodilatation and acute urinary retention, fever, cytopenia, mild renal toxicity, and peripheral sensory neuropathy because of their diverse range. Hence, toxicity investigations and quality control studies for these NPs will serve as a benchmark for the unfulfilled potential of nanotechnology in the diagnostic and therapeutic fields, along with endoscopy.

5.1 Introduction

A requently used medical technique for the diagnosis and treatment of GI diseases include ulcers, polyps, tumours, and inflammatory bowel disease is called a GI endoscopy [1]. It makes imaging, evaluation, and treatment for a range of GI disorders possible. Depending on whether the technique is focused on the upper GI tract (oesophagus, stomach, duodenum, and jejunum) or the lower GI tract (rectum, colon, and terminal ileum), it can be categorized as either an upper endoscopy or a lower endoscopy [2]. When an endoscope is used to examine the lower GI system, the technique is often referred to as a colonoscopy; when the upper GI tract is involved, it is referred to as an esophagogastroduodenoscopy [3].

Colonoscopy is a widely recognized and approved method for bowel cancer screening by various national healthcare systems. This procedure is effective not only in detecting carcinomas but also in identifying early neoplasms and precursors of carcinomas that can be safely removed through endoscopy. In Germany, screening colonoscopy is estimated to prevent around 18 000 cases of colon cancer annually. Additionally, approximately 4000 patients are diagnosed with early-stage cancers that can be effectively treated through endoscopic therapy. Worldwide, colorectal cancer is the most common cancer that develops from benign polyps. In 2020, the United States witnessed 147 000 individuals being diagnosed with the disease, while 53 200 died due to this cancer [4]. It has been demonstrated that colorectal cancer cannot develop as quickly when colorectal polyps are found and removed using a colonoscopy procedure. Screening for colorectal cancer in those at a 2% risk might potentially avert 0–7 cancer cases and 1–3 colorectal cancer-related deaths for every 1000 screened persons. Additionally, for every 1000 people checked, screening for colorectal cancer at a 4% risk may prevent 1–13 occurrences of the disease and 2–7 deaths from the disease [5].

The digestive system's many sections each have their own special traits and difficulties. Effective use of diagnostic or therapeutic techniques is not always feasible, particularly in the lower portion of the small intestine where endoscopy and drug administration are particularly challenging. The design and operation of endoscopes have significantly improved over the last few decades, thanks to developments like narrow-band imaging (NBI) and high-definition imaging. Still, there are issues with standard endoscopes' sensitivity, specificity, and accuracy of diagnosis [6]. With the capabilities of NPs, nanotechnology holds enormous promise for bettering digestive system results. The field of nanotechnology has shown great promise in enhancing the precision and effectiveness of GI endoscopy. Through improved detection and treatment of GI illnesses such hepatitis, inflammatory bowel disease, gastric ulcers, and cancer, nanotechnology can support endoscopy [7]. When materials and devices are designed, created, and used at the nanoscale—typically between 1 and 100 nm—it is referred to as nanotechnology. Certain physical, chemical, and biological characteristics of the materials are displayed at this size, which are absent at the macroscale. Nanotechnology has a number of benefits when it comes to GI endoscopy [8].

Some of the ways nanotechnology can help in endoscopy are: (1) NPs as contrast agents or probes to improve the sensitivity and specificity of endoscopic imaging; (2) nanobiosensors (NBs) or surface-enhanced Raman scattering (SERS) nanoparticles to detect molecular markers or biomarkers of diseases in the GI tract; (3) magnetic nanoparticles (MNPs) or intraoperative imaging nanoparticles (IINPs) to guide endoscopic surgery or biopsy; (4) nanocoatings or nanomaterials to prevent the clogging of plastic stents or enhance the performance of endoscopic devices; (5) capsule endoscopy or microendoscopy to access hard-to-reach regions of the GI tract (figure 5.1) [9].

NPs and nanostructured materials can enhance the contrast of the images, target-specific biomarkers, and deliver therapeutic agents directly to diseased tissues. Several types of NPs and nanostructured materials have been investigated for their potential use in GI endoscopy. For instance, quantum dots (QDs) are fluorescent semiconductor NPs that emit intense and stable fluorescence under excitation with a specific wavelength. QDs have been used to label GI tissues and cells with high sensitivity and specificity [10]. Gold nanoparticles (GNPs) are biocompatible and can be functionalized with various ligands that target-specific receptors or molecules. GNPs have been used to enhance the contrast of endoscopic images and to deliver drugs to cancer cells. Iron oxide nanoparticles (IONPs) are NPs with magnetic properties that are utilized for medication administration and cancer imaging. They are detectable by magnetic resonance imaging (MRI). Applications in biosensing and bioimaging might benefit from the special mechanical, electrical, and optical qualities of carbon-based nanomaterials such as graphene oxide (GO) and carbon nanotubes (CNTs) [11].

Numerous fields, including cell labelling, biological imaging, surgical navigation, early detection of gastrointestinal cancer (GIC), and many others, have shown the great promise of nanotechnology. Nanotechnology is widely used in the diagnosis and treatment of GIC because of its unique advantages in terms of size and wide

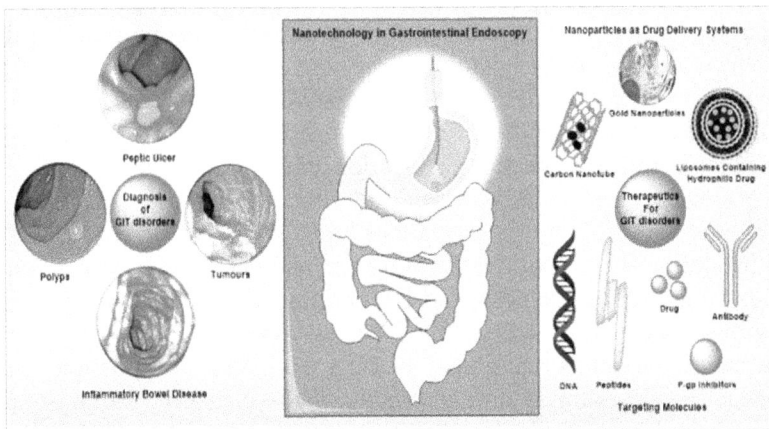

Figure 5.1. Introduction of nanotechnology in GII endoscopy; inflammatory bowel disease, peptic ulcer, tumours, polyps and various NPs as drug delivery system.

range of applications [12]. The use of SERS NPs, electrochemical nanobiosensors, magnetic nanoparticles (MNPs), intraoperative imaging nanoparticles (IINPs), drug delivery systems, and other multifunctional NPs has led to remarkable advancements in clinical GIC. These cutting-edge methods have significantly improved the precision and effectiveness of GIC diagnosis and therapy. To increase the detection rate of early-stage tumours, QDs have been employed, for example, to mark cells squamous cell carcinoma of the oesophagus. GNPs have been utilized to target and visualize pancreatic cancer cells after being functionalized with epidermal growth factor receptor (EGFR) antibodies [13].

Another promising application of nanotechnology in GI endoscopy is targeted drug delivery. Achieving successful targeted drug delivery necessitates the accumulation of drugs within the desired target area and the establishment of specific molecular-level interactions with the target receptor. By using nanocarriers, such as liposomes, micelles, dendrimers, carbon-based nanocarriers, QDs, hydrogels, and exosomes, drugs can be delivered to the tumour site with higher specificity and lower toxicity compared to conventional chemotherapy. Through the increased permeability and retention (EPR) effect, the nanocarriers can shield the medications from deterioration and removal in the systemic circulation while also enhancing their accumulation in the cancer tissue. Additionally, targeting ligands that recognize and attach to tumour cells, including peptides or antibodies, can be added to the nanocarriers to functionalize them and enable more targeted distribution [14]. Among various nanocarriers, liposomes, due to various advantageous attributes such as overall biocompatibility, biodegradability, and the capacity to encapsulate both hydrophilic and hydrophobic compounds, have emerged as the most extensively utilized nanosystems for drug delivery in clinical settings. For instance, paclitaxel has been delivered to stomach cancer cells that exhibit a high level of folate receptors using liposomes conjugated with folate. Micelles are widely used to encapsulate a wide variety of medicinal compounds because of their hydrophilic exterior and hydrophobic centre [15]. Micelles are very promising nanostructure carriers for targeted delivery of hydrophobic anticancer drugs because of their biodegradable, biocompatible, and cell-specific targeting properties. On the other hand, dendrimers have many advantages when it comes to drug delivery, such as longer blood circulation times, better bioavailability, controlled drug molecule release, increased uptake by cancer tissues through the EPR effect, lack of immunogenicity, and remarkable penetration capabilities. The effectiveness and promise of dendrimers as adaptable and effective carriers for drug delivery applications are enhanced by these qualities [16].

Notwithstanding the potential advantages of nanotechnology in gastrointestinal endoscopy, a number of obstacles and restrictions must be overcome before these tools may be applied in clinical settings. For instance, it is important to carefully assess the safety and biocompatibility of NPs, including any possible toxicity or immunogenicity. The stability and specificity of the NPs need to be optimized to ensure reliable and reproducible results. The regulatory and ethical aspects of using nanotechnology in human subjects need to be carefully considered, including informed consent, privacy, and data security [17]. Moreover, the cost-effectiveness and practicality of using nanotechnology in routine clinical settings need to be evaluated, especially in terms of the availability and affordability of the materials and devices. In recent years, researchers and clinicians have explored various strategies to improve the sensitivity, specificity, and accuracy of endoscopic diagnosis and treatment. For example, they have developed fluorescent NPs that can specifically bind to cancer cells or inflamed tissues, enabling early detection and precise resection [18]. They have also designed nanocarriers that can selectively deliver chemotherapeutic agents to the tumour site, reducing the systemic toxicity and improving the efficacy. In addition, they have engineered nano-sensors that can detect and monitor the biomarkers of GI diseases, such as *Helicobacter pylori* infection, celiac disease, and colorectal cancer [19].

As a result, by enabling more sensitive, specific, and precise detection and treatment of GI illnesses, nanotechnology presents significant potential for furthering the discipline of GI endoscopy. Targeted medication administration and enhanced visualization, characterization, and quantification of gastrointestinal lesions and biomarkers are potential benefits of developing new nanomaterials, devices, and tests. To guarantee the safety, effectiveness, and usability of these technologies for clinical applications, more study and development are necessary in order to solve the difficulties and constraints associated with the use of nanotechnology in GI endoscopy.

5.2 Nanotechnology

Modern life is easier because of developments in nanotechnology and nanoscience across almost all scientific fields. Since the arrangement of atoms on the 1–100 nm scale produces devices, systems, and structures with different characteristics and activities, nanotechnology and nanoscience represent an expanding field of research. The field saw a rise in public discussion and awareness in the beginning of the 2000s, which paved the way for the first commercial applications of nanotechnology [20]. Nanotechnologies are beneficial to almost all fields of study, including computer science, biology, chemistry, materials science, physics, and engineering (figure 5.2). Notably, promising advances in cancer treatment have been made recently thanks to the application of nanotechnologies in human health improvement [21].

Nevertheless, despite this restriction, structures as small as a few hundred nanometers can be referred to as 'nanotechnology' and can be produced by either top-down or bottom-up development using standalone components. The conventional food and agricultural sectors have seen significant transformations due to the fast advancement of nanotechnology, as evidenced by the development of innovative and functional packaging, tiny sensors, nanopesticides, and small-molecule fertilisers to name a few. Many innovative nanomaterials have been developed for improving food safety and quality, farming growth, and surveillance of the environment [22].

Although prospective biomaterials and nanotechnology-based uses for wound healing are being developed, there are yet few commercially accessible wound healing solutions that include nanomaterials. The prevalence of chronic wounds is

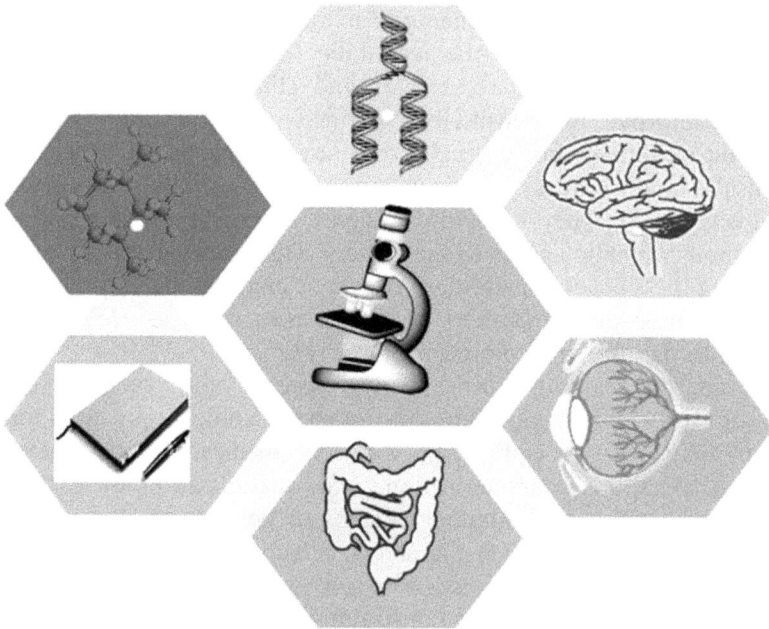

Figure 5.2. Applications of nanotechnology in diverse areas.

rising as our society ages and the number of persons with diabetes rises. With increased understanding of the molecular principles behind these disorders, new medical devices are entering the market for traditional wound treatment. A method to assess intracellular electrical potentials that could be extensively parallelized without interfering with cellular function would revolutionize the field of neuroscience [23]. Although such a technology is not currently available, it may be argued that nanotechnology has made it possible to fabricate solid-state electrical probes with little disruption. Numerous studies have demonstrated that it is feasible to come up with tiny gadgets with qualities that are comparable to those exhibited by biological components, and that nanoscale electrical probes may be used to track the transmembrane electrical potential of electrogenic cell types [24].

Since DNA nanotechnology has established itself as a reliable method for creating a variety of nanoscale structures and devices, it may be useful for achieving the objectives of early cancer diagnosis and prompt cancer therapy. Due to their predictable secondary structures, tiny sizes, great biocompatibility, and programmability, the resulting DNA-based nanoscale structures and devices exhibit outstanding performance in the detection of cancer. Particularly, the fast advancement of molecular assembly technologies and other DNA nanotechnologies has given DNA-based nanomaterials a greater functional and intellectual sophistication [25].

5.3 Nanoparticles

Over the last ten years, the field of the application of nanotechnology has grown dramatically, and numerous substances incorporating nanomaterials are now employed in a variety of sectors, particularly the ones related to nutritional science, cosmetics, skincare, and medication. NPs are units with a single dimension within one nm and one hundred nm. They display a variety of characteristics, which differ depending on their dimensions and interface activities [26]. NPs are widely employed in a variety of sectors, including skincare goods, technology, and both detection and remedial medical applications, because due to their tiny size and vast surface area. The field's exponential growth and increased popularity have been facilitated by the capacity to examine nanomaterials utilizing methods with atomic resolution capabilities, such as scanning tunnelling microscopy, scanning transmission electron microscopy, and tandem electron microscopy. The area's rapid expansion has sparked interest in studying the dangers of NPs and nanotechnology in general [27]. People are exposed to NPs increasingly often, however, research on NP safety has lagged behind NP utilization research. Pharmaceutical carriers of drugs known as NPs are used in therapeutic and diagnostic procedures. These NPs, which include granular NPs, lipid-based, polymer-based NPs, and small emulsions are thought to have potential therapeutic uses. Their therapeutic usefulness is influenced by their chemical and physical properties, drug loading effectiveness, drug release, and—most importantly—minimal or no carrier toxicity. NPs could be therapeutically useful, but some evidence indicates they could also be harmful. These investigations have shown that NPs may build up in cells and cause harm to particular organs. These findings highlight the urgent need to establish safe NPs and stringent standards for their development in relation to toxicity assessment. The fact that humans are subjected to these toxins considerably more often is also emphasized [28].

5.4 Classification of nanoparticles

Due to their unique or improved physical and chemical characteristics relative to bulk material, interest in nanomaterials, and particularly NPs, has grown in recent years (figure 5.3). The domains of healthcare and pharmaceutical industries, technology, farming, chemical catalysis, the food and beverage industry, and many more have all found new uses for these amazing qualities. More recently, physiological procedures using plants or microbes are also being used to create NPs as an ecologically acceptable substitute for the costly, energy-intensive, and possibly hazardous both chemical and physical synthesis processes [29]. In order to characterize these processes effectively, this interdisciplinary strategy for NP manufacturing necessitates that scientists and biotechnology professionals understand how to apply the sophisticated technique. The physicochemical characteristics of NPs and the techniques employed for their characterization are summarized in this older literature, which is geared towards a bio-oriented readership. It demonstrates how NPs differ from small-scale delivery or large-scale substances [30].

5.4.1 Polymer-based nanoparticles

Polymeric NPs have been widely used as drug delivery systems for long-lasting and controlled release. The object that is enclosed may be contained inside the polymer's structure or shell, connected to the outside of a sphere or capsule, or both. Two frequently used polymer compounds, polylactic glycolic acids (PLGA) and

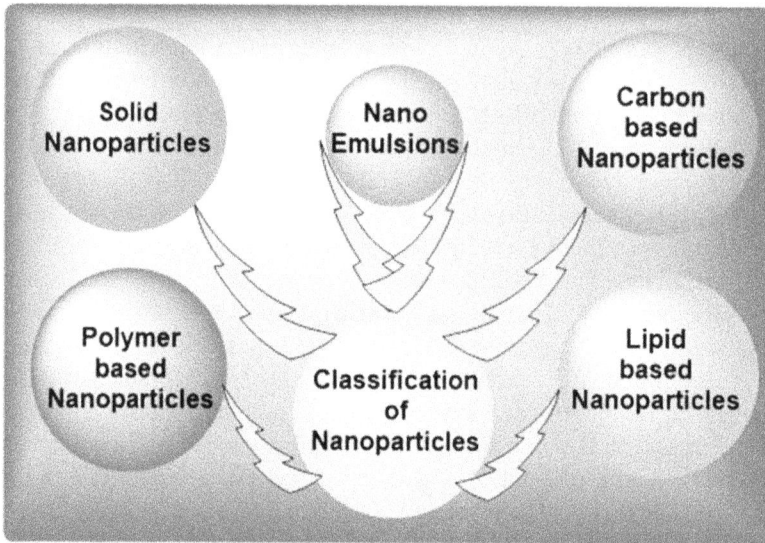

Figure 5.3. Classification of various NPs: solid NPs, carbon-based NPs, polymer-based NPs, lipid-based NPs and nanoemulsions.

polysaccharide-chitosan have both received FDA authorization for therapeutic use since they are biodegradable and biocompatible [31].

5.4.2 Solid nanoparticles

Iron oxides, gold, silver, and various other metal-based NPs are examples of solid NPs. Iron oxide NPs are created by joining a biocompatible polymer to an organic magnetite or magnetite core. Extremely paramagnetic characteristics of iron oxide NPs have received a lot of interest recently. Iron oxide NPs are used as biosensors in magnetic liquid hyperthermia, targeted medication delivery and gene transmission, and MRI. The unique optical features of iron oxide NPs, which allow them to function as biosensors in live cells, have also been employed in a variety of imaging and diagnostic procedures [32]. The NPs of gold have been proposed for use in ionizing radiation treatment, and cancer detection. This is due to a number of variables including their size, shape, and external features. Theranostic systems, which integrate diagnostics, imaging, and drugs for better therapy, can be made using gold NPs. They have been demonstrated to be less harmful than other inorganic NPs, however, their toxicity profile is still not fully understood [33]. A distinct class of solid NPs that has garnered interest are silver NPs. Due to their spectral properties and capacity to catch and distribute light, silver NPs are a prime instance of how NPs may be used as biosensors. Electronics, fabrics, wound dressings, antimicrobial coatings, and medical equipment all often employ silver NPs [34].

5.4.3 Carbon-based nanoparticles

Carbon-based NPs are being used in a range of biological applications, such as drug delivery, gene therapy, and imaging. CNTs, which exist in single-walled and multi-walled types, make up a large class of these NPs. CNTs are good prospects for a variety of biomedical applications, including medication and delivery of genes, biological sensors, and biological tissue engineering because of their distinctive physiochemical properties [35]. They also feature a special surface chemistry that improves the capacity for drug loading and display excellent stability. CNTs' safety is still under question because it has been shown that extended contact with them might injure healthy tissues [36].

5.4.4 Lipid-based nanoparticles

The liposome is the most well-known kind of vesicular lipid-based NP. Liposomes are composed of a bilayer of lipid and sterol that encloses an aqueous core, as was first noted in 1965. There are now several liposome formulations in use that have received FDA approval, and many more are undergoing medical or preliminary research. One of the most popular medication delivery methods is the use of liposomes. Liposomes have been used for drug, nutraceutical, and biological administration because of their excellent encapsulation efficiency and lengthy circulation endurance [37]. Due to the endothelium layer being damaged, the lymphatic system being ineffectual, and a higher permeability and retention effect, liposomes are able to passively aggregate in certain disease areas, such as tumours. A short half-life and rapid circulatory clearance after being opsonized and removed by the reticuloendothelial system are limitations of conventional liposomes from the past [38]. However, sterically stabilized liposomes with better stability and a longer half-life were produced by using saturated high-phase transition lipids and con-jugating polymers like polyethylene glycol with liposomes. These liposomes persist in the systemic circulation for a longer period of time than normal formulations, allowing for altered biodistribution and greater build-up in solid tumours. One advantage of liposomes and other lipid-based NPs is that they have the lowest toxicity for *in vivo* applications [39].

5.4.5 Nanoemulsions

Vaccines and anticancer medications have frequently been delivered using nano-emulsions (NEs). Colloidal dispersions known as NEs are suitable for the usage as medication carriers for compounds with low water solubility. The most common components of NEs are either water nanodroplets scattered in oil or oil nanodroplets spread in water. Usually, surfactants are added to improve their stability. However, a significant drawback of these carriers is that, if their size reaches 500 nm, they become thermodynamically unstable. NEs of a size between 20 and 200 nm, however, are more thermodynamically stable [40]. Parenteral, transdermal, and ocular delivery routes are among the recommended applications for NEs, primarily because of their capacity to shield encapsulated medicines from enzymatic hydrolysis and degradation. NEs may also be modified by conjugating them to different ligands in order to focus on biomolecules that are preferentially abundant in specific diseases, such as cancer. This is similar to how many of the NPs previously described were changed. For instance, ligand-conjugated NEs, which may target receptors with expression that is increased in some malignancies, have been shown to have better absorption into tumour cells, assisting in the reduction of tumour formation [41].

5.4.6 Nanoparticles in biomedical applications

Several NPs, particularly liposomes, metallic NPs, and elastomeric NPs, are being studied in therapeutic and preliminary research to improve the location-specific delivery of medications and genes. Many therapeutically useful drugs have a low water solubility, therefore their entrapment in NPs can boost their stability by lowering precipitation and the need for hazardous cosolvents. The efficacy of the therapy is increased because NPs may alter the rates of drug metabolism and clearance [42]. For instance, the FDA approved the Doxil brand to treat metastatic breast cancer and Kaposi's sarcoma. These NPs are far more effective if compared to a conventional drug. Though specific molecules can be added to NPs to boost delivery to specific cells, traditional or first-generation NPs are unable to target-specific cells. As previously mentioned, illness sites may be actively targeted by utilizing NPs by conjugating them to specific ligands that may identify and attach to proteins in the membrane known to be overproduced in a variety of disorders, such as cancer. Additionally, NPs are used as gene delivery systems, and they have shown success in replacing certain diseased target genes linked to hereditary disorders including malignancy, certain viruses, and others [43]. Sadly, the immunological sensitivities that cationic NPscause may limit their use. Additionally, NPs have been used in cellular imaging to detect cellular changes both *in vivo* and *in vitro*. NPs can be joined with other moieties, such as antibodies and their target, to increase the efficiency of their selection. Despite their potential efficacy as drugs or gene carriers, there are fewer NPs in clinical use than one might predict given the numerous preclinical trials. This is mostly because of potential toxicity brought on by poorly understood mechanisms, which is true in particular for NPs administered repeatedly [44].

5.4.7 Characteristics of nanoparticles

Through molecular level manipulation of a substance's chemical and physical characteristics, nanotechnology creates a variety of nanomaterials with unique features. Because they have higher surface area per volume of smaller particle than larger particles, NPs are more reactive and may be coated with a variety of chemicals. These outperform macroparticles in strength and weight. The electrical, magnetic, and optical characteristics of the inorganic nanomaterials are distinctive [45]. Iron oxide magnetic NPs produce a more powerful more concentrated magnetic field when compared to larger particles since all of their electrons spin in the exact same way. This greater magnetic field may enhance the level of contrast in imaging with magnetic resonance. There are two conceivable energy states for the electrons in metal NPs: the grounded state and an excited state. The variation between these two distinct energy levels determines the fluorescence and colour of any metal NPs [46]. CdSe QDs, sometimes referred to as Qdots, emit significantly more light than organic material fluorescent dye molecules. A blood sample may be quickly and affordably screened for a variety of peptides, infectious agents, and other useful substances using a QD of a certain colour. Unlike microparticles, NPs may cross the blood–brain barrier. Due to their lengthy half-life and ability to avoid immune system detection, they can be used to deliver medications. NPs are useful in the treatment of cancer because tumour cells tolerate them. They may deliver therapeutic and diagnostic agents to specific organelles and cells as well as interact specifically with biological molecules on and inside of cells. Due to the unique properties of NPs and the inherent nanoscale activities of cellular biological components, nanotechnology can be applied in the medical field [47].

5.4.8 Characterization of nanoparticles

At a very small scale, nanotechnology has become extremely prominent in the majority of scientific fields. Atoms and molecules behave differently at this scale and provide a variety of fascinating and enticing uses. NPs, nanospheres, nanocapsules, nanoemulsions, nanoliposomes, and nanoniosomes are examples of pharmaceutical nanocarriers. To achieve particular goals, managing particle size, surface character-istics, and drug release are the main design considerations for nanocarriers. Controlling the desired in-the-laboratory and *in vivo* animal behaviour of tiny carrier molecules is essential because of this [48]. Nanocarriers may be recognized by their size, shape, and surface charge using highly advanced microscopic techniques including microscopy with scanning electrons, electron microscopy with trans-mission, and atomic force microscopy. While the size of particles and size distribution are detected using the dynamic scattering of light and photon-correla-tion spectroscopy, surface shape and size may be examined using electron micro-scopy [49]. Zeta potential, an indirect measurement of surface charge, may be used to determine colloidal stability, and differential scanning calorimetry can be used to characterize particles and study drug interactions. Additionally, cell uptake research might reveal the binding and internalization of targeted carriers to the particular cells. Confocal imaging may be used to analyse the biodistribution of specific nanocarriers and validate their intracellular uptake and subcellular localization [50].

5.5 Intestinal endoscopy

In order to quickly identify malignancies and locate and treat early precursor lesions, endoscopy is a helpful inspection technique utilized in intestinal cancer screening programmes. The intestinal morphology of the tissues surrounding the digestive system may be seen in real time using endoscopic white light imaging, and tissue samples can be collected from highly dubious lesions to aid in the diagnosis. However, endoscopy also has substantial challenges in detecting GIC early on. The prognosis of early microscopic lesions was bad, and lesions that were unseen due to image quality limitations were microscopic [51]. Endoscopy is a useful examination tool used in colorectal tumour detection programmes in order to rapidly detect malignancies and discover and cure early precursor lesions. Endoscopic white light imaging allows for the real-time visualization of the intestinal morphology of the tissues around the digestive system, and tissue samples from highly suspect lesions can be obtained to help with the diagnosis. Endoscopy, however, also has significant difficulties in spotting GIC at an early stage. Early microscopic lesions had a poor prognosis, and microscopic lesions that could not be noticed owing to imaging quality restrictions existed [52]. Early GIC exams are impacted by endoscopy since these semi-invasive procedures frequently leave patients feeling uncomfortable and anxious. Therefore, the primary research focus going forward will be on increasing the comfort and accuracy of endoscopy, which is a crucial diagnostic method for early screening of GI disorders [53].

5.6 Medical nanotechnology

5.6.1 Diagnosis

As completely novel nanomaterials are developed to detect and treat cancer, the discipline of nanomedicine has recently experienced unprecedented progress. Novel biological sensors that utilize nanotechnology have the potential to improve therapeutic investigations' sensitivity in the early diagnosis and monitoring of GIC as well as in the earlier and more accurate identification of specific affected tissues or organs. For example, immuno-microfluidic chips using QDs of semiconductors provide precise identification of cancer markers linked with humans, which may help GIC therapies be more successful. Biocompatible nanodevices include integrated gadgets for cancer detection before it occurs [54].

Nevertheless, despite the discovery of further microscopic cancer lesions in an individual's body, combating treatment resistance and improving the solubility of drugs and utilization efficiency continue to be major challenges in the medical treatment of GIC. The main advantage of employing nanotechnology to develop a drug delivery system is its enormous specific surface area and changeable modification capabilities, which are effective techniques to boost medicine utilization [55].

By modifying the surfaces of NPs to more precisely target tumour tissues, it is feasible to increase the concentrations of pharmaceuticals that are beneficial in treating cancer while reducing the side effects of drugs used for chemotherapy and improving the effectiveness of anticancer drug therapy. NPs' enormous functional surface areas make it possible for them to bind, absorb, and carry small-molecule drugs, RNA and DNA, as well as proteins, and probes [56]. They are also highly sought-after in many medical fields because of their adjustable size, shape, and surface properties, which provide them with good stability, large carrier capacities, their capacity to absorb water-based and hydrophobic agents, and compatibility with different drug delivery paths. Additionally, we may develop detecting and curative NPs that are ideally suited for more targeted and individualized illness treatment by merging diagnostic and therapeutic functionalities into just one biodegradable and biocompatible NP. These NPs have generated a lot of interest since they can increase the effectiveness for GI malignancies [57]. Due to their significant particular surface domains, surface, and interfacial effects, NPs are naturally advantageous as drug carriers. When coupled with bioactive compounds, they can be used for both cancer therapy and imaging. Today's drug delivery alternatives include metallic substances, polymer-based NPs, lipid-based formulations, as well as theranostic NPs. In order to further reduce the negative impacts of intestinal reflex movements on the early diagnosis and treatment of GIC, this data comprehensively explains the uses of the application of nanotechnology in the rapid identification and treatment of GIC as well as the clinical obstacles for GIC therapy. It also covers how to promote the earliest feasible clinical use of lab-developed nanoplatforms [58].

5.6.2 Nanotechnology in the early diagnosis

Medical evidence dating back decades shows that individuals with GIC who have lesions that are precancerous and the initial stages of carcinoma had better forecasts, less mortality, and longer life expectancies than patients with advancing disease. The current main clinical applications of early-diagnosis methods for GIC include an endoscopic examination, growth indicators, MRI, computed tomography, PET, and NIRF detection [59]. Given the development of science and technology as well as the expanding understanding of the aforementioned diagnostic mechanisms, researchers have found that there is room for advancement and refinement of these diagnostic techniques. For instance, the application of endoscope capsules can diminish the discomfort that patients experience during invasive examinations and reduce the risk of inflammation. Contrast chemicals can be administered before to MRI imaging to improve its diagnostic sensitivity. Recent research efforts to combine nanotechnology with the existing imaging technologies have boosted their sensitivity [60].

5.6.3 Theragnostic

To produce separate 'theragnostic' chemical compounds for cancer imaging and medical therapy today, the phase of preclinical development is necessary. A single carrier is used for both therapeutic and diagnostic chemicals in theragnostics. These nanomaterials are intended to make imaging applications more convenient for both clinical and evaluation uses. To put this idea into practice, it is crucial to create important molecules that can react to chemical or physiological stimulus in the treatment zone. A range of triggers, such as pro-inflammatory signs like pH level changes in temperature, an oxygen shortage, or specific binding to an inflamed ligand, may have an impact on the system [61]. Messenger chemicals may be included within or bound to the carrier to help with imaging applications. Molecules may unite instantly through noncovalent or linked contacts during the creation of the nanocarrier, or subsequently through surface modification activities. Noncovalent or covalent interactions are selected depending on the goal and level of specificity of the region that has to be addressed. Under various pH or oxidative regimes, covalent linkages based on carbonyl, amine, or methicone coupling chemistries carry out a range of activities. If chemical adaptability is needed, covalent bonds can be replaced by hydrophobicity, electrostatic attraction, or hydrogen-bonding affinity [62]. There are various potential links between the test substances or curative molecule and the nanocarrier since polymers can be chosen to have a range of functional groups and/or polar sites. Coulomb or hydrophobic bonds (hydrophobic chemical loading) or interactions between ionic compounds (nucleic acids) have been successfully made possible by the use of amide, ester, disulfide, hydrazone, or thioether connections. Yang *et al* showed how a practical approach to treating pancreatic cancers may be used [63]. To prevent the uPA receptor from interacting with its own organic ligand, uPA, this study used the urokinase plasminogen in order stimulating activator amino-terminal disintegration peptide as a substitute ligand with a strong propensity for binding to uPAR. ATF peptides have been shown to suppress angiogenesis and cancer development in a variety of animal carcinoma models. Yang *et al* discovered that cancer cells easily absorbed the ATF-coated NPs, elevating their respective roles in the development of tumour-specific therapeutic medication delivery and carcinoma imaging [64].

5.6.4 Tissue engineering

In tissue engineering, growth factors and scaffolds made of the right materials are combined with cell proliferation. For best effectiveness, biomaterials for biomedical engineering need to have linked pores and a large surface area. By allowing for cell movement, fluid diffusion inside the biological material (such as the diffusion and discharge of nutrients), and electronic and chemical liaison among the cells producing the biomaterial, the holes support proper cell culture development [65]. In the digestive system, gastric ulcers may be treated using tissue engineering procedures. Hassani *et al* claim that polystyrene NPs adhered to the enlarged mucosal regions. This study demonstrated that tiny NPs, which adhered to injured tissue more frequently than healthy tissue, were most closely linked to this relationship. This finding emphasises the notion of using NPs as a technological extension for treating hepatic ulcers [66].

5.6.5 Targeted imaging and therapeutic in colorectal cancer

NPs offer benefits in cancer, particularly imaging, due to their tiny size. When combined with magnetic resonance imaging, QDs, or NPs with quantum confinement qualities like size-tunable light emission, can generate great pictures of cancer locations. These NPs can be activated by any light that is proportionally blue-shifted to the emission spectrum since they are much brighter than organic dyes. When compared to conventional pigments, which are employed as a contrast medium, luminescent QDs may generate pictures with a greater contrast at a lesser cost [67]. The disadvantage is that making QDs typically involves using dangerous substances. For the treatment of cancer, nanotechnology-based treatments have already received approval. NPs like abraxane or liposomes like Doxil are examples of products that have received approval. Small nanocarriers tend to collect at tumour sites because there is ineffective lymphatic drainage there. In photodynamic treatment, particles are supplied to a particular area of the body and illuminated by an external light source [68]. The particle absorbs the light, and if it is made of metal, the light's energy may heat both the metal and the tissue around it. Additionally, by using light to create highly reactive oxygen molecules, it is possible to destroy neighbouring organic molecules by combining them chemically with the oxygen molecules. Photodynamic treatment provides a number of benefits. Chemotherapy does not spread a 'toxic trail' of chemically reactive compounds throughout the body since it only affects the area that has been lit via particle delivery. A noninvasive approach of treating illnesses, growths, and tumours is photodynamic therapy [69]. Recently, Kirui *et al* reported on the creation of advantageous oxide-based gold–iron NPs for the inspection, photothermal stimulation, and focusing of cancer cells utilizing laser light at 800 nm. After the gold NPs had been function-alized using carboxy-terminated phospholipids and linked to the A33 antigen seen in colorectal cancer cells, a single-chain antibody, scFv, was conjugated to them. The A33 antigen is overexpressed on the surface of SW1222 colorectal cancer cells, which led to the NPs becoming particularly immobilized on the cancer cells' surfaces. The NPs were then selectively absorbed by the cancer cells. After 808 nm light was absorbed, malignant tissue was specifically removed, demonstrating the suitability of this technique for cancer diagnosis and therapy [70].

5.6.6 Gene therapy delivery

Due to the ineffectiveness of gene transfection, gene therapy still has significant drawbacks. Vectors produced from viral or nonviral transporters are the two primary kinds employed in gene therapy. Despite having a high transduction yield, the viral gene delivery approach has a variety of undesirable side effects, including immunogenicity and probable carcinogenic consequences. The capacity of cationic polymers, such as chitosan, to bond with DNA or short-interfering RNA to form complexes that might serve as nonviral substitute carriers for gene therapy applications is another advantage [71]. The limited capacity of bare DNA inside cells and siRNA units to enter cell membranes is a significant barrier to DNA and siRNA treatment. As solutions to this issue, several distribution tactics have been studied. Recently made attempts to create synthetic reagent-based tissue-targeted gene transport mechanisms have shown intriguing outcomes. More and more 'targeted NPs' are being developed, which have a surface reconfigured with a synthetic protein, and an attractive substance, or an antibody implanted to the matrix of polymers in order to focus on a specific site before distributing the active agent [72]. This is done to increase the efficacy of siRNA-loaded polymer NPs. Whether biodegradable or not, NPs have demonstrated an intriguing ability to adhere to and disseminate DNA and siRNA among therapeutic carriers. In fact, it has been demonstrated that NPs may protect DNA and siRNA from degradation while also greatly increasing their pharmacological efficacy *in vivo* and *in vitro*. IBD, or inflammatory bowel illness, might make a biocompatible system particularly crucial. The biodegradable polyamide envelope's capacity to safeguard and dissem-inate the siRNA into the cytoplasm may enable a successful *in vivo* transfection [73].

5.6.7 Colitis therapy

Effective, specialized drugs are now available for treating IBD, also known as ulcerative colitis and Crohn's disease, a severe, chronic inflammatory sickness. However, these treatments are often limited by major systemic adverse effects. IBD was treated only with immunosuppressants or anti-inflammatory drugs (5-amino salicylic acid, steroids) up to the past ten years [74]. Although these drugs are effective, their usage has been restricted due to immune system problems that can be extremely hazardous. Despite the therapeutic efficacy of more modern biological therapies, such as monoclonal antibodies that combat tumour necrosis factor (TNF-α), some patients continue to develop antibodies to the medication, raising the risk of infusion reactions and decreasing the response of the individual to the therapy [75].

5.6.8 Oral delivery of vaccines

The delivery of vaccinations to the mucosa via nanocarriers is one of the greatest and most important potential uses for NMs in the future. NPs may be utilized as delivery vehicles, adjuvants, or both. When giving immunizations to the mucosa, nano- or microsized compounds may target certain locations and processes to hasten absorption. The majority of NPs smaller than the wavelengths of 200 nm are absorbed by M cells or the epithelium of the gut at the tips of villi. Large particles that can be consumed by GI macrophages include nano-sized liposomes [76]. The surfaces between NPs and tiny particles now contain a variety of ligands. peptides, such as glandular IgA, aimed at M cells in the rodent Peyer's patch, or immuno-globulins such as mAb 5B11, which engages M cells on polymeric latex particles, can also function as ligands. They can also manifest as other molecules, including the bacterial molecule Invasin-C192, which is involved in the invasion of cells and adhesion. Additionally, ligands can be sugars linked to hydrophobic groups, such as O-palmitoyl the mannan or the B subunit, which is a component of the toxin that causes cholera [77].

5.6.9 Mitigation

An autoimmune illness of the digestive system, this condition affects the whole GI tract, with ulcerative colitis causing specific inflammatory processes in the colon. Serious social, economic, and health issues result from present medications failing and their negative effects. The ideal target for gene therapy delivery vehicles to treat IBD is the gut epithelium. Due to the hydrophilic, negatively charged, and biodegradable properties of nucleic acids (NAs), gene therapy incorporating the use of NA therapies confronts significant difficulties [78]. Scientists are motivated to create gene therapy vehicles that can be readily targeted to the appropriate tissues for IBD by recent success in developing biomaterials for gene therapy and their appearance in clinical trials for diverse illnesses. Nanotechnology advancements have made it possible to construct a variety of NPs for NA administration to treat IBD, which still has issues with targetability, poor therapeutic effectiveness, and GI tract stability [79].

5.6.10 Role in targeted drug delivery

The use of large-sized materials in drug administration also poses a variety of challenges, such as *in vivo* strength, poor bioavailability, and issues with target-specific distribution, in addition to the adverse reactions of the specific medicines (figure 5.4). Therefore, implementing cutting-edge drug delivery techniques to target drugs to a specific area of the body may offer a possibility to address these urgent

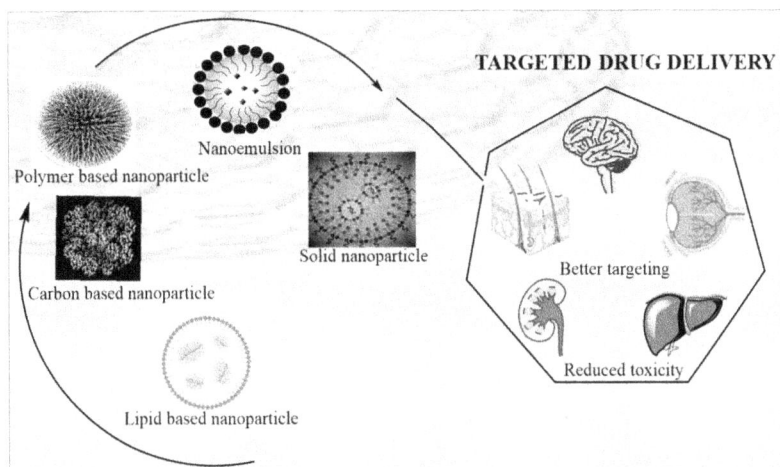

Figure 5.4. Role of NPs in targeted drug delivery.

issues. The field of nanotechnology creates nanoscale-sized materials made of lipids, metals, or natural or synthetic/semi-synthetic polymers [80]. When employed in targeted drug delivery, NPs can increase the bioavailability, biodistribution, and accumulation of treatments, concentrating them mostly in the targeted sick region and serving as stabilizers. The aforementioned variable colloidal systems can deliver drugs to the right places, increasing therapeutic efficacy while reducing side effects and toxicity, protecting the drug from biological degradation, and allowing immediate and physical medicinal properties to control at the exact site of disease.

The early use of nanocarriers for medication administration was founded on an indirect targeting mechanism in order to increase efficiency over traditional free-drug formulations [81]. A unique approach, on the other hand, uses magnetic fields or conjugation procedures to increase medication delivery to target locations while employing active targeting by incorporating specific ligands. Therefore, innovation in drug delivery systems and formulations might result from the use of nano-technology. Effective and site-specific medication delivery makes it simpler to get a therapeutic outcome that can fight immunologic ailments, tumoural diseases, or neurological disorders. This special issue integrates many elements of nanotechnology research in quest of novel therapeutic targets and approaches. The physiological acceptance of layered liposomes and hybrids nanotechnology with surfactant agents, as well as mathematical models to ascertain the body routes of magnetic NPs or to elucidate the molecular make-up of metal-decorated fullerenes, are some examples of these [82].

5.7 Role of nanotechnology in intestinal tract

The digestive system is one among the ways whereby environmental NPs enter the human body. After being consumed, they immediately penetrate into the mucus barrier and engage the enterocytes. They are removed from the intestinal mucosa by

M cells, preventing enterocytes from actively absorbing them. Following cellular trafficking, they can enter the bloodstream and travel throughout the body. A smaller NP's diameter can be used to explain faster diffusion through the mucus layer [83]. Each component of the digestive system has unique characteristics, making the use of diagnostics and therapies challenging since distal small intestine endoscopy or targeted drug administration are still far from optimal. Given the characteristics of NPs, the gastrointestinal tract may be a suitable area for the application of nanotechnology. Numerous gastrointestinal conditions have been tried with varying degrees of success, including the intended application of therapeutic agents in the terminal ileum, gastrointestinal (e.g. inflammatory bowel disease), and stomach (e.g. gastrointestinal ulcer), diagnostic use in tumours (e.g. pancreatic, gastric, and colonic tumours), gene therapy in these conditions, the expression of genes (genomics), production of proteins (proteomics), and gastrointestinal endoscopy [84].

5.8 Nanotechnological aids

5.8.1 Nanopowder

Endoscopic hemostasis utilizing electrical cauterization, implantation tamponade, and hemoclips is the best remedy for peptic ulcer bleeding. However, endoscopic hemostasis can be difficult and ineffectual when there is extensive continuous bleeding and difficult anatomical conditions (figure 5.5) [85]. In a second prospective pilot clinical research, an endoscopic hemospray was administered to 20 individuals with peptic ulcer bleeding during twenty-four hours of hospital admission. Ninety-five percent of patients were in hemostasis. Acute hemostasis was attempted for one patient but failed due to a Forrest Ia ulcer. Two patients experienced recurrent bleeding within 72 h. The 30-day follow-up revealed no significant issues. This study's lone spurter did not get better after receiving therapy, which was a drawback. Hemospray appears to be an easy-to-use, effective endoscopic treatment for continuous bleeding from the GI tract if it is revalidated [86].

5.8.2 Plastic stents

The endoscopic placement of biliary plastic stents is extensively used in the treatment of both malignant and benign biliary disorders. However, the primary disadvantage associated with plastic stents for liver drainage is sludge clogging. Sludge blocks the biliary plastic stents due the outer layer of the stents promotes bacterial, glycoprotein, and protein adherence [87]. Nanotechnology gives up new possibilities for surface modification thanks to the soil-release phenomenon (also referred to as the lotus effect, in which dirt is released from the surface by rapidly flowing water, keeping the lotus petals clean). Sol–gel technique enables the systematic synthesis of impermeable to nanometer-thin coatings with predefined physical and chemical characteristics [88]. According to an *in vitro* experiment, sludge deposition on biliary plastic stents made of synthetic material teflon with sol–gel, the coatings of organic epoxide at 192 g mol^{-1} or 550 g mol^{-1} and

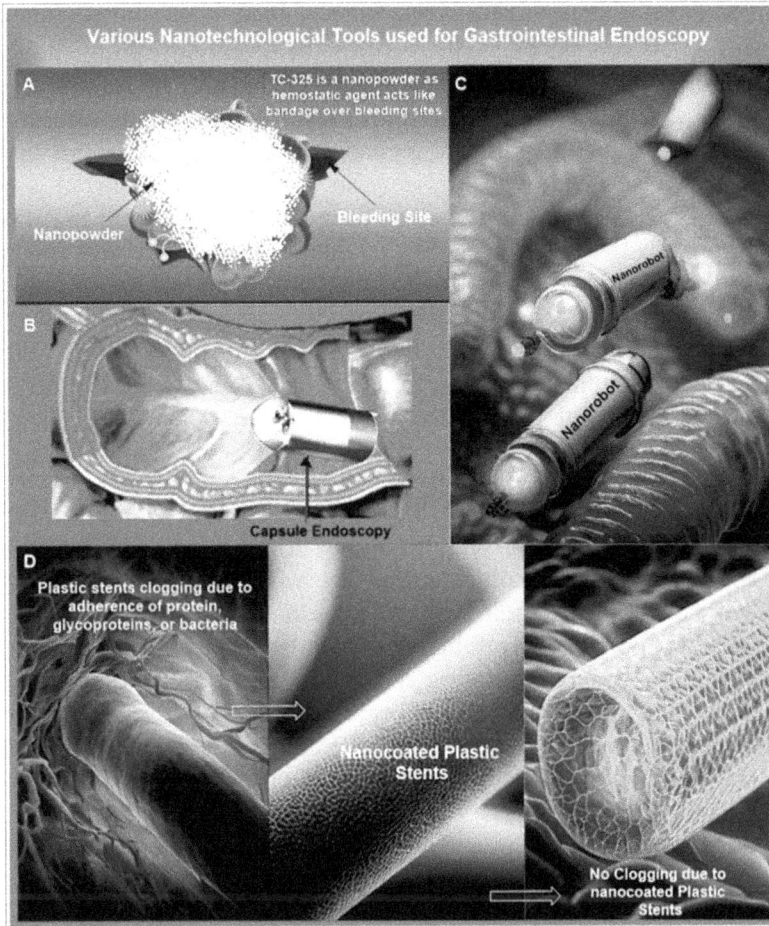

Figure 5.5. Various nanotechnological tools for GI endoscopy: nanopowders, plastic stents, capsule endoscopy, nano-coated plastic stents and nanorobots.

propylaminosilane was reduced when compared with untreated teflon and clear coating. Polymer stents might gain advantage from nanocoating to prevent biliary plastic stent occlusion [89].

5.8.3 Capsule endoscopy

A newly developed tool for diagnosing small-bowel and colonic disorders is capsule endoscopy. The treatment is simple to carry out, and patients generally approve of it. Deep tissue problems cannot be detected by capsule endoscopy, and there is no treatment potential. Recent research has focused on the idea of combining two technological platforms: capsule endoscopy to find the identified abnormality and nanotechnology to target and label the damaged organ [90]. Nano-based capsule endoscopy with biological Imaging and optical biopsy project, which has been funded by the European Union, seeks to combine optical methods with the field of nanotechnology biosensing, and manoeuvring technological advances to create a kind of capsule endoscope that can perform the secretion examination and the identification of declared and deep tissue illnesses. This may be helpful in revealing GI tract lesions that are malignant and at-risk for becoming cancerous [91]. Innovative nanometric robots known as nanorobots may be used for endoscopic treatments. In a capsule endoscopy device (also known as a 'robotic beetle'), robotic arms, bioanalytical sensors, and ultrasonic transducers can be used to collect tissue samples and provide treatments including targeted medication release and hot tissue destruction. The researchers intend to create intelligent endoscopic capsules, which are tiny robotic pills with therapeutic and diagnostic potential. The idea is supported by developments in micro and nanotechnology. The functional units of the vector-based capsule are the fundamental capsule functions, movement systems, screening systems, and therapeutic along with the biopsy systems [92].

5.9 Quality control of nanotechnology

Human exposure to NPs is inevitable as they are used more often, which has increased interest in nanotoxicology study. The varieties and applications of NPs continue to expand, but there is little study to describe the consequences upon access and to tackle their possible harmful effects [93]. Particularly in the medical sector, NPs are being employed in monitoring and therapeutic tools to comprehend better, identify, and treat human ailments. Before clinical use can occur, it is crucial to understand the properties of nanomaterials as well as how they communicate with the body since interacting with NPs for medical purposes necessitates intentional contact or administration [94].

The male reproductive system is now being exposed to more NPs thanks to the science of nanotechnology. Male germ and somatic cells have been observed to be negatively affected by a number of NPs. Many NPs negatively affect male germ and somatic cells, which may have an influence on fertility or the capacity to generate healthy children [95].

The international literature cites many nanoparticle functionalities as the cause of their increased bioefficacy/toxicity. Since different NPs of various shapes and sizes have different surface areas, surface charges, solubilities, and other physicochemical properties, it is clear from the literature on comparative toxicity studies that the toxicity of these particles does not follow a pattern that is determined by their shape, size, surface area, surface charge, and other physicochemical properties. It thus begs the issue of what aspect of an NP is most responsible for its extreme toxicity [96].

The qualities which make NPs so useful for clinical studies could also render them dangerous to people. The epidermis, intestinal tract, bloodstream, nervous system, and airways are among the organs that NPs have been shown to target. Due to the ease of entry, the intestinal tract is frequently exposed to environmental NPs. Environmental variables with nanoscale dimensions are potential contributors to the risk for inflammatory bowel disease [97]. Recent animal and laboratory research demonstrates that nanomaterials can be harmful to the liver. As a result, the probability of human toxicity cannot be discounted. Back pain, vasodilatation, acute retention of urine, a high temperature, cytopenia, hand-foot syndrome, diarrhoea, and mild renal toxicity are some of the negative effects of the tiny substances, which are either accepted for medical use or are participating in clinical trials. Other side effects include dysuria and abdominal pain, peripheral sensory nerve damage, and neutropenia [98].

Since its inception, nanotechnology has had a significant impact on medicines. By generating a wide variety of NPs that can penetrate even highly impenetrable membranes like the blood–brain barrier, it has completely altered traditional approaches to drug development and delivery systems. Similar to how every coin has two sides, nanotechnology also has its share of drawbacks, in this case the toxicity of these NPs. Numerous studies have examined the toxicity of different NPs, and new developments in nanotechnology have been made to make them less harmful. One such method is 'green synthesis' of NPs [99].

5.10 Artificial intelligence in gastrointestinal endoscopy

Artificial intelligence (AI) algorithms began to develop as a result of the constant advancements in information technology and their effects on every aspect of our lives. This was due to the demand for improved machine performance. Human brain performance may be impacted by weariness, stress, and lack of experience, unlike that of computers. AI technology would make up for human limitations, prevent human errors, allow robots some trustworthy autonomy, and boost productivity and efficiency at work. Therefore, AI may be the greatest choice when seeking for a quick and trustworthy assistance to handle the steadily increasing number of patients [100].

GI endoscopy might benefit greatly from the use of AI technology. It can lower inter-operator variability, improve diagnostic accuracy, and support making prompt, correct therapy decisions. AI would also speed up, lower the cost of, and simplify endoscopic treatments.

Based on computer algorithms that function similarly to human brains, AI-assisted endoscopy is performed. When they are constructed, they respond (output) to both what they have learnt and what they are given as information [101]. The principle underpinning this technology is known as 'machine learning' (ML), which is the act of educating computer programmes to spot patterns in data. It offers them the ability to learn new abilities on their own and improve via practice needing explicit programming. AI currently performs equally as well as or even superior to human brains as a result. Among the computerized learning approaches that are growing, the fastest is deep learning (DL). The neural network structure of the human brain served as the model for multi-layered artificial neural networks, a sort of technology [102].

Like our brains, DL models are also capable of logical data analysis, pattern recognition, conclusion drawing, and judgement. DL and AI are therefore much more potent than conventional ML. In essence, the technology known as AI is based on a computer programme that has been trained to do a certain task, such as being able to recognize or characterize specific lesions, like colon polyps. This computer programme is taught utilizing the ML previously described by exposure to various instructional materials, which include a significant amount of recorded video clips containing lesions for the prior example [103].

These computer algorithms will identify and analyse specific characteristics from these footage frames, such as micro-surface topological arrangement, colour differences, microvascular arrangement, pit sequence, physical appearance under light with filters like narrow band image processing, high-magnification, endo cystoscopy physical appearance, and many other features, in order to automate the identification or diagnosis-prediction of infections of interest. After that, either a new test database or impending *in vivo* clinical investigations are used to verify the output algorithm [104].

For a variety of purposes, there are many distinct types of AI systems that are accessible. The two main categories of AI systems are computerized detection for identifying lesion and computerized assistance identification for optical examination and lesion characterization. Lesion delineation for complete endoscopic excision is one example of the therapeutic assistance offered by other AI systems. There are more AI technologies that can offer technical assistance for better gastrointestinal endoscopy efficiency, such as scope insertion guidance, illness detection based on information from patients, and more [105].

5.11 Future perspectives

Traditional endoscopes are now the only devices that can administer and track treatment with any accuracy. Over the last ten years, significant developments in nanomaterials and light-triggered therapy may allow for more precise identification of challenging lesions and customized treatment of GI tumours. Theranostics is a developing area of personalized medicine since it integrates diagnosis and customized therapy delivered in one step using improvements in nanoscale [106].

This field of nanotechnology discusses light-triggered treatments (like photothermal, photodynamic, and photo immunotherapies), nanotechnological advancements with nanostent, nanopowder, nanogels, and NPs, improvements to endoscopic ultrasound, as well as experimental endoscopic techniques, combining both enhanced assessment and treatment therapies, including a developed prototype of a modern multifunctional endoscope for localized gastrointestinal cancer, near-infrared imaging, and other techniques [107]. In order to encompass these techniques, the term 'theranostics gastrointestinal endoscopy' has been suggested. Translational and clinical studies would be the main focus of future efforts to integrate these technologies into medical care, leading to more customized and cross-disciplinary treatment and diagnosis, shorter procedure instances, higher procedural accuracy, higher affordability, and fewer repetitive processes [108].

Nanotechnology and electronics breakthroughs have led to ground-breaking discoveries that will revolutionize the way diagnosis and treatment are currently provided. Medical capsule robots are a new invention that was inspired by the science fiction concept of robots travelling inside the body to detect and treat diseases. A capsule endoscope designed to take pictures of the digestive system was the first capsule robot that was commercially available. There are several different types of capsule endoscopes on the market today [109].

Currently, the absence of movement control is the main issue with all commercial capsule technologies. The doctor will be able to halt and steer the gadget towards places of interest in the future for close examination, diagnosis, and therapeutic delivery thanks to an interface application.

In the clinic, accurate and quantitative tumour marker identification is crucial for cancer diagnosis and subsequent treatment [110]. There has been development of a label-free, real-time, highly sensitive, and direct electrical readout nanobiosensor based on field-effect transistors for the detection of biomarkers [111].

5.12 Limitations of nanotechnology

The use of NPs in biological imaging has a number of attractive advantages. They are able to resist the process of reticuloendothelial ingestion and actively target particular sites for aggregation due to their small size and flexible surfaces [112]. Furthermore, nanomaterials' important parameter improves their durability along with safety while also boosting their capacity to carry pharmaceuticals and contrast agents. Today, a variety of nanoparticle types are available having useful characteristics which are employed in imaging techniques [113]. Iron oxide's magnetic tools modify it the perfect material for MRI. Gold NPs are frequently utilised in CT scan because of their peak imaging attenuation parameter and adaptable physical chemistry. Quantum dots are advantageous for fluorescence imaging due to their varied sizes, predominating imaging characteristics, and ability to produce optical luminescence at a range of wavelengths. Also being researched as prospective novel contenders in visual imaging equipment are up-conversion NPs, which have the ability to convert a number of photons with low energy into high-energy photons. Exosomes can be used with probes that are fluorescent to specifically identify cancers. Exosomes that have been produced with customized modifications enable the exact diagnosis of disorders by specific site delivery of a florescent substance [114]. The application of NP-based visualization methods in the future has a huge potential to identify GI illnesses. Due to this, the application of NP-based diagnostic techniques in the near future has huge potential for GI ailment identification [115]. Even if the impact of research work on the NPs utilized in current scenario scanning technologies is wonderful, they still fall short of being properly translated into imaging substances that may be employed in clinical settings.

When employing nanomaterials as contrast compounds for medical imaging, it is crucial to consider their *in vivo* toxicity [116]. Several animal and in laboratory experiments have proved that there are various degrees of hazard concern associated with NPs. Apoptosis, immunogenicity, and immunogenicity are only a few of the chemical, physical, and immune system processes that NPs may employ when they engage as foreign substances with biological systems to harm them. Nanotoxicity, which may result in issues including capillary blockage, coagulation leading to diminished function, and injury to key organs, can also be brought on by an excessive retention or insufficient elimination of nanomaterials in the body. It comes in addition to some NPs' intrinsic toxicity, such as the cadmium content in QDs. Similar to silica-coated QDs, changing the size, shape, and other characteristics of NPs might reduce the danger of toxicity; nevertheless, converting them into healthcare diagnostic uses is still a highly challenging problem. Therefore, if nanomaterials are not successfully eliminated by the body after parenteral administration, it will require a long time to achieve the impact dosage given after their chronic toxicological effects inside human body. Second, it is important to find out site-specific problems through NPs that are intended for the alimentary canal [117]. During parenteral administration, NPs run across a number of biological barriers in living that prevent them from reaching the area where the GI problem is present. Phagocytosis, which is brought on white blood cells phagocytosis of the liver and spleen, has an impact on non-specific NP dispersion over healthy tissues and non-specific adherence at the tissue sites [118].

The transport of NPs is also severely hampered by vascular rheology and intratumour hypertension. In comparison to injection, mouth administration has several advantages for the GI tract and is more well-liked by patients [119]. It is still challenging for NP-based products to be efficiently absorbed because of the complex nature of the GI tract, which is impacted through many such targets to the mucosal obstacle, many distinct enzymes, gut bacteria, and GI pH. Therefore, for scientists to effectively get around these physiological partitions to NP distribution, a reformation of modern NPs is needed, while expressing the factors like physical shape, dimensions, change in outer surface, along with other key characteristics. Due to this, the biological acceptability of nanomaterials and the byproducts of their breakdown in animals must also be considered in practical diagnostic applications. The fact that organic NPs frequently give better results than heavy complexes emphasises the necessity for modern techniques to favour tissue compatible NPs [120]. The site-specific properties of NPs also improve the results of scanning agents in finding their targets, minimizing undesirable adverse reactions brought on by non-specific build-up in the body. However, NPs or nanocarriers may be destroyed *in vivo* by phagocytosis and enzymatic degradation. As a result, inside intricate physicochemical target in the body, accurately sighting the designated area unless substantial deposition elsewhere achieves a useful impact [121]. It is critical to improve the affinities of compounds and cellular receptors, the long-term viability of NP–ligand relationships, and the negative consequences that might result from deposition of scanning media off-target. Restrictions, for example the dearth of particular requirements, higher manufacturing value, and applications of toxic solvents may potentially hinder the medical uses of NPs [122]. So it is very important to look into the utilization of abundant, safe, and useful renewable resources in the production of NPs. These challenges must be solved in order to fully achieve the enormous potential of NP-based imaging methods for the early detection of GI disorders [123].

The majority of scientific data in the field is presently being done using animal models, and less research work has employed nanomaterial-based scanning technologies in the clinical research area. So it is important to speed up the medical application of NPs. To discover this, we offer some intriguing areas for possible use of NPs in medical practices and GI illness scanning [124]. Firstly, a single imaging method typically cannot show all the specifics of a patient's sickness since patient conditions and disease traits differ. To get over this limitation, it is essential to develop adaptive multimodal imaging approaches based on NPs. By combining various imaging modalities, these techniques can provide substantial amounts of analytical accuracy as well as specificity. Future research should focus on creating NPs with multiple roles that not only make it possible to choose imaging settings that collectively enhance diagnostic performance, but also make it better and part of several scanning media. Site-specific molecular imaging is the second useful change made in recent scientific work [125].

The use of different complexes that target NPs, which can dramatically boost binding affinity and specificity, can help to efficiently accumulate agents for imaging at the region of interest. This allows accurately verifying the tissue, especially in the initial stage of carcinoma, without adverse effects to adjacent organs and tissues. Additionally, due to ability of NPs to image may be enhanced by employing specific triggers like acidity, metabolic enzyme mediators, and power as markers to reactivate them where they are needed [125]. More study into focused biological imaging is therefore necessary, with a focus on selecting the proper compounds for NPs and ensuring that they remain stable in animal studies. In such site-specific drug targets, the difficulties related to GI sites for NPs, a variety of stealth NP approaches have also been developed, such as the deployment of PEG customized NPs that successfully resist clean-up by WBC phagocytic mechanisms. One more method is the GI medication delivery system, which uses a pH dependent biological design to safely maintain the dissolution of drugs in the intestinal environment [126]. This approach similarly employs a new physical surface to penetrate the cell membrane and increase the medication deposition at the carcinoma location [127]. Additionally, hitchhiking nanotechnology that incorporates blood cells, macrophages, neutrophils, and microbes have given their requirement to pass across physiological obstacles and safely assemble at the affected tissue location. These NP techniques will be the main focus of future research to get over delivery limitations. Last but not least, it should go without emphasizing that endoscopy is crucial for GI ailment diagnosis. Utilizing the peculiar physicochemical properties of small particles, such as luminescence, enables the early detection of lesions and the observation of GI disorders [128]. Therefore, we need to do further in-depth research in the field of NP-based endoscopic optical imaging. Instead of being a magic bullet, NPs must be safely created and chosen to function along with certain scanning technologies to assure their optimum functions [129].

5.13 Conclusion

Nanotechnology encompasses all aspects of comprehending, working with, and designing things at the nanoscale. In terms of their physical and chemical characteristics (small measurement, high degree of reactivity, and significant surface area-to-volume ratio), NPs are different from bulk materials with the same composition. Nanotechnology has shown itself to be useful for initial assessment, the field of proteomics scanning examinations, and multifunctional drugs. Recent studies have shown its significance in the early detection and targeted therapy of a range of GI disorders, including cancer, a condition known as inflammatory bowel disease, stomach ulcers, and liver disease caused by the hepatitis B and C viruses. It looks promising to apply this technique for testing and interventional endoscopy, including enhanced capsule endoscopy, avoiding plastic stent obstruction, and endoscopic healing process of haemorrhage from peptic ulcers. The main obstacles, however, are the variety of NPs, the technological hurdles, and potential negative consequences. In conclusion, nanotechnology has become a technological instrument that allows us to keep up with the rapid growth of science and technology while maintaining the speed of innovation in diagnostics and therapies. We can only hope that this technology will help us realise some of our unfulfilled goals in the diagnostic and therapeutic areas of GI sciences.

References

[1] Nguyen V X, Nguyen V T L and Nguyen C C 2010 Appropriate use of endoscopy in the diagnosis and treatment of gastrointestinal diseases: up-to-date indications for primary care providers *Int. J. Gen. Med.* **3** 345

[2] Frøkjaer J B, Drewes A M, Gregersen H, Brøndum Frøkjaer J and Duvnjak M 2009 Imaging of the gastrointestinal tract-novel technologies *World J. Gastroenterol.* **15** 160–8

[3] Overview of upper gastrointestinal endoscopy (esophagogastroduodenoscopy)—UpToDate [Internet]. https://uptodate.com/contents/overview-of-upper-gastrointestinal-endoscopy-esophagogastroduodenoscopy (accessed 6 August 2023)

[4] Young P E and Womeldorph C M 2013 Colonoscopy for colorectal cancer screening *J. Cancer* **4** 217

[5] Qaseem A, Mustafa R A, Hicks L A, Wilt T J, Crandall C J, Fitterman N *et al* 2019 Screening for colorectal cancer in asymptomatic average-risk adults: a guidance statement from the American college of physicians HHS public access *Ann. Intern. Med.* **3002** 643–54

[6] Brenner A T, Dougherty M and Reuland D S 2017 Colorectal cancer screening in average risk patients *Med. Clin. North Am.* **101** 755–67

[7] Alghamdi M A, Fallica A N, Virzì N, Kesharwani P, Pittalà V and Greish K 2022 The promise of nanotechnology in personalized medicine *J. Pers. Med.* **12** 673

[8] Ozak S T and Ozkan P 2013 Nanotechnology and dentistry *Eur. J. Dent.* **7** 145–51

[9] Smolsky J, Kaur S, Hayashi C, Batra S K and Krasnoslobodtsev A V 2017 Surface-enhanced raman scattering-based immunoassay technologies for detection of disease biomarkers *Biosensors* **7** 7

[10] Fang M, Peng C-W, Pang D-W and Li Y 2012 Quantum dots for cancer research: current status, remaining issues, and future perspectives *Cancer Biol. Med.* **9** 151–63

[11] Gil H M, Price T W, Chelani K, Bouillard J S G, Calaminus S D J and Stasiuk G J 2021 NIR-quantum dots in biomedical imaging and their future *iScience* **24** 102189

[12] Choi H K and Yoon J 2023 Nanotechnology-assisted biosensors for the detection of viral nucleic acids: an overview *Biosensors* **13** 208

[13] Ravanshad R, Zadeh A K, Amani A M, Mousavi M, Hashemi A, Dashtaki A S *et al* 2017 Application of nanoparticles in cancer detection by Raman scattering based techniques *Nano Rev. Experiments* **9** 1373551

[14] Nsairat H, Khater D, Sayed U, Odeh F, Al Bawab A and Alshaer W 2022 Liposomes: structure, composition, types, and clinical applications *Heliyon* **8** e09394

[15] Tenchov R, Bird R, Curtze A E and Zhou Q 2021 Lipid nanoparticles from liposomes to mrna vaccine delivery, a landscape of research diversity and advancement *ACS Nano* **15** 16982–7015

[16] Wang Q, Atluri K, Tiwari A K and Babu R J 2023 Exploring the application of micellar drug delivery systems in cancer nanomedicine *Pharmaceuticals* **16** 433

[17] Schulte P A and Salamanca-Buentello F 2007 Ethical and scientific issues of nanotechnology in the workplace *Environ. Health Perspect.* **115** 5

[18] Allhoff F and Henschke A 2018 The internet of things: foundational ethical issues *Internet of Things* **1–2** 55–66

[19] Kocna P, Vanickova Z and Zima T 2013 Laboratory screening markers in gastroenterology--state of the art *Biomed. Pap. Med. Fac. Univ. Palacky Olomouc Czech Repub.* **157** 91–7

[20] Bayda S, Adeel M, Tuccinardi T, Cordani M, Rizzolio F and Baeza A 2020 Molecules the history of nanoscience and nanotechnology: from chemical–physical applications to nanomedicine *Molecules* **25** 112

[21] Rambaran T and Schirhagl R 2022 Nanotechnology from lab to industry—a look at current trends *Nanoscale Adv.* **4** 3664–75

[22] Sahoo M, Vishwakarma S, Panigrahi C and Kumar J 2021 Nanotechnology: current applications and future scope in food *Food Front.* **2** 3–22

[23] Monika P, Chandraprabha M N, Rangarajan A, Waiker P V and Chidambara Murthy K N 2021 Challenges in healing wound: role of complementary and alternative medicine *Front. Nutr.* **8** 791899

[24] Laurano R, Boffito M, Ciardelli G and Chiono V 2022 Wound dressing products: a translational investigation from the bench to the market *Eng. Regen.* **3** 182–200

[25] Ma W, Zhan Y, Zhang Y, Mao C, Xie X and Lin Y 2021 The biological applications of DNA nanomaterials: current challenges and future directions *Signal Transduct. Target. Ther.* **6** 1–28

[26] Cardoza C, Nagtode V, Pratap A and Mali S N 2022 Emerging applications of nanotechnology in cosmeceutical health science: latest updates *Heal. Sci. Rev.* **4** 100051

[27] Gwinn M R and Vallyathan V 2006 Nanoparticles: health effects—pros and cons *Environ. Health Perspect.* **114** 1818

[28] Yildirimer L, Thanh N T K, Loizidou M and Seifalian A M 2011 Toxicology and clinical potential of nanoparticles *Nano Today* **6** 585–607

[29] Bahrulolum H, Nooraei S, Javanshir N, Tarrahimofrad H, Mirbagheri V S, Easton A J *et al* 2021 Green synthesis of metal nanoparticles using microorganisms and their application in the agrifood sector *J. Nanobiotechnol.* **19** 86

[30] Habeeb Rahuman H B, Dhandapani R, Narayanan S, Palanivel V, Paramasivam R, Subbarayalu R *et al* 2022 Medicinal plants mediated the green synthesis of silver nanoparticles and their biomedical applications *IET Nanobiotechnol.* **16** 115

[31] Begines B, Ortiz T, Pérez-Aranda M, Martínez G, Merinero M, Argüelles-Arias F *et al* 2020 Polymeric nanoparticles for drug delivery: recent developments and future prospects *Nanomaterials* **10** 1–41

[32] Nguyen T T, Mammeri F and Ammar S 2018 Iron oxide and gold based magneto-plasmonic nanostructures for medical applications: a review *Nanomaterials* **8** 149

[33] Missaoui W N, Arnold R D and Cummings B S 2018 Toxicological status of nanoparticles: what we know and what we don't know *Chem. Biol. Interact.* **295** 1

[34] Krishnan P D, Banas D, Durai R D, Kabanov D, Hosnedlova B, Kepinska M *et al* 2020 Silver nanomaterials for wound dressing applications *Pharmaceutics* **12** 1–27

[35] Sieber S, Grossen P, Detampel P, Siegfried S, Witzigmann D and Huwyler J 2017 Zebrafish as an early stage screening tool to study the systemic circulation of nanoparticulate drug delivery systems in vivo *J. Control Rel.* **264** 180–91

[36] Maiti D, Tong X, Mou X and Yang K 2018 Carbon-based nanomaterials for biomedical applications: a recent study *Front. Pharmacol.* **9** 1401

[37] Monteiro N, Martins A, Reis R L and Neves N M 2014 Liposomes in tissue engineering and regenerative medicine *J. R. Soc. Interface* **11** 20140459

[38] Jain S, Jain V and Mahajan S C 2014 Lipid based vesicular drug delivery systems *Adv. Pharm* **2014** 1–12

[39] Silva A C, Moreira J N, Manuel J, Lobo S, Subhan A, Filipczak N *et al* 2023 Advances with lipid-based nanosystems for siRNA delivery to breast cancers *Pharm 2023* **16** 970

[40] Attama A A, Agbo C P, Onokala O B, Kenechukwu F C, Ugwueze M E, Mbah C C *et al* 2023 Applications of nanoemulsions as drug delivery vehicle for phytoconstituents *Nanotechnology in Herbal Medicine* (Elsevier) pp 119–94

[41] Yu B, Tai H C, Xue W, Lee L J and Lee R J 2010 Receptor-targeted nanocarriers for therapeutic delivery to cancer *Mol. Membr. Biol.* **27** 286

[42] Yao Y, Zhou Y, Liu L, Xu Y, Chen Q, Wang Y *et al* 2020 Nanoparticle-based drug delivery in cancer therapy and its role in overcoming drug resistance *Front. Mol. Biosci.* **7** 558493

[43] Luo M, Lee L K C, Peng B, Choi C H J, Tong W Y and Voelcker N H 2022 Delivering the promise of gene therapy with nanomedicines in treating central nervous system diseases *Adv. Sci.* **9** 2201740

[44] Sharifi S, Behzadi S, Laurent S, Forrest M L, Stroeve P and Mahmoudi M 2012 Toxicity of nanomaterials *Chem. Soc. Rev.* **41** 2323

[45] Khan I, Saeed K and Khan I 2019 Nanoparticles: properties, applications and toxicities *Arab J. Chem.* **12** 908–31

[46] Sukhanova A, Bozrova S, Sokolov P, Berestovoy M, Karaulov A and Nabiev I 2018 Dependence of nanoparticle toxicity on their physical and chemical properties *Nanoscale Res. Lett.* **13** 1–21

[47] Park H J and Moon D E 2010 Pharmacologic management of chronic pain *Korean J. Pain* **23** 99

[48] Jain A K and Thareja S 2019 *In vitro* and *in vivo* characterization of pharmaceutical nanocarriers used for drug delivery *Artific. Cells Nanomed. Biotechnol.* **47** 524–39

[49] Roobol S J, Hartjes T A, Slotman J A, De Kruijff R M, Torrelo G, Abraham T E *et al* 2020 Uptake and subcellular distribution of radiolabeled polymersomes for radiotherapy *Nanotheranostics* **2020** 14–25

[50] Mandal S, Zhou Y, Shibata A and Destache C J 2015 View online—export citation crossmark confocal fluorescence microscopy: an ultra-sensitive tool used to evaluate intracellular antiretroviral nano-drug delivery in HeLa cells confocal fluorescence micro-scopy: an ultra-sensitive tool used to evaluate intracellular antiretroviral nano-drug delivery in HeLa cells *AIP Adv.* **5** 84803

[51] Lambert R 2012 Endoscopy in screening for digestive cancer *World J. Gastrointest. Endosc.* **4** 518

[52] Ro T H, Mathew M A and Misra S 2015 Value of screening endoscopy in evaluation of esophageal, gastric and colon cancers *World J. Gastroenterol.* **21** 9693

[53] Mcguigan A, Kelly P, Turkington R C, Jones C, Coleman H G and Mccain S Pancreatic cancer: a review of clinical diagnosis, epidemiology, treatment and outcomes

[54] Kher C and Kumar S 2022 The application of nanotechnology and nanomaterials in cancer diagnosis and treatment: a review *Cureus* **14** e29059

[55] Haleem A, Javaid M, Singh R P, Rab S and Suman R 2023 Applications of nano-technology in medical field: a brief review *Glob. Heal. J.* **7** 70–7

[56] Rizvi S A A and Saleh A M 2018 Applications of nanoparticle systems in drug delivery technology *Saudi Pharmaceut. J.* **26** 64–70

[57] Ding Y-N, Xue M, Tang Q-S, Wang L-J, Ding H-Y, Li H *et al* 2022 Immunotherapy-based novel nanoparticles in the treatment of gastrointestinal cancer: trends and challenges *World J Gastroenterol.* **28** 5403–19

[58] Malone J C and Thavamani A 2023 *Physiology, Gastrocolic Reflex* (StatPearls)

[59] Gullo I, Grillo F, Mastracci L, Vanoli A, Carneiro F, Saragoni L *et al* 2020 Precancerous lesions of the stomach, gastric cancer and hereditary gastric cancer syndromes *Pathologica* **112** 166–85

[60] Dessale M, Mengistu G and Mengist H M 2022 Nanotechnology: a promising approach for cancer diagnosis, therapeutics and theragnosis

[61] Hosseini S M, Mohammadnejad J, Salamat S, Beiram Zadeh Z, Tanhaei M and Ramakrishna S 2023 Theranostic polymeric nanoparticles as a new approach in cancer therapy and diagnosis: a review

[62] Cheng Z, Li M, Dey R and Chen Y 2020 Proteolysis-targeting chimera (PROTAC) for targeted protein degradation and cancer therapy *J. Hematol. Oncol.* **14** 85

[63] Cheng Z, Li M, Dey R and Chen Y 2021 Nanomaterials for cancer therapy: current progress and perspectives *J. Hematol. Oncol.* **14** 1–27

[64] Nabil G, Bhise K, Sau S, Atef M, El-Banna H A and Iyer A K 2019 Nano-engineered delivery systems for cancer imaging and therapy: recent advances, future direction and patent evaluation *Drug Discov. Today* **24** 462

[65] Udenni Gunathilake T M S, Ching Y C, Ching K Y, Chuah C H and Abdullah L C 2017 Biomedical and microbiological applications of bio-based porous materials: a review *Polymers (Basel)* **9** 160

[66] Wang L, Hu C and Shao L 2017 The antimicrobial activity of nanoparticles: present situation and prospects for the future *Int. J. Nanomed.* 12–1227

[67] Bera D, Qian L, Tseng T K and Holloway P H 2010 Quantum dots and their multimodal applications: a review *Materials* **3** 2260–345

[68] Singh A, Prasad L B, Shiv K, Kumar R and Garai S 2023 Synthesis, characterization, and *in vitro* antibacterial and cytotoxic study of Co(II), Ni(II), Cu(II), and Zn(II) complexes of N-(4-methoxybenzyl) N-(phenylethyl) dithiocarbamate ligand *J. Mol. Struct.* **1288** 135835

[69] Kumar A, Kumar B, Kumar R, Kumar A, Singh M, Tiwari V *et al* 2022 Acute and subacute toxicity study of ethanolic extract of *Calotropis procera* (Aiton) dryand flower in *Swiss albino* mice *Phytomed. Plus* **2** 100224

[70] Wang J, Sui L, Huang J, Miao L, Nie Y, Wang K *et al* 2021 MoS2-based nanocomposites for cancer diagnosis and therapy *Bioact. Mater.* **6** 4209–42

[71] Naso M F, Tomkowicz B, Perry W L and Strohl W R 2017 Adeno-Associated Virus (AAV) as a vector for gene therapy *Biodrugs* **31** 317

[72] Lee C S, Bishop E S, Zhang R, Yu X, Farina E M, Yan S *et al* 2017 Adenovirus-mediated gene delivery: potential applications for gene and cell-based therapies in the new era of personalized medicine *Genes Diseas.* **4** 43–63

[73] Thomas T J, Tajmir-Riahi H-A and Pillai C K S 2019 Biodegradable polymers for gene delivery *Molecules* **24** 3744

[74] Seyedian S S, Nokhostin F and Dargahi Malamir M 2009 A review of the diagnosis, prevention, and treatment methods of inflammatory bowel disease *J. Med. Life* **12** 113–22

[75] Stezzi T J and Peart W 2009 Product profiler: simponi (golimumab) *MAbs* **5** 422–31

[76] Thakur A and Foged C 2020 Nanoparticles for mucosal vaccine delivery *Nanoeng. Biomater. Adv. Drug Deliv.* **2020** 603–46

[77] Papenfort K and Bassler B 2016 Quorum-sensing signal-response systems in gram-negative bacteria *Nat. Rev.* **14** 576–88

[78] Cojocaru M, Inimioara, Cojocaru M, Silosi I and Doina Vrabie C 2011 Gastrointestinal manifestations in systemic autoimmune diseases *Maedica A J. Clin. Med.* **6** 45–51

[79] Cederbaum A I 2001 Introduction—serial review: alcohol, oxidative stress and cell injury *Free Radic. Biol. Med.* **31** 1524–6

[80] Patra J K, Das G, Fraceto L F, Campos E V R, Rodriguez-Torres M D P, Acosta-Torres L S *et al* 2018 Nano based drug delivery systems: recent developments and future prospects *J. Nanobiotechnol.* **16** 1–33

[81] Din F U, Aman W, Ullah I, Qureshi O S, Mustapha O, Shafique S *et al* 2017 Effective use of nanocarriers as drug delivery systems for the treatment of selected tumors *Int. J. Nanomed.* **12** 7291–309

[82] Riley R S, June C H, Langer R and Mitchell M J 2019 Delivery technologies for cancer immunotherapy HHS public access *Nat. Rev. Drug Discov.* **18** 175–96

[83] Cells E, Brzuszkiewicz E, Gottschalk G, Buchrieser C, Dobrindt U and Oswald E 2006 The mucus and mucins of the goblet cells and enterocytes provide the first defense line of the gastrointestinal tract and interact with the immune system *Immunol. Rev.* **260** 87–107

[84] Johansson M E V, Sjövall H and Hansson G C 2013 The gastrointestinal mucus system in health and disease *Nat. Rev. Gastroenterol. Hepatol.* **10** 352

[85] Baracat F, Moura E, Bernardo W, Pu L Z, Mendonça E, Moura D *et al* 2016 Endoscopic hemostasis for peptic ulcer bleeding: systematic review and meta-analyses of randomized controlled trials *Surg. Endosc.* **30** 2155–68

[86] Ibrahim M, El-Mikkawy A, Hamid M A, Abdalla H, Mostafa I and Devière J 2019 Early application of haemostatic powder added to standard management for oesophagogastric variceal bleeding: a randomised trial *Gut* **68** 844–53

[87] Mangiavillano B, Pagano N, Baron T H and Luigiano C 2015 Outcome of stenting in biliary and pancreatic benign and malignant diseases: a comprehensive review *World J. Gastroenterol.* **21** 9038

[88] Bokov D, Jalil A T, Chupradit S, Suksatan W, Ansari M J, Shewael I H *et al* 2021 Nanomaterial by sol-gel method: synthesis and application *Adv. Mater. Sci. Eng.* **2021** 5102014

[89] Seitz U, Block A, Schaefer A-C, Wienhold U, Bohnacker S, Siebert K *et al* 2007 Clinical-liver, pancreas, and biliary tract biliary stent clogging solved by nanotechnology? *In vitro* study of inorganic-organic sol-gel coatings for teflon stents *Gastroenterology* **133** 65–71

[90] Kopylov U and Seidman E G 2014 Role of capsule endoscopy in inflammatory bowel disease *World J. Gastroenterol.* **20** 1155–64

[91] McAlindon M E, Ching H L, Yung D, Sidhu R and Koulaouzidis A 2016 Capsule endoscopy of the small bowel *Ann. Transl. Med.* **4** 369

[92] Vasilakakis M D, Koulaouzidis A, Marlicz W and Iakovidis D K 2020 The future of capsule endoscopy in clinical practice: from diagnostic to therapeutic experimental prototype capsules *Prz. Gastroenterol.* **15** 179–93

[93] Bahadar H, Maqbool F, Niaz K and Abdollahi M 2016 Toxicity of nanoparticles and an overview of current experimental models *Iran Biomed. J.* **20** 1–11

[94] De Jong W H and Borm P J 2008 Drug delivery and nanoparticles: applications and hazards *Int. J. Nanomed.* **3** 133–49

[95] NazariP M, Reza TalebiP A, Hosseini SharifabadP M, AbbasiP A, KhoradmehrP A, Hossein DanafarP A *et al* 2016 Acute and chronic effects of gold nanoparticles on sperm parameters and chromatin structure in mice *Int. J. Reprod. BioMed.* **14** 637–42

[96] Gupta R and Xie H 2018 Nanoparticles in daily life: applications, toxicity and regulations *J. Environ. Pathol. Oncol.* **37** 209–30

[97] Vitulo M, Gnodi E, Meneveri R and Barisani D 2022 Interactions between nanoparticles and intestine *Int. J. Mol. Sci.* **23** 4339

[98] Marchettini P, Lacerenza M, Mauri E and Marangoni C 2006 Painful peripheral neuropathies *Curr. Neuropharmacol.* **4** 175

[99] Ricciotti E and Fitzgerald G A 2011 Prostaglandins and inflammation *Arterioscler. Thromb. Vasc. Biol.* **31** 986

[100] Song Y-q, Mao X-l, Zhou X-b, He S-q *et al* 2021 Use of artificial intelligence to improve the quality control of gastrointestinal endoscopy *Front. Med.* **1** 709347

[101] Parasher G, Wong M and Rawat M 2020 Evolving role of artificial intelligence in gastrointestinal endoscopy conflict-of-interest statement: specialty type: gastroenterology and hepatology *World J. Gastroenterol.* **26** 7287–98

[102] Sharma N, Sharma R and Jindal N 2021 Machine learning and deep learning applications—a vision *Glob. Transitions. Proc.* **2** 24–8

[103] Alzubaidi L, Zhang J, Humaidi A J, Al-Dujaili A, Duan Y, Al-Shamma O *et al* 2021 Review of deep learning: concepts, CNN architectures, challenges, applications, future directions *J. Big Data* **8** 53

[104] Rey J-F 2023 Artificial intelligence in digestive endoscopy: recent advances *Curr. Opin. Gastroenterol.* **39** 397–402

[105] Hajjar A El and Rey J F 2020 Artificial intelligence in gastrointestinal endoscopy: general overview *Chin. Med. J. (Engl.)* **133** 326

[106] Li Y, Li X, Zhou F, Doughty A, Hoover A R, Nordquist R E *et al* 2019 Nanotechnology-based photoimmunological therapies for cancer *Cancer Lett.* **442** 429

[107] Singeap A M, Stanciu C and Trifan A 2016 Capsule endoscopy: the road ahead *World J. Gastroenterol.* **22** 369

[108] Vélez-Guerrero M A, Callejas-Cuervo M and Mazzoleni S 2021 Design, development, and testing of an intelligent wearable robotic exoskeleton prototype for upper limb rehabilitation *Sensors* **21** 5411

[109] Malik S, Muhammad K and Waheed Y 2023 Nanotechnology: a revolution in modern industry *Molecules* **28** 661

[110] Crew B 2022 The nanoscience revolution *Nature* **608** S1–1

[111] Poghossian A and Schöning M J 2021 Recent progress in silicon-based biologically sensitive field-effect devices *Curr. Opin. Electrochem.* **29** 100811

[112] Zhao X, Huang G, Wu L, Wang M, He X, Wang J R *et al* 2022 Deep learning assessment of left ventricular hypertrophy based on electrocardiogram *Front. Cardiovasc. Med.* **9** 952089

[113] Ather S, Kadir T and Gleeson F 2020 Artificial intelligence and radiomics in pulmonary nodule management: current status and future applications *Clin. Radiol.* **75** 13–9

[114] Patel U K, Anwar A, Saleem S, Malik P, Rasul B, Patel K *et al* 2021 Artificial intelligence as an emerging technology in the current care of neurological disorders *J. Neurol.* **268** 1623–42

[115] Belić M, Bobić V, Badža M, Šolaja N, urić-Jovičić M and Kostić V S 2019 Artificial intelligence for assisting diagnostics and assessment of Parkinson's disease—a review *Clin. Neurol. Neurosurg* **184** 105442

[116] Stidham R W and Takenaka K 2022 Artificial intelligence for disease assessment in inflammatory bowel disease: how will it change our practice? *Gastroenterology* **162** 1493–506

[117] Pei Q, Luo Y, Chen Y, Li J, Xie D and Ye T 2022 Artificial intelligence in clinical applications for lung cancer: diagnosis, treatment and prognosis *Clin. Chem. Lab. Med.* **60** 1974–83

[118] Wells A, Patel S, Lee J B and Motaparthi K 2021 Artificial intelligence in dermatopathology: diagnosis, education, and research *J. Cutan. Pathol* **48** 1061–8

[119] Mirbabaie M, Stieglitz S and Frick N R J 2021 Artificial intelligence in disease diagnostics: a critical review and classification on the current state of research guiding future direction *Health Technol.* **11** 693–731

[120] Kumar Y, Koul A, Singla R and Ijaz M F 2023 Artificial intelligence in disease diagnosis: a systematic literature review, synthesizing framework and future research agenda *J. Ambient. Intell. Humaniz Comput.* **14** 8459–86

[121] Schmidt-Erfurth U, Sadeghipour A, Gerendas B S, Waldstein S M and Bogunović H 2018 Artificial intelligence in retina *Prog. Retin. Eye Res.* **67** 1–29

[122] Nagarajan V D, Lee S L, Robertus J L, Nienaber C A, Trayanova N A and Ernst S 2021 Artificial intelligence in the diagnosis and management of arrhythmias *Eur. Heart J.* **42** 3904–16

[123] Kaplan A, Cao H, FitzGerald J M, Iannotti N, Yang E, Kocks J W H *et al* 2021 Artificial intelligence/machine learning in respiratory medicine and potential role in asthma and COPD diagnosis *J. Allergy Clin. Immunol. Pract.* **9** 2255–61

[124] Huang X, Wang H, She C, Feng J, Liu X, Hu X *et al* 2022 Artificial intelligence promotes the diagnosis and screening of diabetic retinopathy *Front. Endocrinol. (Lausanne)* **13** 1–12

[125] Kamdar J H, Jeba Praba J and Georrge J J 2020 Artificial intelligence in medical diagnosis: methods, algorithms and applications *Machine Learning with Health Care Perspective. Learning and Analytics in Intelligent Systems* vol 13 (Springer) pp 27–37

[126] Lim C T 2020 Future of health diagnostics *View* **1** 2–4

[127] Misawa M, Kudo S-Ei, Mori Y, Maeda Y, Ogawa Y, Ichimasa K *et al* 2021 Current status and future perspective on artificial intelligence for lower endoscopy *Dig. Endosc* **33** 273–84

[128] Alsharif W and Qurashi A 2021 Effectiveness of COVID-19 diagnosis and management tools: a review *Radiography* **27** 682–7

[129] Balyen L and Peto T 2019 Promising artificial intelligence–machine learning–deep learning algorithms in ophthalmology *Asia-Pac. J. Ophthalmol.* **8** 264–72

IOP Publishing

Nanobiotechnology and Artificial Intelligence in Gastrointestinal Diseases

Vivek K Chaturvedi, Anurag Kumar Singh, Jay Singh and Dawesh P Yadav

Chapter 6

Nano-biotechnology in gastrointestinal cancer

Mohammad Zafaryab, Mazharul Haque and Komal Vig

Gastrointestinal malignancies cause 35% of all cancer related fatalities as well as 26% of the world cancer incidence. Gastrointestinal cancer, which includes tumors of the stomach, esophagus, liver, biliary system, pancreas, and colon, is one of the most common cancers and the largest cause of cancer-related death worldwide. Gastrointestinal related cancer has the same weightage in term of diagnosis and therapeutics as well. Developments in nanotechnology have explored new frontiers in the diagnosis and treatment of cancer. Nanobiotechnology is an emerging field that utilizes the optimized nanoscale system to overcome issues related to diagnostics and therapeutics of cancer. As far as diagnosis of gastroinstestinal cancer is concerned, routine systematic imaging such as magnetic resonance imaging, computed tomography (CT) and positron emission tomography, local imaging that covers endoscopy and ultrasound has wide application. Conventional use of contrast agents in this imaging system has low specificity, quick maintenance time period, but also severe side effects. Currently, the advancements in the field of nanotechnology, contributing nanoparticles like quantum dots, gold nanoparticles and iron oxide nanoparticles, have presented many aids in gastroinstinal cancer imaging as bearing nano size, manipulative surface properties and having good retention time in the body. There is ongoing research to combine the existing traditional diagnostic method with nanoparticles, significantly improving the imaging of the digestive tract for early diagnosis and prediction accuracy of cancer stages. Traditional drugs have a large number of side effects due to their low specificity and non-targeted delivery. However, there is extensive study demonstrating that nano-sized drugs were found effective against gastrointestinal cancer as its optimized nano system in order to improve specificity, targeted delivery and reduce toxicity as well. Here, we discuss the most recent research on the application of nanoparticles for the detection and treatment of gastrointestinal cancer.

6.1 Introduction

The study of materials and systems with the lowest feasible functional organization on a nanoscale is the focus of the science and engineering discipline known as nanotechnology. Nanotechnology now offers a new treatment possibility for several compounds that cannot be used effectively in conventional formulations because of their poor functionality. Agents vulnerable to degradation are protected by nano-particle formulations, also help to prevent denaturation in harsh pH and extend the drug exposure time by improving formulation retention time through bio-adhesion [1]. Engineers have spent more than thirty years attempting to make manufactured structures smaller in order to enable quicker and denser electronic circuits, which have reached feature sizes as small as 20 nm. In addition, for many years, molecular biologists have worked in the field of molecular and cellular biology to study dimensions ranging from nanometers to micrometers [2]. Nanobiotechnology is combining engineering and molecular biology to build a new class of multifunc-tional devices and systems for biological and chemical testing with improved sensitivity, specificity, and recognition rates. The numerous significant analytical uses of nano-objects include nanotubes, nanochannels, nanoparticles, nanoporous materials, nanocapacitors, and nanofibers [3]. Analyzing signaling pathways using nanobiotechnology approaches may offer fresh perspectives on how diseases develop, helping to find more accurate biomarkers and comprehend therapeutic action mechanisms. It is anticipated that these fields can effectively work together to produce a new class of multifunctional tools and systems for biological and chemical analysis that are more sensitive, specific, and able to achieve greater identification rates than those currently in use [4]. Nanomaterials have the ability to be manipulated easily in different forms that can allow for binding to a diverse range of biomolecules, including bacteria, poisons, proteins, and nucleic acid [5]. Nanotechnology has produced a number of promising outcomes in the management of treatments such as drug delivery, gene therapy, monitoring, diagnostics, medi-cation carrying, biomarker tracing, histopathological imaging and medications. Quantum dots)/gold nanoparticles are frequently used in molecular level detection of cancer. Molecular diagnostic techniques based on these nanoparticles, especially biomarker identification, can quickly and effectively diagnose tumors. Drug delivery at the nanoscale is one example of a therapeutic based on nanotechnology that will ensure that malignant tissues are appropriately targeted while reducing potential dangers. Nanomaterials' biological characteristics allow them to easily overcome cell barriers. As a result of their active and passive targeting, nanomaterials have long been used in the treatment of cancer [6].

6.2 Global burden of gastric cancer

According to the most recent predictions made public by GLOBOCAN, the yearly incidence of gastric cancer reached 1 089 000 cases worldwide in 2020 and incident rate 11.1 per hundred thousand as equating to an age, placing it fifth among all malignant tumors. Including lung, colorectal, and liver cancers, gastric cancer had

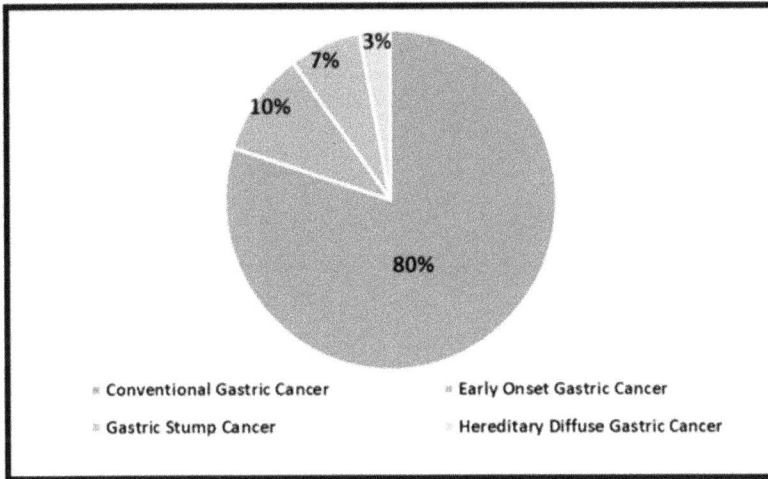

Figure 6.1. Onsets of gastric cancer development.

769 000 fatalities in the same year, ranking it fourth overall with a 7.7 per hundred thousand age-standardized mortality rate. Despite a general drop in incidence rates around the world, regional variations continue to exist in gastric cancer incidence and fatality rates. The number of new cases is anticipated to increase globally by 62% to 1.77 million by 2040, according to research published in 2022. High or very high HDI countries have greater rates of gastric cancer incidence but also lower rates of gastric cancer-related death in comparison to countries with medium or low HDI, where gastric related cancer is one of the leading causes of cancer-related mortality [7] (figure 6.1).

6.3 Gastric cancer risk factors

The main risk factors for gastric cancer development are shown in figure 6.2.

6.3.1 Infection with *Helicobacter pylori*

Based on epidemiological data, *Helicobacter pylori* was identified by the International Agency for Research on Cancer (IARC) in 1994 as a group 1 agent (carcinogen) for non-cardia stomach cancer [8]. Intestinal and non-cardia stomach cancers are primarily caused by chronic *H. pylori* infection. *H. pylori* infection is the root cause of most (90%) of all gastric cancers worldwide, with a reported sensitivity of 95.6% and specificity (92.6%), according to immunoblot-based studies [9, 10]. Most people who get infected with *H. pylori* do so as a child, and if the illness is not treated, it can last a lifetime. China and South Korea have the highest prevalence of *H. pylori* infection globally, with rates of roughly 55% and 60%, respectively, in Central and South America and Asia. Eastern Europe has the lowest incidence (50%) overall [11].

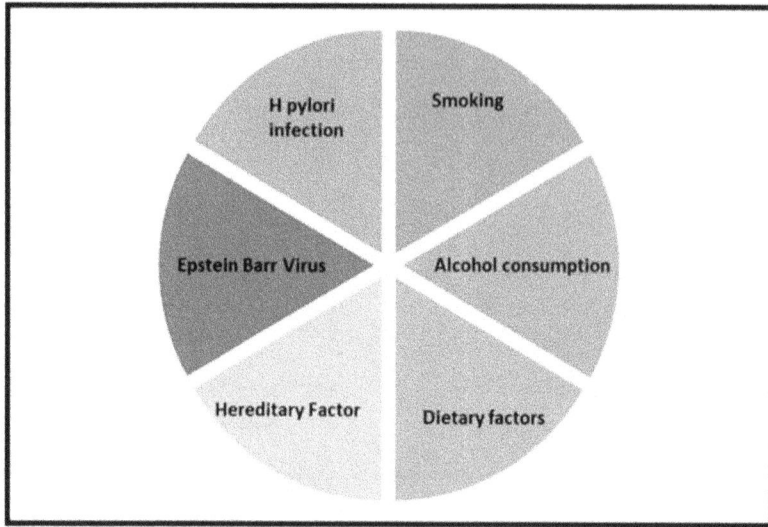

Figure 6.2. Main risk factors for gastric cancer development.

6.3.2 Age and sex

The risk of stomach cancer rises with age, just like that of other cancers. Additionally, compared to women, men have a two- to three-fold higher risk of developing stomach cancer [12]. With incidence rates of 15.8 per million for women and 7.0 per hundred thousand for men, respectively, stomach cancer was the fourth most frequent disease worldwide in 2020 [12].

6.3.3 Cigarette smoking

There is adequate evidence to infer that smoking promotes gastric cancer, according to a 2002 IARC assessment [13]. According to a meta-analysis of information from 32 research (27 group and 5 embedded case–control) published up through 2007, current smokers were more likely than non-smokers to develop both cardia and non-cardia kinds of gastric cancer [13].

Additionally, current smokers had a larger risk than former smokers (OR relative to never smokers 1.12, 95% CI 0.99–1.27), who had a reduced risk (OR relative to non-smokers 1.25, 95% CI 1.11–1.40). This risk rises in direct proportion to both the number of cigarettes smoked daily (OR 1.32 for >20 cigarettes/day) and the length of time a person has smoked continuously (OR 1.33 for >40 years of use) [14].

6.3.4 Obesity and metabolic dysfunction

Studies looking at the connection between gaining weight and the risk of stomach cancer have produced mixed results. A meta-analysis of 24 prospective research papers published till 2012 found no association between having a BMI of 25–30 kg m^{-2} or higher with developing stomach cancer [15].

6.3.5 Dietary factors

There are still issues with the planning and execution of nutritional epidemiology research, which is likely the cause of the conflicting published data on food and the risk of gastric cancer. For instance, a 2017 meta-analysis based on 24 case–control studies indicated that eating more red meat increased the risk of gastric cancer (RR 1.67, 95% CI 1.36–2.05) [16]. In a meta-analysis of data from 9 case–control studies, white meat consumption was associated with a lower risk of gastric cancer (RR 0.75, 95% CI 0.61–0.93), but not in a meta-analysis of data from five cohort studies (RR 0.85, 95% CI 0.63–1.16) [17]. However, research linking processed beef to a higher risk of stomach cancer offers more convincing evidence. Case–control studies (RR 2.17, 95% CI 1.51–3.11; 12 studies) and cohort studies (RR 1.21, 95% CI 1.04–1.41; 7 studies) have both found this connection [17].

6.3.6 Alcohol use

Both preclinical and clinical studies have linked drinking alcohol to an increased risk of gastric cancer because it increases the production of reactive oxygen species (ROS), which help to activate carcinogens, and because it promotes folate deficiencies, which alter DNA methylation and result in gastric cancer [18]. A meta-analysis of data from 81 epidemiological studies (68 case–control and 13 cohort studies) found that people who drink alcohol at any level had a higher chance of developing stomach cancer than people who don't (OR 1.20, 95% CI 1.12–1.27) [19].

6.3.7 Medications

Aspirin and other nonsteroidal anti-inflammatory medicines (NSAIDs) have been proposed to lower the risk of gastric cancer by inhibiting the activity of cyclo-oxygenase 2, which is overexpressed during gastric carcinogenesis [20]. According to another meta-analysis, those who use any NSAID had a decreased chance of having gastric cancer compared to people who don't (observational studies: RR 0.78, 95% CI 0.72–0.85; 24) [21].

6.3.8 Host genetics

Despite the fact that most cases of gastric cancer are random, they occasionally run in families and are linked to particular mutational patterns. Families with a history of the condition have a higher risk of developing stomach cancer (OR 2–10 depending on location) [9]. Strong links exist between the following three heritable disorders and stomach cancer: diffuse gastric cancer that is inherited (CDH1 or CTNNA1 mutations); gastric adenocarcinoma, proximal gastric poly-posis, and familial intestine gastric cancer are all linked to mutations in the APC104 promoter 1B region [22]. Gastric cancer is more likely to arise as part of a familial cancer syndrome such as Lynch syndrome in people who have MLH1 or MSH2 germline mutations [23], familial adenomatous polyposis, Peutz-Jeghers syndrome, or Li–Fraumeni syndrome [24].

6.4 Other risk factors

Around the world, 10% of gastric cancers are caused by other risk factors. The primary risk factor is highlighted in the following (figure 6.3).

6.4.1 Epstein–Barr virus infection

Approximately 8% of the 5081 gastric cancer patients in a global pooled study of 15 cross-sectional studies harbored Epstein–Barr virus (EBV) in tumor tissue. However, there is currently insufficient epidemiological evidence to conclusively link EBV infections to the development of gastric cancer [25].

6.4.2 Autoimmune disorders

As a result of autoimmune gastritis, which also goes by the names intestinal metaplasia and spasmolytic polypeptide-expression metaplasia, the parietal and principal cells of the gastric mucosa are altered by cells that resemble intestinal cells that secrete mucus [26]. The oxyntic mucosa in the stomach body fully atrophies as a result of these processes, making it more likely that gastric cancer would occur [27].

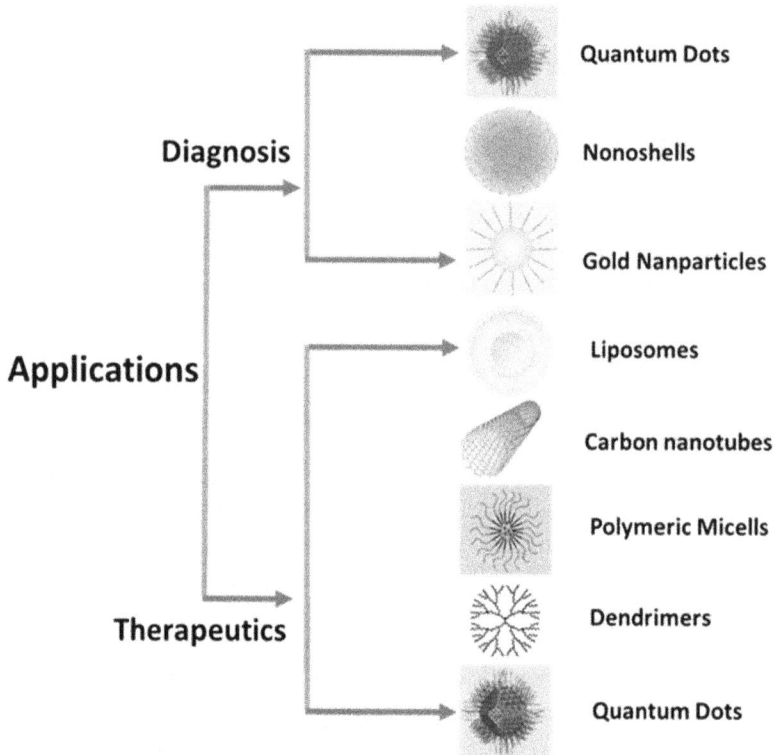

Figure 6.3. Applications of nanomaterial in cancer diagnosis and therapeutics.

Intestinal metaplasia patients had a 0.72 per thousand person-years incidence risk of gastric adenocarcinoma, whereas intestinal metaplasia plus low-grade dysplasia patients had a 7.7 per thousand person-years incidence rate. Women are more than twice as likely to have autoimmune gastritis than men [28], and in more than 10% of males it is linked to the condition developing into gastric carcinoid tumors or gastric adenocarcinomas [29].

6.4.3 Ménétrier's disease

The oxyntic gland mucosa atrophy, tortuous and cystic gland enlargement, smooth muscle hyperplasia, and foveolar hyperplasia are all signs of Ménétrier's disease. There is no information on the prevalence or incidence of this uncommon acquired stomach illness called hypertrophy gastropathy [30]. The cause of childhood Ménétrier disease is unknown, despite a link between the illness and CMV infection being found in a small cohort of patients. In addition, it has been suggested that *H. pylori* infection may increase the likelihood of developing Ménétrier disease [31].

6.5 Nanotechnology in cancer diagnostic and therapeutics

Different types of nanomaterials use in diagnostic and therapeutics mentioned in figures 6.3. Since numerous types of nanoparticles are being employed for molecular imaging, the use of nanoparticles in cancer diagnosis and monitoring has attracted a lot of attention. Recent advancements in cancer research and diagnostics have made them important due to their benefits, including their small size, good biocompatibility, and high atomic number. A few examples of nanoparticles with distinctive structural, optical, or magnetic features that are used in the diagnosis of cancer are iron oxide nanocrystals, semiconductors, and quantum dots [32]. Nanoparticles can be marked or coated with very specific malignancies using a variety of anti-tumor medicines and biomolecules, such as peptides, antibodies, or other compounds. It may be possible to identify cancer in its earliest stages by using nanoparticle imaging of tumor tissue for cancer diagnostics or early cancer cell identification and screening. The development of immunological superparamagnetic iron oxide nanoparticles (SPIONs) that can be employed in MRI imaging and target certain cancer cell types has enabled the detection of metastases in lung cancer [33, 34]. Due to their great specificity and lack of known adverse effects, recent investigations have demonstrated that SPIONs are suitable building blocks for aerosols in MRI imaging of lung cancer [35]. Regarding their potential use in cancer treatment, numerous nanotechnology tools, including dendrimers, nanotubes, and liposomes, each with their own distinct properties, have been studied. For instance, nanotubes, which are carbon cylinders formed of benzene rings, can enter the cell through passive diffusion and endocytosis [36]. Additionally, their dynamic chemical characteristics enable the adjustment of their solubility, enabling the drugs held inside the tubes to be released at a predetermined rate. Instead, liposomes, which can form lipid bilayers, are promising delivery methods for combination drugs because they can transport both hydrophilic and hydrophobic substances simultaneously [37].

The most recent classes of dendrimers have also been developed to carry a therapeutic medication, a diagnostic agent, and an active targeting molecule all in one dendrimer therapy. They are characterized by their inner core and tree-like branches that offer enormous amounts of surface area for drug attachment [37, 38]. In order to achieve targeted drug administration, it is clear that nanotechnology, which involves the generation of numerous nanoparticles with different shapes and behaviors, can open up a vast range of options. Numerous techniques have been used to demonstrate how nanotechnology can be used to cure cancer. They include, but are not limited to: photothermal cancer cell elimination, gene therapy, and intracellular drug delivery for therapeutic purposes [39, 40]. Angiogenesis is used in the delivery of intracellular chemotherapy. Angiogenesis, the formation of new blood vessels used by tumor cells to expand by taking nutrients and oxygen from surrounding cells, is one of the traits of cancer. Angiogenesis blood vessels form unevenly and are more leaky than typical healthy vasculature as a result of their fast, uncontrolled growth [41]. These vessels have pores that are between a few hundred nanometers to several microns in size, as opposed to ordinary vessels, which only have pores that are 2–6 nm in size. Nanoparticles' diameter, which ranges from 10 to 300 nm, makes them the ideal size for entering tumor cells' blood arteries without significantly damaging healthy tissues [41]. This Trojan horse approach offers an attractive way to reduce harm to neighboring cells. Another approach is photo-thermal ablation makes use of the difference between the average apoptotic temperature of cancer cells, which occurs at about 42 °C, and normal cells, which occur at about 46 °C. Gold nanoparticles that are made to only excite at particular light frequencies have been used in multiple studies to target and kill specific tumor cells while sparing the surrounding healthy cells [42]. Nanotechnology has the ability to overcome the shortcomings of current methods, such as reducing the health risks associated with treatments depending on viruses. Researchers successfully developed nanoparticles using a synthetic delivery method and small interfering ribonucleic acid (siRNA) to reduce the expression of RRM2, a known anticancer target [43].

6.6 Nanotechnology and gastric cancer diagnostic

In clinical settings, the detection of stomach cancer typically involves the use of conventional imaging techniques such CT, PET, MRI, PET-CT and SPECT. The only imaging modality, poorly targeted biodistribution, fast clearance, and other unfavorable side effects are all drawbacks of contrast agents. It is clear from the various types of nanoparticles that have built-in characteristics or functional modifications that new, better imaging techniques are being created for the diagnosis of gastric cancer. They most typically have real-time imaging, specific tumor accumulation and local metastasis, a low tumor-background ratio, high sensitivity, and high resolution [44].

6.6.1 Fluorescence imaging and gastric cancer detection

Fluorescence imaging, a beautiful imaging method, has wonderful benefits including real-time mode, quick imaging, adaptable equipment, great safety, and low cost [45].

The visible spectrum is inferior to the 700–1300 nm near-infrared (NIR) window. Hemoglobin and other endogenous substances greatly absorb and scatter imaging light with wavelengths below 700 nm in human tissues. The lipid and water absorption hinders imaging at wavelengths above 1300 nm [46]. The FDA-approved NIR fluorophore indocyanine green (ICG) stands out among the others because of its higher quantum yield and much lower tissue absorption [47]. The use of *in vivo* imaging in the human body is being adopted for the first time [48]. Hironori *et al* investigated the theranostic potential of the ICG-loaded lactosome (ICGm) nano-particle using a murine draining lymph node metastasis model for gastric cancer [49]. The presence of metastatic lymph nodes was found to be reported in the ICGm-treated mice but not in the ICG-treated mice using *in vivo* imaging. Wang *et al* developed unique ICG conjugated gold nanoshells that efficiently gathered in peritoneal metastasis models as well as subcutaneously transplanted models [50]. For surgical excision and preoperative guiding, near-infrared imaging provided sufficient optical contrast and accurate detection of visible and microtumor lesions (3 mm). The FDA-approved 5-aminolevulinic acid (5-ALA) and other cyanine-based fluorophores have been created for the diagnosis of gastric cancer, however, there are still certain inherent limitations that need to be taken into account. Due to the fluorophores' visible emission profile, imaging light scattering and tissue penetration are still anticipated to be enhanced. In actuality, the NIR window has further divisions called NIR I and NIR II. Because the quantity of scattering is inversely linked to the wavelength of light, NIR II fluorophores are of interest to researchers [51, 52]. Additionally, tissue autofluorescence, scattering, and photon attenuation all drasti-cally degrade with increasing imaging wavelengths [53]. Despite the fact that many NIR II nanoparticles have been investigated for tumor imaging, their usage for stomach malignancies is now quite limited [54].

6.6.2 Photoacoustic imaging and gastric cancer detection

One of the promising imaging modalities that can produce incredibly accurate and detailed 2D and 3D images is photoacoustic (PA) imaging. When biological tissue is subjected to non-ionizing pulse lasers directly for PA imaging, exogenous nano-particles or endogenous molecules like hemoglobin absorb the energy. When energy is transformed into heat and causes thermal expansion, which is related to the physiological properties of the tissue, an ultrasound transducer measures the resulting ultrasonic waves. In the end, these outcomes are assessed and recreated as PA photos [55]. Animal models with gastric cancer were subjected to carbon nanotubes coated with RGD-conjugated silica by Wang *et al*. Results from an optoacoustic imaging system demonstrated that the stomach cancer cells were successfully targeted by the nanotubes *in vivo* and that the nude model produced powerful PA imaging [56].

Another set of researchers described the use of iron oxide nanoparticles coated with anti-HER2 moieties for PA tumor imaging. The nanoparticles could be used as a PA contrast agent for the imaging of gastric cancer since they specifically identified HER2-positive tumors in PA imaging experiments [57]. According to Liang *et al* targeted ligands were CD44v6 monoclonal antibodies coupled to gold nanostar-based PEGylated nanoprobes. PA imaging shown that the nanoprobes could effectively target the vascular system of gastric cancer 4 h following injection [58].

6.6.3 Computed tomography and gastric cancer detection

A common non-radioactive diagnostic for detecting malignancies is CT. Although secure and cutting-edge imaging technologies have been created for clinical usage, the main drawbacks of inadequate targeting and poor sensitivity continue to exist. Nanotechnology is recognized as a magnificent development approach. In a clinical experiment, Zhang *et al* employed targeted nanoparticle contrast agents and contrast-enhanced CT to find early-stage stomach cancer [59]. Contrast-enhanced CT with targeted nanoparticles enhances not only CT accuracy but also diagnostic confidence in people with suspected stomach cancer as compared to a single CT detection. It was discovered that esophageal carcinoma had similar consequences [60].

6.6.4 Magnetic resonance imaging and gastric cancer detection

The majority of the inorganic nanoparticles used in magnetic resonance imaging (MRI), another popular method of detection, are superparamagnetic iron oxide nanoparticles (SPIONs) [61]. A molecular probe with MRI and optical dual-modality was disclosed by Yan *et al* [62]. Cyclopeptide GX1 and the near-infrared fluorescent dye Cy5.5 were attached to the nano-Fe_3O_4 that had been altered by polyethylene glycol (PEG) to create the nanoprobe. Iron oxide-gold nanoclusters (Fe_3O_4@Au@-CD) are coated with -CD to provide a biological nanoprobe with great biocompatibility [63].

This nanoprobe displayed red fluorescence in the cells and could be selectively picked up by the MGC-803 gastric cancer cells. Although various types of nano-particles have been investigated for MRI, it is important to keep in mind SPIONs' drawbacks, such as their genotoxicity [64].

6.6.5 Multimodal imaging and gastric cancer detection

The aforementioned imaging modalities undoubtedly improved the ability to detect gastric cancer, however, each imaging strategy was constrained by its own draw-backs. A single imaging method cannot, however, provide all the information needed. Clinicians can access diverse, complementary, and integrated diagnosis signals by combining several imaging strategies, and they can simultaneously highlight the benefits of various tools while also minimizing any potential draw-backs. For example, despite having a low depth of detection, real-time modalities like fluorescence imaging and PA imaging can export high contrast pictures for intraoperative use. Nanoparticles are highly suited to act as the carrier in multi-modal imaging because of their capacity to transport a variety of payloads. There have been numerous investigations into nanoparticles with the potential for multi-modal imaging [65, 66]. False signal reduction is possible with SPECT/CT with dual validation as compared to a single imaging equipment. A unique targeted nuclear imaging agent called DTPA/glucose-regulated protein 78 (GRP78BP) displayed greater radioactive signals than non-targeted 111In-labeled micelles [67]. Micelles conjugated with 111In and DTPA/GRP78BP showed a 93% efficiency. Additional perfluoropentane (PFP)-labeled copper-64 (64Cu) nanodroplets with phospholipid shells were examined for PET/CT and ultrasonic imaging [68].

These nanoparticles help in diagnosis by combining the technology and science with multiple imaging modalities. Additionally, mesoporous silica gap-enhanced Raman tags (Gd-GERTs) loaded with gadolinium are designed specifically for preoperative and intra-operative imaging. High MRI T1 relaxivity, multi-mode imaging performance, and remarkable surface-enhanced Raman spectroscopy (SERS) signal with extraordinary dispersity and stability were also displayed [69].

6.7 Nanotechnology and gastric cancer management

6.7.1 Nanomaterial and chemotherapy

Nanomedicines are practical for the delivery of chemotherapeutics due to benefits such as reliable biocompatibility and biodegradability. Due to its severe lipophilicity and inability to be supplied via injection, PTX is only used as a second-line treatment for locally advanced or metastatic gastric cancer. The primary components of abraxane are albumin nanoparticles and PTX with a particle size of about 130 mm. The nanoformulation concurrently reduces toxicity while maintaining the therapeutic benefits. Additionally, transendothelial transport via albumin-binding protein causes nanoparticles to accumulate more in tumor tissue in addition to the enhanced permeability and retention effect [70]. Abraxane underwent clinical trials to determine its efficacy and safety in treating gastric cancer, which showed promising action and moderate toxicity. Lung, pancreatic, and metastasized breast cancer are among the tumors for which the FDA has approved the use of Abraxane [71]. Shi *et al* introduced a brand-new form of PTX nanoparticle with RGD decoration and a disulfide connection, giving the polymer-PTX an active target and environment response capability. The nanoparticles effectively suppressed the growth of the tumor by releasing PTX as demonstrated by *in vivo* studies, and with little adverse effect [72].

Tetrandrine (Tet), an alkaloid of the bisbenzylisoquinoline class, has been shown to increase the anticancer activity of PTX in cases of stomach cancer. By encasing Tet inside self-assembling PTX nanofibers, Li *et al* reported novel PTX and Tet co-loaded nanofibers. The self-assembled nanofibers showed an improvement in the therapeutic efficiency and side effects of PTX in treating gastric cancer, as well as an increase in mitochondrial apoptosis levels and a substantial anti-tumor effect both *in vitro* and *in vivo* [73].

One of the first-line therapies for gastric cancer is 5-fluorouracil (5-FU), a fluorinated pyrimidine uracil analog. Its cytotoxicity is caused by the binding and inhibition of thymidylate synthase [74]. In the studies by Elisabete *et al* a monoclonal antibody against sialyl-Lewis A, a glycan that encourages hematogenous metastasis, was used to functionalize the surface of nanoparticles co-loaded with 5-FU and PTX. As a result, a nano-vehicle that successfully delivered the therapeutic medications 5-FU and PTX to metastatic gastric cancer cells was developed. It is hoped that the use of nanoparticles will lead to the development of better therapies for the treatment of gastric associated cancer.

Additionally, doxorubicin (DOX) and irinotecan both have single-agent activity and have been widely used in clinical practice. In slightly acidic conditions, gastric cancer cells demonstrated higher absorption and greater toxicity to nanoparticles than single components of an irinotecan hydrochloride curcumin nano system [75]. For chemo-photothermal synergistic therapy, Zhou and his team encapsulated DOX in a pH-sensitive, long-circulation nanoparticle [76]. Yang and his associates showed how to treat gastric tumors that overexpress Her2 and CD44 using dual-targeting hybrid nanoparticles [77]. Delivering the nanoparticle to stomach cancer cells preferentially is made possible by the anti-Her2 peptide and hyaluronic acid on the surface of NPs that carry the SN38 agent. Treatment for stomach cancer is still hampered by the persistence of chemotherapy resistance, which results in tumor recurrence and chemotherapy failure [78].

Because of their unique physicochemical features resulting from their nanoscale size, nanoparticles have the potential to be used in the battle against drug resistance since they can pass through cell membranes and concentrate more in tumor areas than traditional drugs [79]. TiO_2 nanoparticles were used by Azimee et al to enhance the therapeutic effects of 5-FU in human AGS gastric cells [80].

TiO_2 nanoparticles increase the generation of ROS, inhibit autophagy flux, and raise the level of ROS, which induce 5-FU improvement to have cytotoxic and apoptotic effects on AGS cells. Yang et al demonstrated a different strategy to deal with medication resistance by preventing the expression of P-glycoprotein (Pgp). To deliver the anticancer medicine DOX to multidrug resistant gastric cancer cells (SCG 7901/VCR), the SPION functionalized with chemosensitizing chemical XMD8-92 may be employed. Both in vitro and in vivo, the nanoparticles showed greater tumor suppression power than DOX therapy alone. Utilizing nanoparticles could pave the way for a new treatment for chemotherapy resistance in stomach cancer [81].

6.7.2 Nanomedicine and radiotherapy

High-energy radiation therapy that produces ionizing radiation has the potential to kill tumor cells, stop the growth of tiny tumors, and extend local lymph nodes [82].

Nanoparticles contributed significantly to radiotherapy together with advancements in tumor imaging. When used as radiosensitizers, nanoparticles could provide more therapeutic advantages than radiation alone [83].

Using chitosan-modified gold nanoparticles (CS-GNPs), Zhang et al studied how gastric cancer cells respond to x-ray irradiation. The biocompatibility of CS-GNPs was shown by MTT findings, and survival rates under radiation compared to radiation alone showed an enhancement in cell radiation therapeutic sensitivity, suggesting a possible use in radiation therapy for gastric cancer [84]. Similar techniques were employed by Huang et al to produce biocompatible Ag microspheres using BSA (bovine serum albumin). Compared to Ag microspheres, individual nanoscale Ag assemblies showed higher radiation effects on gastric cancer cells [85]. Due to their high atomic number and electron density, gold and silver nanoparticles have been used frequently as radiation sensitizers to improve energy deposition into tumor areas and boost the effectiveness of radiotherapy [86].

Adjuvant chemotherapy and radiation therapy appeared to be an effective treatment for advanced gastric cancer that possessed the characteristic of a strong propensity for invasion and metastasis. A significant amount of general toxicity, however, has slowed down the use of traditional chemo-radiotherapy in clinical settings. Because of this, new therapeutic approaches were created in response to the need for treatments with increased efficacy and fewer adverse effects [87].

6.7.3 Phototherapy and gastric cancer detection

The two primary forms of phototherapy, or photo-triggered therapeutic modalities, are photodynamic treatment (PDT) and photothermal therapy (PTT), which have the advantages of being repeatable, non-invasive, and selective. Additionally, in recent years, photoimmunotherapy and photo-induced chemotherapy have garnered a lot of interest [88, 89].

Nanoparticles may be the finest carriers to carry photosensitizers implanted in tumor sites and enhance their biodistribution due to the hydrophobic nature of the majority of photosensitizers, which limits their systemic administration. Additionally, light may be easily adjusted and focused to offer precise treatment while causing the least amount of damage to healthy tissue. A common photosensitizer, IR780 produces ROS and heat in response to exposure to light. However, because of its excellent photosensitivity and hydrophobicity, IR780 cannot be dissolved in water and must instead be encapsulated. In order to encapsulate IR780, Deng *et al* used an amphiphilic macromolecular molecule (sericin-cholesterol) with folic acid as the target ligand. The solubility and photo-stability of IR780 were significantly improved by using an amphiphilic macromolecule that could self-assemble into stable micelles [90]. After being exposed to an 808 nm laser, these nanoparticles aggregated in tumor tissues and produced ROS, metformin, and IR780. Consequently, complex I in the mitochondrial electron transport chain can be directly inhibited by metformin. Thus, cell respiration prevented tumor hypoxia and improved PDT and PTT for stomach cancer. These studies showed that phototherapy for stomach cancer can be promoted by using nanoparticles to deliver photosensitizers. Other forms of nanomaterials, including CuS, graphene, and gold nanoparticles, were created for photothermal therapy in addition to organic nanoparticles [51, 91, 92]. The tumor-targeting nanoparticles developed by Yang *et al* include 17AAG, iRGD, and carboxyl-functionalized W18O49 nanoparticles. The W18O49 nanoparticles had outstanding PTT and CT imaging contrast, and 17AAG's ability to avoid thermoresistance and block the heat-shock response enhanced the therapeutic effects of PTT and decreased the likelihood of tumor recurrence. W18O49 nanoparticles can greatly increase PTT *in vivo* and *in vitro*, target gastric cancer, and offer dual-modality imaging [66].

Gold nanoparticles are particularly efficient in converting optical energy to heat. Mesoporous carbon–gold hybrid nanoprobes for real-time imaging, PTT/PDT, and nanozyme oxidative treatment were described by Zhang *et al.* Due to the wide surface area and multiple –COOH groups of the carbon–gold hybrid nanoparticles, surface chemical modification with different targeting molecules was possible. This resulted in outstanding tumor-targeting efficacy, longer tumor retention, and a helpful therapeutic impact for gastric tumor [93].

6.7.4 Combination therapies and theranostics for gastric cancer detection

Recent years have seen the emergence of novel therapeutics that support anticancer treatments, including targeted, gene and immune-therapy. Although most patients do not benefit, the FDA and the European Union have approved ramucirumab and tratuzumab for targeted therapy against advanced gastric cancer [94].

In clinical research, the addition of trastuzumab to chemotherapy dramatically boosted overall survival, suggesting that combination therapies may be the most effective option for better outcomes. In addition, the use of gene therapy in conjunction with anticancer drugs has enhanced the effectiveness of treatment [95].

A collagen membrane with an aptamer-siRNA chimera/5-FU combination, for instance, may precisely latch on to gastric cancer cells, transport 5-FU to the desired location, and silence a drug-resistant gene [96]. Another fascinating potential therapeutic approach is the combination of immunotherapy and chemotherapy. In clinical gastric cancer, TfR1 binding with H-ferritin nanocarrier may be a novel approach that enhances treatment effectiveness and prognostic prognosis [97]. A PTT/PDT combination with chemotherapy and adjuvant immunotherapy was also created, strengthening the immune responses against cancer [98].

In addition to multimodal imaging and combination therapy, theranostic nano-particles, which combine co-delivery of an imaging unit and a therapeutic unit, are being used in an increasing number of nano-based designs. Prior to the development of theranostic nanoparticles, doctors could only detect tumors either before or after therapeutic interventions. Additionally, a number of nanoparticle frameworks with integrated imaging capabilities, such as SPIONs for MRI and gold nanoparticles for CT, make excellent candidates for the development of theranostic systems. And most photosensitizers, notably IR780 and chlorin E6, exhibited both tumor toxicity and imaging capabilities. This is due to the fact that photosensitizers can act as a vector to produce heat and/or ROS in addition to excitation of fluorescence and absorption of NIR. The other kind of theranostic nanoparticles combine the payloads for diagnosis and treatment into a single nanoparticle. However, more intricate quality control comes at a higher price. Theranostic systems based on nanotechnology have been created and have shown promise in the treatment of gastric cancer [99].

6.8 Challenges and prospectives

There are only a few FDA-approved nanomedicines for treating gastric cancer out of the more than 50 that have been approved [100]. The complexity of patients' aberrant molecular traits in gastric cancer patients continues to be a major barrier. The gastric cancers papillary, tubular, mucinous, and poorly cohesive carcinomas were classified by the World Health Organization. But there is currently no defined system for classifying biologics, and the clinical applicability is quite modest [101]. Additionally, it is still unknown how gastric cancer develops on a molecular level. Theranostic performance is believed to be aided by knowledge of molecular pathways and the discovery of potent biomarkers for gastric cancer. The limitations of the accessible nanoparticles are mentioned, along with the aforementioned uses. NIR dyes were not as effective because of insufficient tissue penetration. Quantum dots can detect a signal at a deeper level, however, safety and biocompatibility are concerns. To clear the way for improved performance, some strategies have been put out. Donor–acceptor–donor (DAD) dyes and NIR-II imaging probes are combined to form multiplexed NIR-II probes, which have been described by Rui *et al* as an excellent imaging approach for directing sentinel lymph node excision in a variety of cancer models [102]. On the one hand, tissue autofluorescence and scattering are diminished by longer wavelength NIR-II fluorescence imaging. Bright-light dual-NIR II imaging-guided surgery has greater clinical potential and is more practical. Another fluorescence dual-mode imaging agent has been developed to diagnose lymph node tumor metastasis without the use of a microscope. However, there are not many pertinent studies focused on gastric cancer [103].

Although there are numerous studies in this area, the majority of them involve *in vivo* research. The biodistribution and targeting capabilities of nanoparticles may differ between preclinical investigations and clinical practice due to changes in the body's metabolisms, the characteristics of the nanoparticles, and the significant degree of tumor heterogeneity. For instance, proteins, such as antibodies, may be taken up by nanoparticle surfaces and form the protein corona [104]. The targeting and anticancer actions *in vivo* are impacted by denatured proteins in the corona of nanoparticles. These problems are supposed to be addressed by biomimetic nano-particles [105]. Natural nanoscale membrane vesicles are found outside of cells. Tumor image monitoring and therapy are made possible by extracellular vesicles with special physiological and biochemical characteristics, such as prolonged retention circulation duration, higher tissue and organ targeting specificity, and improved cytoplasmic delivery effectiveness [106]. Nanoparticles with membrane coatings have also shown to be efficient nanocarriers. For minimizing the off-target effect and extending *in vivo* circulation, the gold standard is to combine biomimetic nanoplatforms with RGD peptide or HER-2 antibodies [107]. Multifunctional nanoparticles now have the ability to target and improve image contrast. But more functionality necessitates more expensive and time-consuming synthetic processes. Additionally, there are more complicated *in vivo* behavior and impacts, as well as greater regulatory obstacles [108].

Gastric cancer is one of the most common malignant tumors in the world, and nanotechnology offers a practical option for early detection and therapy that is guided by imaging. Nanoparticle design and synthesis involved a number of materials with various imaging and therapeutic properties, and the results were encouraging. A thorough knowledge and rigorous approach may stimulate rational planning and translational medical research, even though there are still some obstacles to be addressed and a long way to go before preclinical investigations can be transferred into clinical practice. We believe that nanotechnology has a bright future and advances both imaging and treatments.

Acknowledgments

One of the authors MZ thanks NSF (USA), EIR (USA) and FTTP as seed grant fund for providing financial support in the form Postdoctoral Research Associate fellowship.

References

[1] Sahoo S K, Parveen S and Panda J J 2007 The present and future of nanotechnology in human health care *Nanomedicine* **3** 20–31

[2] Whitesides G M 2003 The right size: nanobiotechnology *Nat. Biotechnol.* **21** 1161–5

[3] Fortina P, Kricka L J, Surrey S and Grodzinski P 2005 Nanobiotechnology: the promise and reality of new approaches to molecular recognition *Trends Biotechnol.* **23** 168–73

[4] Fakruddin M, Hossain Z and Afroz H 2012 Prospects and applications of nanobiotechnology: a medical perspective *J. Nanobiotechnol.* **10** 31

[5] Crean C, Lahiff E, Gilmartin N, Diamond D and O'Kennedy R 2011 Polyaniline nanofibres as templates for the covalent immobilisation of biomolecules *Synth. Met.* **161** 285–92

[6] Jin C, Wang K, Oppong-Gyebi A and Hu J 2020 Application of nanotechnology in cancer diagnosis and therapy—a mini-review *Int. J. Med. Sci.* **17** 2964–73

[7] Aaron P T, Theresa N W and Hashem B E 2023 Global burden of gastric cancer: epidemiological trends, risk factors, screening and prevention *Nat. Rev. Clin. Oncol.* **20** 338–49

[8] IARC Working Group on the Evaluation of Carcinogenic Risk to Humans 1994 *Schistosomes, Liver Flukes and Helicobacter pylori (IARC Monographs on the Evaluation of Carcinogenic Risks to Humans* **vol 61** (IARC)

[9] Gonzalez C A and Agudo A 2012 Carcinogenesis, prevention and early detection of gastric cancer: where we are and where we should go *Int. J. Cancer.* **130** 745–53

[10] Plummer M, Franceschi S, Vignat J *et al* 2015 Global burden of gastric cancer attributable to *Helicobacter pylori Int. J. Cancer* **136** 487–90

[11] Zamani M, Ebrahimtabar F, Zamani V *et al* 2018 Systematic review with meta-analysis: the worldwide prevalence of *Helicobacter pylori* infection *Aliment. Pharmacol. Ther.* **47** 868–76

[12] Morgan E, Arnold M, Camargo C *et al* 2022 The current and future incidence and mortality of gastric cancer in 185 countries, 2020–40: a population-based modelling study *eClinicalMedicine* **47** 101404

[13] Karimi P, Islami F, Anandasabapathy S *et al* 2014 Gastric cancer: descriptive epidemiology, risk factors, screening, and prevention *Cancer Epidemiol. Biomarkers Prev.* **23** 700–13

[14] Praud D, Rota M, Pelucchi C *et al* 2018 Cigarette smoking and gastric cancer in the stomach cancer pooling (StoP) project *Eur. J. Cancer Prev.* **27** 124–33

[15] Chen Y, Liu L, Wang X *et al* 2013 Body mass index and risk of gastric cancer: a meta-analysis of a population with more than ten million from 24 prospective studies *Cancer Epidemiol. Biomarkers Prev.* **22** 1395–408

[16] Zhao Z, Yin Z and Zhao Q 2017 Red and processed meat consumption and gastric cancer risk: a systematic review and meta-analysis *Oncotarget* **8** 30563–75

[17] Kim S R, Kim K, Lee S A *et al* 2019 Effect of red, processed, and white meat consumption on the risk of gastric cancer: an overall and dose–response meta-analysis *Nutrients* **11** 826

[18] Na H K and Lee J Y 2017 Molecular basis of alcohol-related gastric and colon cancer *Int. J. Mol. Sci.* **18** 1116

[19] Deng W, Jin L, Zhuo H *et al* 2021 Alcohol consumption and risk of stomach cancer: a meta-analysis *Chem. Biol. Interact.* **336** 109365

[20] Oba M, Miwa K, Fujimura T *et al* 2008 Chemoprevention of glandular stomach carcinogenesis through duodenogastric reflux in rats by a COX-2 inhibitor *Int. J. Cancer* **1123** 1491–8

[21] Huang X Z, Chen Y, Wu J *et al* 2017 Aspirin and non-steroidal anti-inflammatory drugs use reduce gastric cancer risk: a dose-response meta-analysis *Oncotarget* **2003** 4781–95

[22] Gullo I, van der Post R S and Carneiro F 2021 Recent advances in the pathology of heritable gastric cancer syndromes *Histopathology* **78** 125–47

[23] Capelle L G, Van Grieken N C, Lingsma H F *et al* 2010 Risk and epidemiological time trends of gastric cancer in Lynch syndrome carriers in the Netherlands *Gastroenterology* **138** 487–92

[24] Oliveira C, Seruca R and Carneiro F 2006 Genetics, pathology, and clinics of familial gastric cancer *Int. J. Surg. Pathol* **14** 21–33

[25] Camargo M C, Murphy G, Koriyama C *et al* 2011 Determinants of Epstein–Barr virus-positive gastric cancer: an international pooled analysis *Br. J. Cancer* **105** 38–43

[26] Bizzaro N and Antico A 2014 Diagnosis and classification of pernicious anemia *Autoimmun. Rev.* **13** 565–8

[27] Zamcheck N *et al* 1955 Occurrence of gastric cancer among patients with pernicious anemia at the Boston City hospital *N. Engl. J. Med.* **252** 1103–10

[28] Lahner E, Dilaghi E, Cingolani S *et al* 2022 Gender-sex differences in autoimmune atrophic gastritis *Transl Res.* **248** 1–10

[29] Landgren A M, Landgren O, Gridley G *et al* 2011 Autoimmune disease and subsequent risk of developing alimentary tract cancers among 4.5 million US male veterans *Cancer* **117** 1163–71

[30] Wolfsen H C, Carpenter H A and Talley N J 1993 Menetrier's disease: a form of hypertrophic gastropathy or gastritis? *Gastroenterology* **104** 1310–9

[31] Madsen L G, Taskiran M, Madsen J L and Bytzer P 1999 Ménétrier's disease and *Helicobacter pylori*: normalization of gastrointestinal protein loss after eradication therapy *Dig. Dis. Sci.* **44** 2307–12

[32] Popescu R C, Fufă M O and Grumezescu A M 2015 Metal-based nanosystems for diagnosis *Rom. J. Morphol. Embryol* **56** 635–49

[33] Singh R 2019 Nanotechnology based therapeutic application in cancer diagnosis and therapy *3 Biotech* **9** 415

[34] Wan X, Song Y, Song N *et al* 2016 The preliminary study of immune superparamagnetic iron oxide nanoparticles for the detection of lung cancer in magnetic resonance imaging *Carbohydr. Res.* **419** 33–40

[35] Jafari A, Salouti M, Shayesteh S F *et al* 2015 Synthesis and characterization of Bombesin-superparamagnetic iron oxide nanoparticles as a targeted contrast agent for imaging of breast cancer using MRI *Nanotechnology* **26** 075101

[36] Parhi P, Mohanty C and Sahoo S K 2012 Nanotechnology-based combinational drug delivery: an emerging approach for cancer therapy *Drug Discov. Today* **17** 1044–52

[37] Alexis F, Rhee J W, Richie J P *et al* 2008 New frontiers in nanotechnology for cancer treatment *Urol. Oncol.* **26** 74–85

[38] Kim K Y 2007 Nanotechnology platforms and physiological challenges for cancer therapeutics *Nanomedicine* **3** 103–10

[39] Kawasaki E S and Player A 2005 Nanotechnology, nanomedicine, and the development of new, effective therapies for cancer *Nanomedicine* **1** 101–9

[40] Bourzac K 2012 Nanotechnology: carrying drugs *Nature* **491** S58–60

[41] Grossman J H and McNeil S E 2012 Nanotechnology in cancer medicine *Phys. Today* **65** 38–42

[42] Vines J B, Yoon J H, Ryu N E *et al* 2019 Gold nanoparticles for photothermal cancer therapy *Front. Chem.* **7** 167

[43] Davis M E, Zuckerman J E, Choi C H *et al* 2010 Evidence of RNAi in humans from systemically administered siRNA via targeted nanoparticles *Nature* **464** 1067–70

[44] Li X, Ai S, Lu X *et al* 2021 Nanotechnology-based strategies for gastric cancer imaging and treatment *RSC Adv.* **11** 35392–407

[45] Gao H, Bao P, Dai S *et al* 2019 Far-red/near-infrared emissive (1,3-dimethyl)barbituric acid-based AIEgens for high-contrast detection of metastatic tumors in the lung *Chem. Asian J.* **4** 871–6

[46] Chen Y, Wang S and Zhang F 2023 Near-infrared luminescence high-contrast *in vivo* biomedical imaging *Nat. Rev. Bioeng* **1** 60–78

[47] Aya M, Eiichi T, Hak Soo C *et al* 2010 Real-time intra-operative near-infrared fluorescence identification of the extrahepatic bile ducts using clinically available contrast agents *Surgery* **148** 87–95

[48] Ishizawa T, Fukushima N, Shibahara J *et al* 2009 Real-time identification of liver cancers by using indocyanine green fluorescent imaging *Cancer* **115** 2491–504

[49] Tsujimoto H, Morimoto Y, Takahata R *et al* 2015 Theranostic photosensitive nanoparticles for lymph node metastasis of gastric cancer *Ann. Surg. Oncol.* **2** S923–8

[50] Wang S H, Chi C W, Cheng H D *et al* 2018 Photothermal adjunctive cytoreductive surgery for treating peritoneal metastasis of gastric cancer *Small Methods* **2** 7

[51] Shi H, Yan R Q, Wu L Y *et al* 2018 Tumor-targeting CuS nanoparticles for multimodal imaging and guided photothermal therapy of lymph node metastasis *Acta Biomater.* **72** 256–65

[52] Li X J, Zhou J J, Liu C R *et al* 2017 Stable and biocompatible mushroom beta-glucan modified gold nanorods for cancer photothermal therapy *J. Agric. Food Chem.* **65** 9529–36

[53] Zhu S J, Tian R, Antaris A L *et al* 2019 Near-infrared-II molecular dyes for cancer imaging and surgery *Adv. Mater.* **31** 25

[54] Tian R, Ma H L, Yang Q L *et al* 2019 Rational design of a super-contrast NIR-II fluorophore affords high-performance NIR-II molecular imaging guided microsurgery *Chem. Sci.* **10** 326–32

[55] Ku G and Wang L H V 2005 Deeply penetrating photoacoustic tomography in biological tissues enhanced with an optical contrast agent *Opt. Lett.* **30** 507–9

[56] Wang C, Bao C C, Liang S J *et al* 2014 RGD-conjugated silica-coated gold nanorods on the surface of carbon nanotubes for targeted photoacoustic imaging of gastric cancer *Nanoscale Res. Lett.* **9** 10

[57] Kanazaki K, Sano K, Makino A *et al* 2015 Development of anti-HER2 fragment antibody conjugated to iron oxide nanoparticles for *in vivo* HER2-targeted photoacoustic tumor imaging *Nanomedicine* **11** 2051–60

[58] Liang S J, Li C, Zhang C L *et al* 2015 CD44v6 monoclonal antibody-conjugated gold nanostars for targeted photoacoustic imaging and plasmonic photothermal therapy of gastric cancer stem-like cells *Theranostics* **5** 970–84

[59] Hang K M, Du X J, Yu K H *et al* 2018 Application of novel targeting nanoparticles contrast agent combined with contrast-enhanced computed tomography during screening for early-phase gastric carcinoma *Exp. Ther. Med.* **15** 47–54

[60] Gai J J, Gao Z L, Song L *et al* 2018 Contrast-enhanced computed tomography combined with Chitosan–Fe_3O_4 nanoparticles targeting fibroblast growth factor receptor and vascular endothelial growth factor receptor in the screening of early esophageal cancer *Exp. Ther. Med.* **15** 5344–52

[61] Bakhtiary Z, Saei A A, Hajipour M J *et al* 2016 Targeted superparamagnetic iron oxide nanoparticles for early detection of cancer: possibilities and challenges *Nanomedicine* **12** 287–307

[62] Yan X J, Song X Y and Wang Z B 2017 Construction of specific magnetic resonance imaging/optical dual-modality molecular probe used for imaging angiogenesis of gastric cancer *Artif. Cells, Nanomed. Biotechnol.* **45** 399–403

[63] Guo H E, Zhang Y X, Liang *et al* 2019 An inorganic magnetic fluorescent nanoprobe with favorable biocompatibility for dual-modality bioimaging and drug delivery *J. Inorg. Biochem.* **192** 72–81

[64] Mahmoudi M, Hofmann H, Rothen-Rutishauser B *et al* 2012 Assessing the *in vitro* and *in vivo* toxicity of superparamagnetic iron oxide nanoparticles *Chem. Rev.* **112** 2323–38

[65] Li Z, Yin S, Cheng L *et al* 2014 Magnetic targeting enhanced theranostic strategy based on multimodal imaging for selective ablation of cancer *Adv. Funct. Mater.* **24** 2312–21

[66] Yang Z Y, Wang J F, Liu S *et al* 2019 Tumor-targeting W18O49 nanoparticles for dual-modality imaging and guided heat-shock-response-inhibited photothermal therapy in gastric cancer *Part. Part. Syst. Charact.* **36** 12

[67] Cheng C C, Huang C F, Ho A S *et al* 2013 Novel targeted nuclear imaging agent for gastric cancer diagnosis: glucose-regulated protein 78 binding peptide-guided 111In-labeled polymeric, micelles *Int. J. Nanomed.* **8** 1385–91

[68] Shin U, Kim J, Lee J *et al* 2020 Development of (Cu)–C-64-loaded perfluoropentane nanodroplet: a potential tumor theragnostic nano-carrier and dual-modality pet-ultrasound imaging agents *Ultrasound Med. Biol.* **46** 2775–84

[69] Shi B W, Zhang B Y, Zhang Y Q *et al* 2020 Multifunctional gap-enhanced Raman tags for preoperative and intraoperative cancer imaging *Acta Biomater.* **104** 210–20

[70] Jang K, Yoon S, Kim S E *et al* 2014 Novel nanocrystal formulation of megestrol acetate has improved bioavailability compared with the conventional micronized formulation in the fasting state *Drug Des. Dev. Ther.* **8** 851–8

[71] Bando H, Shimodaira H, Fujitani K *et al* 2018 A phase II study of nab-paclitaxel in combination with ramucirumab in patients with previously treated advanced gastric cancer *Eur. J. Cancer.* **91** 86–91

[72] Shi J W, Liu S P, Yu Y *et al* 2019 RGD peptide-decorated micelles assembled from polymer-paclitaxel conjugates towards gastric cancer therapy *Colloids Surf. B* **180** 58–67

[73] Li X L, Yu N, Li J *et al* 2020 Novel 'carrier-free' nanofiber codelivery systems with the synergistic antitumor effect of paclitaxel and tetrandrine through the enhancement of mitochondrial apoptosis *ACS Appl. Mater. Interfaces* **12** 10096–106

[74] Fernandes E, Ferreira D, Peixoto A *et al* 2019 Glycoengineered nanoparticles enhance the delivery of 5-fluorouracil and paclitaxel to gastric cancer cells of high metastatic potential *Int. J. Pharm.* **570** 12

[75] Liu H M, Yuan M H, Liu Y S *et al* 2021 Self-monitoring and self-delivery of self-assembled fluorescent nanoparticles in cancer therapy *Int. J. Nanomed.* **16** 2487–99

[76] Zhou Y, Sun X Z, Zhou L S and Zhang X Z 2020 pH-sensitive and long-circulation nanoparticles for near-infrared fluorescence imaging-monitored and chemo-photothermal synergistic treatment against gastric cancer *Front. Pharmacol.* **11** 14

[77] Yang Z, Luo H Y, Cao Z *et al* 2016 Dual-targeting hybrid nanoparticles for the delivery of SN38 to Her2 and CD44 overexpressed human gastric cancer *Nanoscale* **8** 11543–58

[78] Chang H J, Choi M Y, Cho M *et al* 2019 Molecular mechanism of chemoresistance and restoration in human gastric cancer cells *J. Clin. Oncol.* **37** 1

[79] Vinardell M P and Mitjans M 2015 Antitumor activities of metal oxide nanoparticles *Nanomaterials* **5** 1004–21

[80] Azimee S, Rahmati M, Fahimi H and Moosavi M A 2020 TiO$_2$ nanoparticles enhance the chemotherapeutic effects of 5-fluorouracil in human AGS gastric cancer cells via autophagy blockade *Life Sci.* **248** 9

[81] Yang C X, Pang X, Chen W H *et al* 2019 Environmentally responsive dual-targeting nanotheranostics for overcoming cancer multidrug resistance *Sci. Bull.* **64** 705–14

[82] Liu Y, Zhang P, Li F, Jin X, Li J, Chen W and Li Q 2018 Nanoenhancersmetal-based for future radiotherapy: radiosensitizing and synergistic effects on tumor cells *Theranostics* **8** 1824–49

[83] Azizi S, Ghasemi A, Asgarian-Omran H *et al* 2019 Cerium oxide nanoparticles sensitize non-small lung cancer cell to ionizing radiation *Marmara Pharm. J.* **822** 307–13

[84] Zhang C, Huang P, Bao L, He M *et al* 2011 Enhancement of gastric cell radiation sensitivity by chitosan-modified gold nanoparticles *J. Nanosci. Nanotechnol.* **11** 9528–35

[85] Huang P, Yang D P, Zhang C L *et al* 2011 Protein-directed one-pot synthesis of Ag microspheres with good biocompatibility and enhancement of radiation effects on gastric cancer cells *Nanoscale* **3** 3623–26

[86] Batooei S, Khajeali A and Khodadadi Islamian J P 2020 Metal-based nanoparticles as radio-sensitizer in gastric cancer therapy *J. Drug Deliv. Sci. Technol.* **56** 6

[87] Ju C Y, Wen Y J, Zhang L P *et al* 2019 Neoadjuvant chemotherapy based on abraxane/human neutrophils cytopharmaceuticals with radiotherapy for gastric cancer *Small* **15** 10

[88] Wang Y B, Wu W B, Mao D, Teh C, Wang B and Liu B 2020 Metal-organic framework assisted and tumor microenvironment modulated synergistic image-guided photo-chemo therapy *Adv. Funct. Mater.* **30** 2002431

[89] Zuo W, Chen D, Fan Z *et al* 2020 Design of light/ROS cascade-responsive tumor-recognizing nanotheranostics for spatiotemporally controlled drug release in locoregional photo-chemotherapy *Acta Biomater.* **111** 327–40

[90] Yang Z, Wang J, Li X *et al* 2020 Defeating relapsed and refractory malignancies through a nano-enabled mitochondria-mediated respiratory inhibition and damage pathway *Biomaterials* **229** 119580

[91] Chen J, He G M, Xian G Y *et al* 2020 Mechanistic biosynthesis of SN-38 coated reduced graphene oxide sheets for photothermal treatment and care of patients with gastric cancer *J. Photochem. Photobiol., B* **204** 7

[92] Singh M, Harris-Birtill D C C, Zhou Y *et al* 2016 Application of gold nanorods for photothermal therapy in *ex vivo* human oesophagogastric adenocarcinoma *J. Biomed. Nanotechnol.* **12** 481–90

[93] Zhang A M, Pan S J, Zhang Y H *et al* 2019 Carbon–gold hybrid nanoprobes for real-time imaging, photothermal/photodynamic and nanozyme oxidative therapy *Theranostics* **9** 3443–58

[94] Apicella M, Corso S and Giordano S 2017 Targeted therapies for gastric cancer: failures and hopes from clinical trials *Oncotarget* **8** 57654–69

[95] Dai X and Tan C 2015 Combination of microRNA therapeutics with small-molecule anticancer drugs: mechanism of action and co-delivery nanocarriers *Adv. Drug Deliv. Rev.* **81** 184–97

[96] Chen W, Yang S, Wei X *et al* 2020 Construction of aptamer-siRNA Chimera/PEI/5-FU/ carbon nanotube/collagen membranes for the treatment of peritoneal dissemination of drug-resistant gastric cancer *Adv. Healthcare Mater.* **9**

[97] Cheng X J, Fan K L, Wang L *et al* 2020 TfR1 binding with H-ferritin nanocarrier achieves prognostic diagnosis and enhances the therapeutic efficacy in clinical gastric cancer *Cell Death Dis* **11** 13

[98] Meng X B, Wang K, Lv L *et al* 2019 Photothermal/photodynamic therapy with immune-adjuvant liposomal complexes for effective gastric cancer therapy *Part. Part. Syst. Charact.* **36** 9

[99] Deng L Z, Guo W H, Li G X *et al* 2019 Hydrophobic IR780 loaded sericin nanomicelles for phototherapy with enhanced antitumor efficiency *Int. J. Pharm.* **566** 549–56

[100] Farjadian F, Ghasemi A, Gohari O *et al* 2019 Nanopharmaceuticals and nanomedicines currently on the market: challenges and opportunities *Nanomedicine* **14** 93–126

[101] Nagtegaal I D, Odze R D, Klimstra D *et al* 2020 Edito WHOCT: the 2019 WHO classification of tumours of the digestive system *Histopathology* **76** 182–8

[102] Tian R, Ma H L, Zhu S J *et al* 2020 Multiplexed NIR-II Probes for lymph node-invaded cancer detection and imaging-guided surgery *Adv. Mater.* **32** 10

[103] Zhang W J, Song S C, Wang H X *et al* 2019 *In vivo* irreversible albumin-binding near-infrared dye conjugate as a naked-eye and fluorescence dual-mode imaging agent for lymph node tumor metastasis diagnosis *Biomaterials* **217** 11

[104] Liu S, Jiang X, Tian X *et al* 2020 A method to measure the denatured proteins in the corona of nanoparticles based on the specific adsorption of Hsp90ab1 *Nanoscale* **12** 15857–68

[105] Yoo J W, Irvine D J, Discher D E and Mitragotri S 2011 Bio-inspired, bioengineered and biomimetic drug delivery carriers *Nat. Rev. Drug Discovery* **10** 521–35

[106] Wu P, Zhang B, Ocansey D K W, Xu W and Qian H 2020 Extracellular vesicles: a bright star of nanomedicine *Biomaterials* **269** 120467

[107] Alipour M, Baneshi M, Hosseinkhani S *et al* 2020 Recent progress in biomedical applications of RGD-based ligand: from precise cancer theranostics to biomaterial engineering: a systematic review *J. Biomed. Mater. Res.* A **108** 839–50

[108] Cheng Z, Al Zaki A, Hui J Z, Muzykantov V R and Tsourkas A 2012 Multifunctional nanoparticles: cost versus benefit of adding targeting and imaging capabilities *Science* **338** 903–10

IOP Publishing

Nanobiotechnology and Artificial Intelligence in Gastrointestinal Diseases

Vivek K Chaturvedi, Anurag Kumar Singh, Jay Singh and Dawesh P Yadav

Chapter 7

Role of nanoparticles for the treatment of gastric cancer

Ravi Kumar Yadav, Shefali Singh, Zeba Azim, Niraj Kumar Goswami and Navneet Yadav

The second-leading cause of cancer-related fatalities worldwide is gastric cancer (GC). The advancement in medicine will probably be linked to the research of cancer biology, followed by the formation of a customized and molecular-based method for the administration of anticancer medications. Proper medications for cancerous diseases rely highly on their timely diagnosis for which *in vivo* molecular imaging technique is popular but a trend for a more feasible approach is seen as molecular imaging requires specialized molecular probes. The use of nanoparticles (NPs) is the current paradigm for diagnosing and treating GC. With the advent of extensive explorations in the field of nanotechnology (NT), NPs have been realized to have proficient curative properties for GC. Since the past decade, extensive research work has been allocated to applications of NPs in the direction of therapeutics and diagnosis. Several reports have documented that NPs-based therapeutic agents overcome problems associated with conventional therapy. However, it seems that perusal of the characteristics of NPs and their interactive efficacies with biological entities is vital to analyze the potential of NPs-based nanomedicines and NPs-based diagnostic protocols. Today green synthesized NPs are also used as a potential agent for GC treatment. This study is significant since NPs might also pose certain side effects and toxicity and these aspects should be well addressed prior to the utilization of NPs in biological systems. This chapter will encompass the diverse purview of NPs and how this can be a plausible alternative in the diagnosis and therapeutic treatment of gastric cancer.

7.1 Introduction

Biotic and abiotic variables contribute to a variety of diseases that impact humans. These illnesses not only have an effect on day-to-day life but also result in fatalities

doi:10.1088/978-0-7503-6134-7ch7

for people. As a result of the way we live, cancer is increasingly the most common life-threatening illness in the world. According to Piazuelo and Correa [1], one of the most prevalent cancer kinds worldwide is GC. Despite the anticipated drop in incidence, GC still ranks third in mortality and fifth in morbidity among all diagnosed malignancies, making it a major cause of cancer-related fatalities [2]. The high prevalence and poor prognosis of stomach cancer is a public health concern, particularly in East Asia [3]. The majority of patients are diagnosed at an advanced stage, with a poor prognosis and quality of life. The World Health Organisation (WHO) categorises GC as papillary, tubular, mucinous, or poorly cohesive carcinomas. However, no accurate biological categorization approach has been established, and clinical relevance is restricted [4].

Currently, the most common clinical treatments for GC are surgical resection, chemotherapy, radiation, and molecular targeted therapy [5]. With the discovery of various molecular pathways in malignancy, molecular targeted therapy has seen significant progress in recent years. However, only a few targets, like VEGFR-2, HER2, PD-1, and others, are utilized to create GC medicines [6]. Furthermore, the most classic small molecule inhibitors act on the active site of the target to impede its action. The development of targeted therapy for GC is currently limited due to the scarcity of pharmacological targets and related technology. NT is a novel and promising technology and its application in various areas like agriculture, industrial, medicinal, and energy production is appreciable. NT in medicine and healthcare is referred to as nanomedicine, and it has been utilized to combat some of the most common ailments, viz., heart-related disease and cancer. Due to its diverse imaging and therapeutic capabilities, the nano platform has emerged as a potential technique for cancer theranostics and surgery guidance [7]. Because of their distinctively small sizes, NPs are used as contrast agents and as carriers for the administration of medications. For instance, cancer tissue has poor lymphatic drainage and leaky vasculature, NPs are more likely to infiltrate the interstitium and prolong tumor retention [8]. Addressing concerns including *in vivo* stability, rapid clearance of contrast agents, and the limited effectiveness and adverse effects of the usual treatment are crucial [9]. Specific ligands were also used to functionalize and modify some nanomaterials (NMs) (figure 7.1). NPs have diverse application in medicine and ever

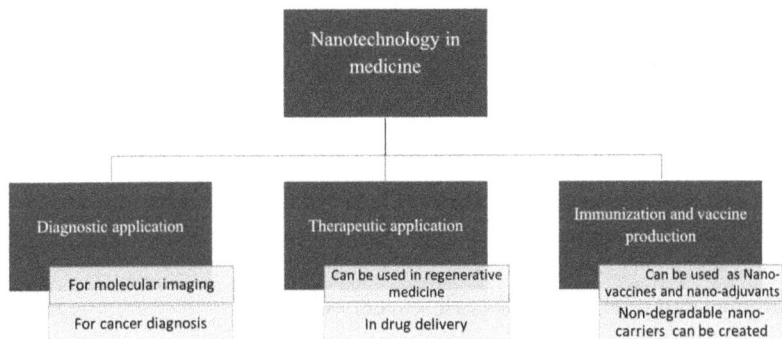

Figure 7.1. Applications of NPs in the field of medicine.

since their pioneering work in the field of medicine, they have performed substantially in easing several complex protocols of cancer diagnosis, have complemented well for therapeutics and can prove remarkable in the field of immunization.

7.2 Nanoparticles as drug delivery systems

NPs are regarded as magic bullets due to their special size and shape. Paul Ehrlich's idea of a miraculous cure has been refined into nanomedicine. To prepare a targeted-delivery system, a wide range of NPs can be utilized. NPs enable the modification of parameters such as the solubility, diffusivity, half-life, toxicity, pharmacokinetics, pharmacodynamics, and biodistribution of medications and therapeutic agents, adding a new level of engineering and control to medicine.

7.2.1 Advantages of nanoparticles for drug delivery

NT has the potential to aid in the treatment of chronic human ailments by delivering medications to particular places. In recent decades, effective and safe drug delivery via nanocarriers has been created. Drug delivery systems (DDSs) based on NMs can deliver drugs to diseased cells in a controlled releasing way. NMs are nanoscale materials (sizes ranging from 1 to 100 nm) [10]. NMs and NPs have diverse physicochemical, optical, conductive, and biological properties that can be adjusted. These distinguishing characteristics are owing to their small size and vast surface area. NMs display quantum qualities and unique features due to their huge surface area-to-volume ratio [11]. The use of NMs and nanostructures as DDSs has sparked interest in nanomedicine [12]. DDS can deliver medications to specific tissues in a regulated manner. In these nanocarriers, medications can be chemically conjugated or physically enclosed [13]. Because of their nanoscale size and vast surface area, NMs can easily permeate cells and interact with biomolecules. The use of NT in drug delivery can increase absorption, bioavailability, and stability while addressing the drawbacks of standard DDSs.

7.2.2 Types of nanoparticles used in gastric cancer treatment

In order to promote human health, NPs are increasingly being used in medical research. Using nanosize materials like biocompatible NPs [14] and nanorobots [15] for various applications, such as diagnosis, delivery, sensory, or actuation purposes in a living entity, nanomedicine uses NT to prevent and treat various diseases [16].

Today, the different metallic NMs viz., old, iron, and others, are used for treatment of GC. Drugs with very low solubility have a number of biopharmaceutical delivery problems, including limited bioaccess after oral intake, decreased ability to diffuse into the outer membrane, a higher dosage needed for intravenous administration, and unfavourable side effects occurring before the conventionally formulated vaccination process.

7.2.3 Targeted drug delivery to gastric cancer cells

Delivery systems have seen tremendous progress in transporting curative agents or bio-active chemicals to their target site to heal different diseases [17]. There have been many successful DDSs in recent years. However, some obstacles must be addressed, and novel technology must be created to ensure successful drug delivery to its targeted and specific location [9]. The standard and simple drug delivery pattern is not fully functioned to remedy GC cells. The target drug delivery is considered a boon for GC cell diagnosis. As a result, nano-based DDSs are currently being researched to support the enhanced DDS. Only a handful of NP-based therapies have been approved for clinical use [18].

7.3 Nanoparticles for imaging and diagnosis

Diagnostic imaging refers to numerous procedures for in-depth study of the body to determine the causes of sickness or damage and confirm a diagnosis. Developing unique detection techniques helps early cure of different diseases [19]. The pressing need for early disease identification and diagnosis drives the improvement of imaging techniques and contrast agents. Current problems include quick and comprehensive imaging of tissue microstructures and lesion characterization, which could be accomplished by developing nontoxic contrast agents with longer circulation duration [20]. NPs-based technology opens a new window for the curing of diseases. This is made possible via NP-based technology [21]. The novel NP-based contrast agents working in most common biomedical imaging modalities and fluorescence imaging are considered essential tools. These traditional tools and techniques like magnetic resonance imaging (MRI), computerized tomography (CT), positron emission tomography (PET) and single-photon emission computed tomography (SPECT) are helpful for detection [22].

7.3.1 Nanoparticles in gastric cancer imaging

The imaging of GC also uses nano-based techniques. Traditional imaging techniques, such as MRI, CT, PET, SPECT, and PET-CT, are frequently utilized in clinical practise for GC detection and diagnosis. Contrast agents, on the other hand, are constrained to a single imaging modality, a rapid clearance, and other unfavourable side effects, as well as poorly tailored biodistribution. The different NPs with built-in characteristics or functional modifications provide insight into the creation of new, more effective imaging techniques for the detection of stomach cancer. The same advantages apply to all of them: real-time imaging, targeted accumulation in tumors and local metastases, improved tumor-background ratio, excellent sensitivity, and high resolution. Biomarkers were employed in the instance of GC tissue to create new NPs. Transmembrane receptors called integrins are involved in cellular interactions with the extracellular matrix. On the surface of several cancer cells, particularly stomach cancer, and activated endothelial cells of tumorneovasculature, $\alpha v\beta 3$ integrin is overexpressed. In contrast, it expresses itself at a remarkably low level in healthy cells [23].

7.3.2 Contrast agents and theranostic nanoparticles

Recently, there has been increased interest in integrating contrast and therapy. Theranostic medicine is a novel discipline of medicine that incorporates diagnostic and focused therapy into a single drug. Theranostic agents provide both imaging and treatment. These characteristics of theranostic agents provide synergistic benefits over standard contrast agents, which are used to see inside the body. To boost theranostic agent efficiency, the contrasting effect at the target site must be increased, or the desired therapeutic effect must be achieved. A number of compounds are used in theranostic technology. Various ways on theranostic compounds have been used to improve target-specific imaging. To boost contrast effect at target sites, targeting antibodies, peptides, aptamers, siRNAcodelivery, pH-sensitive polymers, temperature-sensitive polymers, catalyst-responsive polymers, light-sensitive polymers, ultrasound sensitive polymers, and magnetic stimuli polymers have been studied. Furthermore, many treatment strategies for different disease types, including chemotherapy, radiation, nucleic acid therapy, phototherapy, and hyperthermia treatment, have been developed to improve therapeutic efficacy.

7.3.3 Molecular imaging and targeting approaches

Mankoff [24] defined molecular imaging as the capacity to see and assess cellular and biological activities *in vivo*. The rapidly developing field of molecular imaging offers advancements in specificity and quantitation for screening and early diagnosis, focused and individualized therapy, and earlier treatment follow-up. Anatomical imaging is helpful for diagnosis, surgical guidance and treatment. *In vivo* molecular imaging's main benefit is its ability to diagnose diseases in diseased tissues without invasive biopsies or surgical procedures. Along with this data, a more individualized treatment planning regimen can be used.

7.4 Therapeutic applications of nanoparticles in gastric cancer

NPs have found their way into therapeutics, more specifically in the case of cancer treatments. For therapeutics, certain properties of NPs such as specific sizes, shapes, and surface characteristics are crucial in determining the efficiency of the nano-drug delivery and thus control therapeutic efficacy, as highlighted by Bahrami *et al* [25]. Size specificity is an important criterion for NPs-based drugs as NPs within 10–100 nm diameter range can effectively deliver drugs and achieve enhanced permeability and retention effect [26]. Li *et al* [27] also supported using NPs in GC treatment owing to their high efficacy. Figure 7.2 displays multifarious applications of NPs in augmenting therapeutic potentials.

7.4.1 Chemotherapy with nanoparticle formulations

Chemotherapy is the most widely used treatment for tumor cells. But the idea of non-selective killing of all growing cells in the affected area, be it a tumor or normal cells, threatens serious adverse effects on vital activities such as hair loss, suppression of bone marrow and various gastrointestinal reactions [28]. NP-based medicines have substantially helped find better target-specific drug delivery machinery. NPs have been extensively used recently for targeted drug delivery in cancer treatment and chemotherapy based on their high reliability, biocompatibility and biodegradability [29]. NP-based chemotherapy offers an advantage in efficiently crossing the

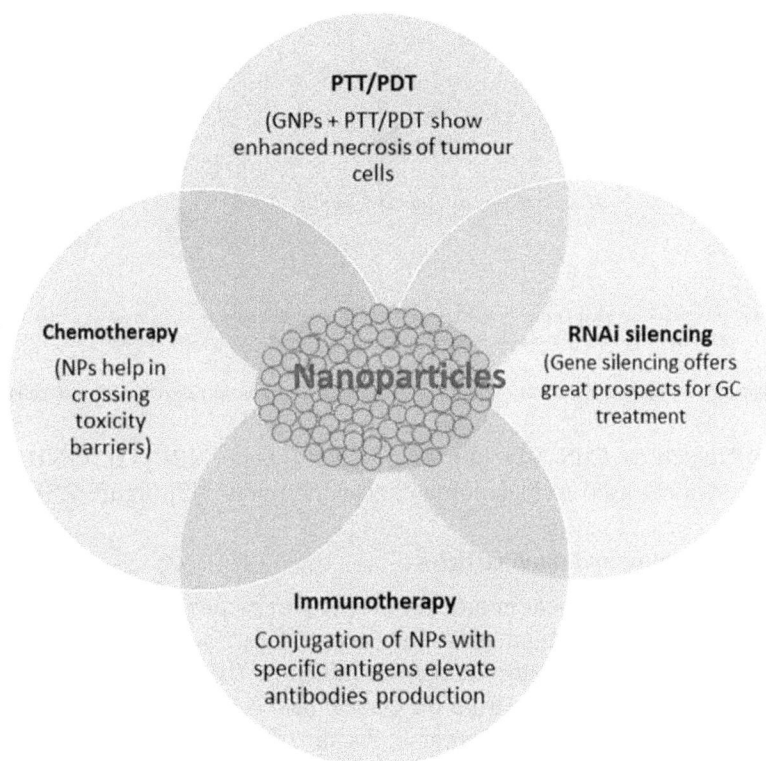

PTT/PDT
(GNPs + PTT/PDT show enhanced necrosis of tumour cells

Chemotherapy
(NPs help in crossing toxicity barriers)

Nanoparticles

RNAi silencing
(Gene silencing offers great prospects for GC treatment

Immunotherapy
Conjugation of NPs with specific antigens elevate antibodies production

Figure 7.2. Applications of NPs in various facets of therapeutics.

toxicity barriers of therapeutics. For instance, a chemomedicine PTX is highly unsuitable for injection owing to its lipophilic properties, but when it is formulated with Abraxanealbumin NPs, this drug formulation exhibits stability and decreases the toxicities simultaneously [30]. Clinical trials on Abraxane deduced promising results for GC treatment; thus, the drug was approved by the FDA for GC therapy [31]. Jain [32] established the use of magnetic fields for NP-based chemotherapic formulations.

7.4.2 Photothermal and photodynamic therapy

In the quest to find suitable therapeutic protocols, photo-triggered based therapies have evolved in the form of photothermal therapy and photodynamic therapy to fight against human malignancies. Mocan *et al* [33] gave a detailed account of photothermal treatment by center-focusing on the use of GNPs. GNPs based-photothermal therapy that employs GNPs can potently destroy tumor/cancerous cells via selective necrosis at cellular levels [34–36]. GNPs are highly promising for photothermal therapies for gastrointestinal tumors. Singh *et al* [37] and Batooei *et al* [38] highlighted that photothermal treatment could target tumor tissue to heat it while sparing healthy tissues. Different types of NPs are employed in PTT, but GNPs specifically accumulate in tumor tissue [39]. Several workers have designed

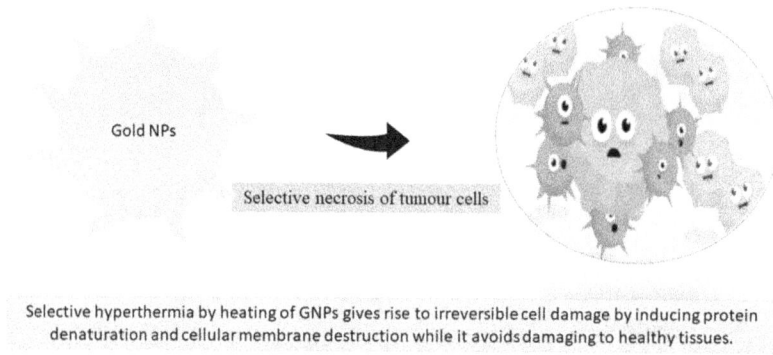

Gold NPs

Selective necrosis of tumour cells

Selective hyperthermia by heating of GNPs gives rise to irreversible cell damage by inducing protein denaturation and cellular membrane destruction while it avoids damaging to healthy tissues.

Figure 7.3. GNPs are used in photothermal therapy for induced necrosis of tumor cells.

metallic NPs such as CuS NPs [40, 41], and graphene NPs [42]. GNPs are also known to be widely used in melanoma cancer treatment [43] (figure 7.3).

7.4.3 Immunotherapy and nanoparticles

NPs have proven to be efficient in targeted chemotherapy procedures. Immunotherapy is considered as a quintessential pillar for cancer. This novel idea evolved with the realization of the role of immune checkpoint inhibitors (ICIs) in treating tumor cells. ICIs have gained good reception from the clinical field because of their high efficacy in several malignancies, such as GC. Recent works have documented extensive research on the changing trends in the field of immunotherapy [44, 45].

7.4.4 RNA interference (RNAi) and gene therapy

Fire *et al* [46] discovered a revolutionizing technique of RNA interference that opened new prospects in the field of oncology, as described by Wang *et al* [47]. RNAi is involved in post-transcriptional modification and gene silencing. This technique has immense possibilities in health as RNAi exclusively represses the target gene expression of the concerned genes by blocking their translation into proteins. That RNA-induced silencing complex (RISC), which functions as an endonuclease on target messenger RNA (mRNA), specifically uses RNAi to silence genes is a likely explanation. As a result, RNAi regulates gene expression via influencing the post-transcriptional stage by identifying and cleaving mRNA in conjunction with RISC [48–50]. Several classical works of deploying RNAi technique for GC treatment are reported. The homoeobox Nanog protein (an integral part of pluripotent stem cells) seems to be associated with GC invasion in cells [51]. The small hairpin loop RNA suppresses the Nanog gene expression. The expression of Nanog is silenced by this shRNA, which prevents cancer cells from proliferating, migrating, and invading [52]. This methodology might serve as an experimental foundation for a gene therapy strategy to treat GC. Tian *et al* [53] reviewed a multitude of prospects RNAi in cancer therapy. They opined that compared with traditional gene therapy, RNAi has more promising outcomes owing to its high efficiency and stability. This states the reason for RNAi being one of the widely used tumor gene therapy strategies. RNAi-based gene therapy is used in various cancer diseases, such as breast cancer. Zuo *et al* [54] reviewed and opined that regulation of defective gene expression through gene therapy is emerging as a promising strategy for treating breast cancer, a prevalent ailment in females. Genetic modification of target cells using siRNAs and miRNAs has shown promising results [55]. Several antiapoptotic miRNAs such as miR-17–92, miR-21, miR-214, miR-221 and miR-222 have been shown to directly down-regulate the expression of pro-apoptotic molecules such as PTEN. PTEN is a critical tumor suppressor molecule that often gets mutated in cancerous cells [56, 57]. Some essential drugs have been designed against cancer diseases using RNAi technique, such as Ampligen[58], Genasense [59], IMO-2125 [60] LY-900003 [61]. Tam *et al* [62] described the efficacy of long-coding RNA(lncRNA) combined with miRNAs in synergistic regulation of gastric and colorectal cancers.

7.5 Nanoparticles for combination therapy

In present times, our situation to fight with life-threatening cancerous cells has achieved an appreciable benchmark with the arrival of novel protocols for cancer diagnosis and treatment. However, there is still room for improvement. Patients often require more sophisticatedly planned medication strategies such as a combination of gene therapy, immunotherapy, PTT and PDT.

7.5.1 Synergistic effects of nanoparticle-based combination therapies

So far, we have discussed individual methods such PTT/PDT, chemotherapy, immunotherapy and RNAi as tools for oncogene cells. However, recent trends direct for adopting better synergistic efforts for simultaneous diagnosis and medication protocols. NPs DOX-IR820 was combined with PTT/chemotherapy for enhanced tumor combatting strategies, as reported by Zhou *et al* [63]. In this study, NPs were trained to treat GC using chemo-photothermal synergistic therapy and continuous imaging. After one therapy shot, the fluorescent signal persisted in the cancer tissues for almost a week. The results gave concrete findings of the synergistic effects of PCC NPs in suppression of tumors, which was more significant than that of single chemotherapy or photothermal treatment [63]. For instance, Meng *et al* [64] reported a combination of PTT/PDT with chemotherapy and adjuvant immunotherapy established and promoted strong antitumor immune responses. Dai *et al* [65] reviewed combination strategies of miRNAs with small anticancer drugs that were fabricated with sophisticated NP carriers for efficient co-delivery. Several reports have presented this combination therapy [66–68]. Immunotherapy in combination with PTT/PDT chemotherapy has also been shown to substantially elevate the therapeutic potential in the case of cancer biology, as underlined by Meng *et al* [64]. Similarly, the synergistic effect of chemotherapy and immunotherapy also offers promising potential against tumors, as Davern and Lysaght [69] reported. Their findings show that, in addition to immune evasion, immune checkpoint-intrinsic signaling in cancer cells promotes proliferation, metastasis, glycolysis, DNA repair, and chemoresistance. Combining ICIs with chemotherapy can emerge as an attractive putative therapeutic strategy.

A combination of Pembrolizumab (a humanized IgG4 monoclonal antibody) with trastuzumab received accelerated approval by the FDA. It addressed for first-line chemotherapy for patients with HER2-positive GC, as reported by Janjigian *et al* [70].

7.5.2 Sequential and simultaneous delivery of therapeutics

The use of NPs in drug design and therapy has been covered in detail thus far. NT genuinely contributes to medicine delivery. Drugs can be loaded onto nanodevices and delivered with fewer adverse effects to specific locations. The main type of vector for gene therapy may be cationic polymers like chitosan, which can form complexes with DNA or siRNA. For siRNA administration *in vivo*, liposomes and cationic polymers are most frequently utilized [71, 72]. The science of theranostics NPs enables pairing diagnostic biomarkers with therapeutic agents so that target diseased tissues can be directly studied and treated. Theranostic nanoplex with advanced multimodality imaging reporters such as fluorescent dyes, radioisotopes and PSMA-targeting moiety were developed for delivering small interfering RNA (siRNA) and a prodrug enzyme to PSMA-expressing tumors [73].

7.6 Challenges and limitations of nanoparticle-based therapy

7.6.1 Biocompatibility and toxicity concerns

NPs along with the pre-requisite medicine, get access to living cells, and therefore, all the pros and cons associated with its biocompatibility and toxicity concerns must be critically assessed. NPs have been extensively approved and validated for their biocompatibility by various studies [72, 74–76]. Nanodevices and nano-based medicines are highly biocompatible, nontoxic and of high specificity. GNPs have attracted considerable attention due to their proficient biocompatibility and ease of synthesis [77, 78]. Blum and Saltzman [79] also approved GNPs as highly biocompatible but reported a certain level of nephrotoxicity. There are certain complications in combination treatment due to the different pharmacokinetic properties of certain drugs. For example, Doxorubicin, a chemotherapy drug, is combined with IR-820, a drug used in tumor photothermal therapy. The combination of DOX and IR-820 has a lot of potential, but each of these medications has unique pharmacokinetic characteristics that make it challenging to obtain good accumulation and performance in cancer tissues at the same time. Therefore, there are certain critical technical concerns with *in vivo* delivery and stability of the two medicines that must be further overcome before clinical trials [80]. Since NPs are directly used in drug delivery, molecular visualization and imaging, hence NPs-associated cellular toxicity should also be discussed. Some seminal research papers have heavily focused on this parameter. Manke *et al* [81] discussed multiple facets of NP-induced toxicity, such as increased production of reactive oxygen species (ROS) as well as depletion of antioxidant reservoirs by inducing cellular oxidative stress. Excessive oxidative stress causes mitochondrial membrane damage and electron chain malfunction, which finally leads to DNA damage and apoptosis [81]. Silica or silicon dioxide (SiO_2) NPs induce oxidative stress in human umbilical vein endothelial cells (HUVECs) [82].

7.6.2 Nanoparticle clearance and stability

Optimal and reasonable utilization of NPs can be accomplished only when we intimately follow and unravel the whole passage of NPs from their inception to their exit in the human body or living cellular entities. Researchers must increase our understanding of how physicochemical qualities may affect the fate and consequences of rational NPs on the body [76] before creating them. While more significant-sized NPs can accumulate in the organs and increase toxicity levels in prolonged exposure, inorganic NPs with hydrodynamic sizes of less than 5 nm can be efficiently removed from the body through renal clearance and still maintain efficient tumor targeting.

7.6.3 Regulatory aspects and clinical translation

Studies on NPs-based therapeutics are state-of-the-art, and witnessing continuous revival and novel ideas. Some of these studies are in a very nascent stage, but these need to be explored here as these techniques have enough potential to bring a paradigm shift in the field of cancer biology. Chen *et al* [83] performed a meta-analysis of clinical trials for a testing combination of immunotherapy and chemotherapy to the efficacy of anti-PD1 (anti-programmed cell death-1), anti-PD-L1 and anti-CTLA-4 ICIs in advanced GC which demonstrated that the addition of ICIs to the second- and third-line setting for treating gastric ovarian cancer improves some, but not all survival end points. NPs develop a positive charge on their surface, which implicitly hinders cellular adsorption and leads to toxicity. This issue has been raised in the case of GNPs coated with amphiphilic polymers having different surface charges since such particles have a positive charge and are more toxic [84]. This issue can be solved by altering the surface with zwitterionic or neutral organic coatings while also achieving minimal hydrodynamic size and great stability in biological conditions [85]. Similarly, toxicity concerns and leaching of ions from inorganic NPs of a heavy metal atom can be reduced by sophisticated NP engineering by coating the surface with biocompatible molecules [86]. Coating GNPs with polyethylene glycol (PEG) avoided immunotoxic responses, as reported by Chen and Gao [87]. Problems also arise owing to different chemical composition, size and structure of NPs. The new technology of *in silico* method is developing to answer this concern.

7.7 Preclinical and clinical studies with nanoparticles for gastric cancer

GC is generally the most common malignant tumor, and the fourth (after lungs, breast, and colorectal) leading cause of death related to cancer worldwide [88]. Adenocarcinomas are the common type of GC and more than 95% of cases are adenocarcinoma type [89] gastro-oesophageal-junction adenocarcinomas [90]. The heterogeneous group of malignant lesions with a range of etiologic factors related to stomach are adenocarcinomas. The potential applications of NMs in medicine are increasingly being explored day by day. Due to unique characteristics such as high sensitivity, permeability and specificity, NPs have been used in the early diagnosis of GI cancers. Nanotechnologies have been used for the detection of tumors and as contrasting agent in MRI-based clinical applications. The application of NT in drugs or gene delivery systems in GC shows tremendous relevance for high therapeutic efficacy in cancer treatment.

7.7.1 Preclinical studies and animal models

Preclinical experimental models are decisive towards the development and promotion in oncological studies. Currently, experimental tumors are generally constructed on the basis of many factors such as xenograft, genetic engineering, editing and toxicity induction [91]. The mouse model is the most frequently used model organism in research of human cancer. They have passable physiological characteristics, complete genome sequencing, high fertility and growth, and high-efficiency experiments can be carried out in relatively little time [92]. In comparison to normal cells and blood vessels, the expression tissue factor was higher in human vascular endothelium and lung cancer cells of transplanted tumors in nude mice [93]. Zebrafish, a non-mammalian animal model, has an early-stage non-specific immunity, which is used to create the xenograft model of cancer [94]. Zebrafish tumor models have been successfully constructed and used through targeted gene regulation in lung cancer and GC [95, 96].

7.7.2 Clinical trials and human studies

Recently, in clinical treatments of GC, some target drugs are used. On the basis of overall survival and progression free survival, trastuzumab is the pioneer therapy for the patient of epidermal growth factor receptor (HER 2). Besides, ramucirumab and apatinib are second- and third-line therapies, respectively. TAS 102 is also used in GC patients. New target drugs are the way for improving therapeutic impact of GC [97].

7.7.3 Promising results and future directions

NPs are a potential avenue for developing current prophetic and GC therapeutic approaches. NPs are beneficial for imaging and drug delivery to specific target locations, as well as serving as delivery carriers that improve the pharmacological and therapeutic properties of cancer therapies. Incorporating NPs into drug molecules can shield a drug from degradation while also ensuring systematic drug targeting and release. But the long-term effects and potential toxicity of NPs exposure need to be carefully evaluated. Beyond this, the development of effectual and safe methods for the synthesis and functions of NPs is necessary for their clinical translation.

7.8 Nanoparticles in personalized medicine for gastric cancer

NT has revolutionized the field of oncology; NPs are successfully used in imaging, diagnosis, and tumor therapies. NPs are also used in drug delivery to improve administration methods that upgrade traditional modalities in anticancer therapies [98]. The use of NPs in drug delivery is one of the potential applications because the surface properties of NPs allocate them to the target diseased cells selectively without harming close healthy cells. NPs can also be used for diagnostic functions (such as in biological recognition of specific bimolecular or contrast agents in medical imaging) and also designed in such a way that can allow sustained drug delivery over time. NMs also act as carrier for signaling molecules that endorse tissue repair and regeneration. NPs are also used in drug delivery, to improve administration methods that upgrade traditional modalities in anticancer therapies [98]. The strategies of using NMs have numerous advantages over chemotherapeutic drugs. NPs protect the therapeutic compounds in the bloodstream from increased level of enzymes and proteases from the highly acidic environment in stomach. The application of NPs is also useful in co-delivery of multiple diagnostic agents, controlled delivery of drugs over a fixed time period, for efficient treatment [99, 100].

7.8.1 Biomarker-driven nanoparticle therapies

The complicacy of aberrant molecular uniqueness of GC patients remains a hurdle and the molecular pathway of GC is still unclear. To explore the potent biomarkers and deciphering molecular mechanisms of GC that uphold the ratio of signal background and assisted theranostic performance. With adequate response following neoadjuvant treatment, the organ-sparing surgery seems feasible and acceptable for patients with advanced proximal GC. Cheng *et al* [101] developed a molecular probe with a surgical navigation system RGD-indocyanine green targeting integrin. HER2 is the overexpressed human epithelial growth factor related to chemoresistance, tumor invasion, metastasis in cancers. According to Kanazaki *et al* [102], iron oxide NPs containing anti-HER2 moieties include entire IgG, single fragment variable, and peptides. Tanaka *et al* [103] created a cisplatin-encapsulated transferrin-PEG liposome for peritoneal distribution of GC, and Iinuma *et al* [104] created CEA-targeted adenovirus-mediated gene delivery.

7.8.2 Individualized treatment approaches

The development of advanced accrual technologies such as genomics, transcriptomics, proteomics, metabolomics, etc is to comprehensively analyze DNA, RNA, protein, and metabolites endowed with novel kinds of cancer detection [105]. At present, this omics technology has emerged as a new area in the molecular imaging field [106]. The molecular imaging (noninvasive medical imaging method) term can be defined as visualization, characterization, measurement and quantification of biological processes at the molecular, cellular and sub-cellular in oncology [107]. Molecular imaging plays a crucial role in earlier cancerous tumor detection, targeted drug delivery and imaging-based therapy [108]. At the early stage of tumor formation, molecular imaging can be assisted to detect malignant cells at cellular levels without any invasive operations like surgery or biopsy [109, 110]. SPECT, PET, optical frequency-domain imaging, fluorescence reflectance imaging, fluorescence-mediated tomography (FMT), bioluminescence imaging, multiphoton microscopy, and laser-scanning confocal microscopy are a few emerging molecular imaging technologies applied in preclinical and clinical stage [111–113]. Drug delivery is one of the most promising applications of NPs to overcome complicated barriers in the treatment of obstinate diseases. It appreciably improved their potential in therapy, and drugs with capabilities that are unfeasible to achieve via drug optimization.

7.9 Nanoparticle-based theranostics for gastric cancer

In recent years, many novel therapies (gene therapy, targeted therapy, etc) have emerged to endorse the treatment of cancer. For better results, combination therapies may prevail. By taking advantage of the flexibility of NPs there are myriads of nano-based designs that refer to theranostic NPs. Theranostic NPs provide the opportunity of synchronous diagnosis and treatment. NPs are known to act as contrasting agents, for example, combining chemotherapy immunotherapy with immunotherapy is an unprecedented opportunity to obtain better results [69]. To improve the therapeutic effectiveness in clinical GC and also achieve prognostic diagnosis, the combination of H-ferritin (nanocarrier) and TfR1 may also be a useful strategy [114]. However, several NP frameworks by themselves that have imaging capabilities, such as GNPs paired with CT and SPIONs for MRI, have been effectively exploited in theranostic system development. The therapeutic effects of SATB1 siRNA for GC therapy were studied using CD44-STAB1-ILNP immuno-liposomes and it was discovered that SATB1 protein production was suppressed by CD44 by delivery of SATB1 siRNA to CD44s on GCICs [115]. CT and MRI contrast agents frequently use inorganic NPs that comprise SPIONs (supermagnetic iron oxide NPs). As MRI contrast agents, SPIONs (ferumoxides and ferucarbotran) have received clinical approval. Magnetic fluorescent NPs containing BRCAA1 antibody have been used in models to target GC cells *in vivo*. This improves screening precision through visualizing GC cells by fluorescent MRI [116]. *In vitro* experiments, for targeted imaging of GC CD44v6 antibody tagged with poly-ethylene glycol (PEG). This signaling modality help in identifying the GC stem and prevent the recurrence of GC [117].

7.9.1 Diagnostic and therapeutic integration

The use of NPs in GC imaging opens up significant options for clinical strategy-based medication, formulation and diagnosis. MRI, PET, fluorescence imaging, CT etc are the notable imaging techniques for whole-body scan. Fluorescence imaging holds excellent qualities like quick imaging, high sensitivity, fast imaging, maximum safety, and low cost [118]. Besides their novelty, these techniques have non-specific distribution, hasty clearance, differences in imaging, and also adverse effects, that limit these wonderful techniques [119]. The unique size, surface properties, increased signal density, permeability etc are some features that make NPs a useful tool in the diagnosis of tumor [120]. CT (non-radioactive diagnosis) is extensively used in tumor detection. CT and MRI are combined with inorganic NPs for GC diagnosis. For the diagnosis of early-stage of GC, contrast-enhanced CT with targeting NPs contrast agent is used, and that improves accuracy [41]. Davis *et al* [121] documented that fluorescent substrate was cleaved by using Gd-doping CuS NPs fuses with a metal-loprotease-2 (MMP-2) and cRGD and Wu *et al* [122] reported optical or dual-modality MRI molecular probe.

7.9.2 Multifunctional nanoparticle platforms

Recently, owing to unique characteristics of NPs, NT has drawn a lot of scientific interest. The distinctive physical, chemical, and functional properties of NPs include their minute size, vast surface area, chemical composition, and structure [123]. In the bloodstream, NPs enhance the time of drug, they also increase the access and accumulation of pharmaceuticals at tumor sites, which increases the safety and acceptability of medications [124, 125]. Iron oxide NPs exhibit the unique property of superparamagnetism, belonging to the ferrimagnetic class [126]. Iron oxide NPs are used in biomedical applications [127] like MRI contrast, antigen/receptor ligand, magnetic targeting; lymph nodes etc. The low cost and high reproductibility are the the advantage of iron oxide NPs, but they have some limitations [128]. Carbon NPs are light weight, high tensile strength, chemically and thermally stable, easily penetrate into the tissue, and are used in active and passive targeting and therapeutic drug delivery [129]. Carbon nanotubes are used in initialization for the detection of lymph nodes and tumor localization [130]. GNPs are applied in MRI contrast, fluorescence, and multiple treatment opportunities. Dendrimers and nanoshells are used in boron neutron capture therapy, target drugs delivery and gene therapy [131, 132]. Polymers that have high thermal stability and biocompatibility are used in ligand antigen/receptor targeting, tumor micro-environment-dependent drug release [133].

7.10 Future perspectives and concluding remarks

NT, that entitled adaptable and immense modifications, helps in achieving specific and efficient tumor therapy. More precise cancer treatments with gene expression specificity can be accomplished through the targeted therapies that increase the survival rates of cancer patients. Nevertheless, the development of drug resistance and the absence of a regulated release impact remains a challenge. The main obstacles in mass production, however, that necessitated facilitating the clinical application of nanotherapeutics, are attaining storage and enhancing reducibility.

Acknowledgments

The authors are thankful to the colleagues of Department of Botany, K N Government P G College for their supreme cooperation and help. One of the authors, Z A, expresses gratitude to Department of Botany, University of Allahabad.

References

[1] Piazuelo M B and Correa P 2013 Gastric cancer: overview *Colomb. Med.* **44** 192–201
[2] Arnold M, Park J Y, Camargo M C, Lunet N, Forman D and Soerjomataram I 2020 Is gastric cancer becoming a rare disease? A global assessment of predicted incidence trends to 2035 *Gut* **69** 823–9

[3] Leake P A, Cardoso R, Seevaratnam R, Lourenco L, Helyer L, Mahar A and Coburn N G 2012 A systematic review of the accuracy and indications for diagnostic laparoscopy prior to curative-intent resection of gastric cancer *Gastric Cancer* **15** 38 47

[4] Nagy G A, Neag M A, Drasovean R, Crisan D and Chira R I 2022 Duodenal ampulla neuroendocrine tumor with GISTs of the proximal jejunum: a case report *Int. J. Mol. Sci.* **23** 10351

[5] Drossman D A and Hasler W L 2016 Rome IV—functional G.I. disorders: disorders of gut-brain interaction *Gastroenterology* **150** 1257–61

[6] Cetin B, Gumusay O, Cengiz M and Ozet A 2016 Advances of molecular targeted therapy in gastric cancer *J. Gastrointest. Cancer* **47** 125–34

[7] He S, Song J, Qu J and Cheng Z 2018 Crucial breakthrough of second near-infrared biological window fluorophores: design and synthesis toward multimodal imaging and theranostics *Chem. Soc. Rev.* **47** 4258–78

[8] Wong C, Stylianopoulos T, Cui J, Martin J, Chauhan V P, Jiang W and Fukumura D 2011 Multistage nanoparticle delivery system for deep penetration into tumor tissue *Proc. Natl Acad. Sci.* **108** 2426–31

[9] Li C, Wang J, Wang Y, Gao H, Wei G, Huang Y and Jin Y 2019 Recent progress in drug delivery *Acta Pharm. Sin.* B **9** 1145–62

[10] Sajid M 2016 Toxicity of nanoscale metal organic frameworks: a perspective *Environ. Sci. Pollut. Res.* **23** 14805–7

[11] Cheng L C, Jiang X, Wang J, Chen C and Liu R S 2013 Nano-bio effects: interaction of nanomaterials with cells *Nanoscale* **5** 3547–69

[12] Singh S 2010 Nanomedicine–nanoscale drugs and delivery systems *J. Nanosci. Nanotechnol.* **10** 906–7918

[13] Aryal S, Hu C M J, Fang R H, Dehaini D, Carpenter C, Zhang D E and Zhang L 2013 Erythrocyte membrane-cloaked polymeric nanoparticles for controlled drug loading and release *Nanomedicine* **8** 1271–80

[14] McNamara K and Tofail S A 2015 Nanosystems: the use of nanoalloys, metallic, bimetallic, and magnetic nanoparticles in biomedical applications *Phys. Chem. Chem. Phys.* **17** 27981–95

[15] Saadeh Y and Vyas D 2014 Nanorobotic applications in medicine: current proposals and designs *Am. J. Robot. Surg* **1** 4–11

[16] Golovin Y I, Gribanovsky S L, Golovin D Y, Klyachko N L, Majouga A G, Master A M and Kabanov A V 2015 Towards nanomedicines of the future: remote magneto-mechanical actuation of nanomedicines by alternating magnetic fields *J. Control. Release* **219** 43–60

[17] Garg T, Bhandari S, Rath G and Goyal A K 2015 Current strategies for targeted delivery of bio-active drug molecules in the treatment of brain tumor *J. Drug Target.* **23** 865–87

[18] Sahu T, Ratre Y K, Chauhan S, Bhaskar L V K S, Nair M P and Verma H K 2021 Nanotechnology based drug delivery system: current strategies and emerging therapeutic potential for medical science *J. Drug Deliv. Sci. Technol.* **63** 102487

[19] Hussain S, Mubeen I, Ullah N, Shah S S U D, Khan B A, Zahoor M and Sultan M A 2022 Modern diagnostic imaging technique applications and risk factors in the medical field: a review *BioMed Res. Int.* **2022** 5164970

[20] Han X, Xu K, Taratula O and Farsad K 2019 Applications of nanoparticles in biomedical imaging *Nanoscale* **11** 799–819

[21] Sim T M, Tarini D, Dheen S T, Bay B H and Srinivasan D K 2020 Nanoparticle-based technology approaches to the management of neurological disorders *Int. J. Mol. Sci.* **21** 6070

[22] Anttinen M, Ettala O, Malaspina S, Jambor I, Sandell M, Kajander S and Boström P J 2021 A prospective comparison of 18F-prostate-specific membrane antigen-1007 positron emission tomography computed tomography, whole-body 1.5 T magnetic resonance imaging with diffusion-weighted imaging, and single-photon emission computed tomography/computed tomography with traditional imaging in primary distant metastasis staging of prostate cancer (PROSTAGE) *Eur. Urol. Oncol* **4** 635–44

[23] Jin C, Zhang B N, Wei Z, Ma B, Pan Q and Hu P 2017 Effects of W.D.-3 on tumor growth and the expression of integrin αvβ3 and ERK1/2 in mice bearing human gastric cancer using the 18F-RGD PET/CT imaging system *Mol. Med. Rep.* **16** 9295–300

[24] Mankoff D A 2007 A definition of molecular imaging *J. Nucl. Med.* **48** 18N

[25] Bahrami B, Hojjat-Farsangi M, Mohammadi H, Anvari E, Ghalamfarsa G, Yousefi M et al 2017 Nanoparticles and targeted drug delivery in cancer therapy *Immunol. Lett.* **190** 64–83

[26] Yao Y, Zhou Y, Liu L, Xu Y, Chen Q, Wang Y, Wu S, Deng Y, Zhang J and Shao A 2020 Nanoparticle-based drug delivery in cancer therapy and its role in overcoming drug resistance *Front. Mol. Bioscie* **7** 193

[27] Li R, Liu B and Gao J 2017 The application of nanoparticles in diagnosisandtheranostics of gastric cancer *Cancer Lett.* **386** 123–30

[28] Zitvogel L, Apetoh L, Ghiringhelli F and Kroemer G 2008 Immunological aspects of cancer chemotherapy *Nat. Rev. Immunol.* **8** 59–73

[29] Li X, Ai S, Lu X, Liu S and Guan W 2021 Nanotechnology-based strategies for gastric cancer imaging and treatment *RSC Adv.* **11** 35392–407

[30] Li X, Wang L, Fan Y, Feng Q and Cui F Z 2012 Biocompatibility and toxicity of nanoparticles and nanotubes *J. Nanomater.* **2012** 548389

[31] Jang K, Yoon S, Kim S E, Cho J Y, Yoon S H, Lim K S, Yu K S, Jang I J and Lee H 2014 Novel nanocrystal formulation of megestrol acetate has improved bioavailability compared with the conventional micronized formulation in the fasting state *Drug Des. Devel. Ther* **2014** 851–8

[32] Jain K K 2017 Biomarkers of cancer In *The Handbook of Biomarkers* (New York: Humana Press) pp 273–462

[33] Mocan L et al 2016 Selective *in vitro* photothermal nano-therapy of MRSA infections mediated by IgG conjugated gold nanoparticles *Sci. Rep.* **6** 39466

[34] Iancu C, Ilie I R, Georgescu C E, Ilie R, Biris A R, Mocan T et al 2009 Applications of nanomaterials in cell stem therapies and the onset of nanomedicine *Particul. Sci. Technol.* **27** 562–74

[35] Akhter S, Ahmad M Z, Ahmad F J, Storm G and Kok R J 2012 Gold nanoparticles in theranostic oncology: current state-of-the-art *Expert Opin. Drug Deliv* **9** 1225–43

[36] Huo S, Ma H, Huang K, Liu J, Wei T, Jin S et al 2013 Superior penetration and retention behavior of 50 nm gold nanoparticles in tumors *Cancer Res.* **73** 319–30

[37] Singh M, Harris-Birtill D C, Markar S R, Hanna G B and Elson D S 2015 Application of gold nanoparticles for gastrointestinal cancer theranostics: a systematic review *Nanomedicine* **11** 2083–98

[38] Batooei S, Khajeali A, Khodadadi R and Islamian J P 2020 Metal-based nanoparticles as radio-sensitizer in gastric cancer therapy *J. Drug Deliv. Sci. Technol.* **56** 101576

[39] Wan Z, Zhang P, Lv L and Zhou Y 2020 NIR light-assisted phototherapies for bonerelated diseases and bone tissue regeneration: a systematic review *Theranostics* **10** 11837

[40] Shi H, Yan R, Wu L, Sun Y, Liu S, Zhou Z and Ye D 2018 Tumor-targeting CuS nanoparticles for multimodal imaging and guided photothermal therapy of lymph node metastasis *Acta Biomater.* **72** 256–65

[41] Shi H, Sun Y, Yan R, Liu S, Zhu L, Liu S and Ye D 2019 Magnetic semiconductor Gd-doping CuS nanoparticles as activatable nanoprobes for bimodal imaging and targeted photothermal therapy of gastric tumors *Nano Lett.* **19** 937–47

[42] Chen J, He G M, Xian G Y, Su X Q, Yu L L and Yao F 2020 Mechanistic biosynthesis of SN-38 coated reduced graphene oxide sheets for photothermal treatment and care of patients with gastric cancer *J. Photochem. Photobiol., B* **204** 111736

[43] Bagheri S, Yasemi M, Safaie-Qamsari E, Rashidiani J, Abkar M, Hassani M, Mirhosseini S A and Kooshki H 2018 Using gold nanoparticles in diagnosis and treatment of melanoma cancer *Artif. Cells Nanomed. Biotechnol.* **46** 462–71

[44] Avgustinovich A V, Bakina O V, Afanas' ev S G, Cheremisina O V, Spirina L V, Dobrodeev A Y, Buldakov M and Choynzonov E L 2021 Nanoparticles in gastric cancer management *Curr. Pharm. Des* **27** 2436–44

[45] Takei S, Kawazoe A and Shitara K 2022 The new era of immunotherapy in gastric cancer *Cancers* **14** 1054

[46] Fire A, Xu S, Montgomery M K *et al* 1998 Potent and specific genetic interference by double-stranded RNA in caenorhabditis elegans *Nature* **391** 806–11

[47] Wang Z, Rao D D, Senzer N, Nemunaitis J and Nemunaitis J 2011 RNA interference and cancer therapy *Pharm. Res.* **12** 2983–95

[48] Bader A G, Brown D and Winkler M 2010 The promise of microRNA replacement therapy *Cancer Res.* **70** 7027–30

[49] Wilson P A and Plucinski M 2011 A simple Bayesian estimate of direct RNAi gene regulation events from differential gene expression profiles *BMC Genomics* **12** 250

[50] Felipe A V, Oliveira J D, Chang P Y J, Moraes A A D F S, Silva T D D, Tucci-Viegas V M and Forones N M 2014 RNA interference: a promising therapy for gastric cancer *Asian Pac. J. Cancer Prev.* **15** 5509–15

[51] Lin T, Ding Y Q and Li J M 2012 Overexpression of Nanog protein is associated with poor prognosis in gastric adenocarcinoma *Med. Oncol* **29** 878–85

[52] Ji W and Jiang Z 2013 Effect of shRNA-mediated inhibition of Nanog gene expression on the behavior of human gastric cancer cells *Oncol Lett.* **6** 367–74

[53] Tian Z, Liang G, Cui K, Liang Y, Wang Q, Lv S and Zhang L 2021 Insight into the prospects for RNAi therapy of cancer *Front. Pharmacol* **12** 644718

[54] Zuo Y, Li Y, Zhou Z, Ma M and Fu K 2017 Long non-coding RNA MALAT1 promotes proliferation and invasion via targeting miR-129-5p in triple-negative breast cancer *Biomed. Pharmacother.* **95** 922–8

[55] Bottai G, Truffi M, Corsi F and Santarpia L 2017 Progress in nonviral gene therapy for breast cancer and what comes next? *Expert Opin. Biol. Ther.* **17** 595–611

[56] Pezzolesi M G, Platzer P, Waite K A and Eng C 2008 Differential expression of PTEN-targeting microRNAs miR-19a and miR-21 in Cowden syndrome *Am. J. Hum. Genet* **82** 1141–9

[57] Wang F, Li T, Zhang B, Li H, Wu Q, Yang L, Nie Y, Wu K, Shi Y and Fan D 2013 MicroRNA-19a/b regulates multidrug resistance in human gastric cancer cells by targeting PTEN *Biochem. Biophys. Res. Commun.* **434** 688–94

[58] Jiang Q, Wei H and Tian Z 2008 Poly I:C enhances cycloheximide-induced apoptosis of tumor cells through TLR3 pathway *BMC Cancer* **8** 12

[59] Han Z, Liang J, Li Y and He J 2019 Drugs and clinical approaches targeting the antiapoptotic protein: a review *BioMed Res. Int.* **2019** 1212369

[60] Wang D, Jiang W, Zhu F, Mao X and Agrawal S 2018 Modulation of the tumor microenvironment by intratumoral administration of IMO-2125, a novel TLR9 agonist, for cancer immunotherapy *Int. J. Oncol.* **53** 1193–203

[61] Villalona-Calero M A, Ritch P, Figueroa J A, Otterson G A, Belt R, Dow E *et al* 2004 A phase I/II study of LY900003, an antisense inhibitor of protein kinase C-alpha, in combination with cisplatin and gemcitabine in patients with advanced non-small cell lung cancer *Clin. Cancer Res.* **10** 6086–93

[62] Tam C, Wong J H, Tsui S K W, Zuo T, Chan T F and Ng T B 2019 LncRNAs with miRNAs in regulation of gastric, liver, and colorectal cancers: updates in recent years *Appl. Microbiol. Biotechnol.* **103** 4649–77

[63] Zhou Y, Sun X, Zhou L and Zhang X 2020 pH-sensitive and long-circulation nanoparticles for near-infrared fluorescence imaging-monitored and chemo-photothermal synergistic treatment against gastric cancer *Front. Pharmacol.* **11** 610883

[64] Meng X, Wang K, Lv L, Zhao Y, Sun C, Ma L and Zhang B 2019 Photothermal/photodynamic therapy with immune-adjuvant liposomal complexes for effective gastric cancer therapy *Part. Part. Syst. Charact.* **36** 1900015

[65] Dai X and Tan C 2015 Combination of microRNA therapeutics with small-molecule anticancer drugs: mechanism of action and codelivery nanocarriers *Adv. Drug Deliv. Rev.* **81** 184–97

[66] Mittal A, Chitkara D, Behrman S W and Mahato R I 2014 Efficacy of gemcitabine conjugated and miRNA-205 complexed micelles for treatment of advanced pancreatic cancer *Biomaterials* **35** 7077–87

[67] Qian X, Long L, Shi Z, Liu C, Qiu M, Sheng J and Kang C 2014 Star-branched amphiphilic PLA-b-PDMAEMA copolymers for codelivery of miR-21 inhibitor and doxorubicin to treat glioma *Biomaterials* **35** 2322–35

[68] Deng X, Cao M, Zhang J, Hu K, Yin Z, Zhou Z, Xiao X *et al* 2014 Hyaluronic acid-chitosan nanoparticles for codelivery of MiR-34a and doxorubicin in therapy against triple negative breast cancer *Biomaterials* **35** 4333–44

[69] Davern M and Lysaght J 2020 Cooperation between chemotherapy and immunotherapy in gastroesophageal cancers *Cancer Lett.* **495** 89–99

[70] Janjigian Y Y, Kawazoe A, Yañez P, Li N, Lonardi S, Kolesnik O, Barajas O, Bai Y, Shen L, Tang Y *et al* 2021 The KEYNOTE-811 trial of dual PD-1 and HER2 blockade in HER2-positive gastric cancer *Nature* **600** 727–30

[71] Whitehead K A, Langer R and Anderson D G 2009 Knocking down barriers: advances in siRNA delivery *Nat. Rev. Drug Discov.* **8** 129–38

[72] Liang M, Li L D, Li L and Li S 2022 Nanotechnology in diagnosis and therapy of gastrointestinal cancer *World J. Clin. Cases* **10** 5146

[73] Chen Z, Penet M F, Nimmagadda S, Li C, Banerjee S R, Winnard P T Jr, Artemov D, Glunde K, Pomper M G and Bhujwalla Z M 2012 PSMA-targeted theranosticnanoplex for prostate cancer therapy *ACS Nano* **6** 7752–62

[74] Xing H, Zhang S, Bu W, Zheng X, Wang L, Xiao Q, Ni D, Zhang J, Zhou L, Peng W *et al* 2014 Ultrasmall NaGdF4 nanodots for efficient MR angiography and atherosclerotic plaque imaging *Adv. Mater.* **26** 3867–72

[75] Miao X *et al* 2018 Stable and non-toxic ultrasmall gadolinium oxide nanoparticle colloids (coating material= polyacrylic acid) as high-performance T 1 magnetic resonance imaging contrast agents *RSC Adv.* **8** 3189–97

[76] Damasco J A, Ravi S, Perez J D, Hagaman D E and Melancon M P 2020 Understanding nanoparticle toxicity to direct a safe-by-design approach in cancer nanomedicine *Nanomaterials* **10** 2186

[77] Cole L E, Ross R D, Tilley J M, Vargo-Gogola T and Roeder R K 2015 Gold nanoparticles as contrast agents in X-ray imaging and computed tomography *Nanomedicine* **10** 321–41

[78] Gao Y, Kang J, Lei Z, Li Y, Mei X and Wang G 2020 Use of the highly biocompatible Au nanocages@PEG nanoparticles as a new contrast agent for *in vivo* computed tomography scan imaging *Nanoscale Res. Lett.* **15** 53

[79] Blum J S and Saltzman W M 2008 High loading efficiency and tunable release of plasmid DNA encapsulated in submicron particles fabricated from PLGA conjugated with poly-L-lysine *J. Control. Rel.* **129** 66–72

[80] Xiong X B, Ma Z S, Lai R and Lavasanifar A 2010 The therapeutic response to multifunctional polymeric nano-conjugates in the targeted cellular and subcellular delivery of doxorubicin *Biomaterials* **31** 757–68

[81] Manke A, Wang L and Rojanasakul Y 2013 Mechanisms of nanoparticle-induced oxidative stress and toxicity *BioMed. Res. Int.* 1–15

[82] Guo C, Xia Y, Niu P, Jiang L, Duan J, Yu Y, Zhou X, Li Y and Sun Z 2015 Silica nanoparticles induce oxidative stress, inflammation, and endothelial dysfunction *in vitro* via activation of the MAPK/Nrf2 pathway and nuclear factor-kappa-signaling *Int. J. Nanomed.* **10** 1463–77

[83] Chen C, Zhang F, Zhou N, Gu Y M, Zhang Y T, He Y D, Wang L, Yang L X, Zhao Y and Li M 2019 Efficacy and safety of immune checkpoint inhibitors in advanced gastric or gastroesophageal junction cancer: a systematic review and meta-analysis *Oncoimmunology* **8** 1581547

[84] Hühn D *et al* 2013 Polymer-coated nanoparticles interacting with proteins and cells: focusing on the sign of the net charge *ACS Nano* **7** 3253–63

[85] Hsu J C, Cruz E D, Lau K C, Bouché M, Kim J, Maidment A D A and Cormode D P 2019 Renally excretable and size-tunable silver sulfide nanoparticles for dual-energy mammography or computed tomography *Chem. Mater.* **31** 7845–54

[86] Kinnear C, Moore T L, Rodriguez-Lorenzo L, Rothen-Rutishauser B and Petri-Fink A 2017 Form follows function: nanoparticle shape and its implications for nanomedicine *Chem. Rev.* **117** 11476–521

[87] Chen X Y and Gao C Y 2017 Influences of size and surface coating of gold nanoparticles on inflammatory activation of macrophages *Colloid Surf.* B **160** 372–80

[88] Zhang X Y and Zhang P Y 2016 Gastric cancer: somatic genetics as a guide to therapy *J. Med. Genet.* **54** 305–12

[89] Ferlay J, Colombet M, Soerjomataram I, Parkin D M, Piñeros M, Znaor A and Bray F 2021 Cancer statistics for the year 2020: an overview *Int. J. Cancer* **149** 778–89

[90] Van Cutsem E, Sagaert X, Topal B, Haustermans K and Prenen H 2016 Gastric cancer *Lancet* **388** 2654–64

[91] Silva Z S Jr, Bussadori S K, Fernandes K P S, Huang Y Y and Hamblin M 2015 Animal models for photodynamic therapy (PDT) *Biosci. Rep.* **35** e00265

[92] Mendes N, Dias Carvalho P, Martins F, Mendonça S, Malheiro A R, Ribeiro A and Velho S 2020 Animal models to study cancer and its microenvironment *Tumor Microenvironment: The Main Driver of Metabolic Adaptation* (Springer) pp 389–401

[93] Cheng J, Xu J, Duanmu J, Zhou H, Booth J, Hu C and Z 2011 Effective treatment of human lung cancer by targeting tissue factor with a factor VII-targeted photodynamic therapy *Curr. Cancer Drug Targets* **11** 1069–81

[94] Fior R, Póvoa V, Mendes R V, Carvalho T, Gomes A, Figueiredo N and Ferreira M G 2017 Single-cell functional and chemosensitive profiling of combinatorial colorectal therapy in zebrafish xenografts *Proc. Natl. Acad. Sci.* **114** 8234–43

[95] Ablain J, Xu M, Rothschild H, Jordan R C, Mito J K, Daniels B H and Yeh I 2018 Human tumor genomics and zebrafish modeling identify SPRED1 loss as a driver of mucosal melanoma *Science* **362** 1055–60

[96] Zhang Q, Hou D, Luo Z, Chen P, Lv B, Wu L and Liu J 2015 The novel protective role of P27 in MLN4924-treated gastric cancer cells *Cell Death Dis.* **6** 1867–7

[97] Jiang L, Gong X, Liao W, Lv N and Yan R 2021 Molecular targeted treatment and drug delivery system for gastric cancer *J. Cancer Res. Clin. Oncol.* **147** 973–86

[98] Abdul Kuddus S 2017 Nanoparticles to deal with gastric cancer *J Gastrointest. Cancer Stromal Tumors* **2** 112

[99] Sun Z, Yi Z, Zhang H, Ma X, Su W, Sun X and Li X 2017 Bio-responsive alginate-keratin composite nanogels with enhanced drug loading efficiency for cancer therapy *Carbohydr. Polym.* **175** 159–69

[100] Farokhzad O C and Langer R 2009 Impact of nanotechnology on drug delivery *ACS Nano* **3** 16–20

[101] Cheng H, Chi C, Shang W, Rengaowa S, Cui J, Ye J and Tian J 2017 Precise integrin-targeting near-infrared imaging-guided surgical method increases surgical qualification of peritoneal carcinomatosis from gastric cancer in mice *Oncotarget* **8** 6258

[102] Kanazaki K, Sano K, Makino A, Shimizu Y, Yamauchi F, Ogawa S and Saji H 2015 Development of anti-HER2 fragment antibody conjugated to iron oxide nanoparticles for *in vivo* HER2-targeted photoacoustic tumor imaging *Nanomed. Nanotechnol. Biol. Med.* **11** 2051–60

[103] Tanaka T, Huang J, Hirai S, Kuroki M, Kuroki M, Watanabe N and Hamada H 2006 Carcinoembryonic antigen–targeted selective gene therapy for gastric cancer through FZ33 fiber-modified adenovirus vectors *Clin. Cancer Res.* **12** 3803–13

[104] Iinuma H, Maruyama K, Okinaga K, Sasaki K, Sekine T, Ishida O and Yonemura Y 2002 Intracellular targeting therapy of cisplatin-encapsulated transferrin-polyethylene glycol liposome on peritoneal dissemination of gastric cancer *Int. J. Cancer* **99** 130–7

[105] Ghasemi M, Nabipour I, Omrani A, Alipour Z and Assadi M 2016 Precision medicine and molecular imaging: new targeted approaches toward cancer therapeutic and diagnosis *Am. J. Nucl. Med. Mol. Imaging* **6** 310

[106] Katrib A, Hsu W, Bui A and Xing Y 2016 RADIOTRANSCRIPTOMICS': a synergy of imaging and transcriptomics in clinical assessment *Quant. Biol.* **4** 1–12

[107] Ametamey S M, Honer M and Schubiger P A 2008 Molecular imaging with PET *Chem. Rev.* **108** 1501–16

[108] Smith A M, Mancini M C and Nie S 2009 Second window for *in vivo* imaging *Nat. Nanotechnol.* **4** 710–1

[109] Hricak H 2011 Oncologic imaging: a guiding hand of personalized cancer care *Radiology* **259** 633–40

[110] Kircher M F, Hricak H and Larson S M 2012 Molecular imaging for personalized cancer care *Mol. Oncol.* **6** 182–95

[111] Chen Z Y, Wang Y X, Lin Y, Zhang J S, Yang F, Zhou Q L and Liao Y Y 2014 Advance of molecular imaging technology and targeted imaging agent in imaging and therapy *BioMed. Res. Int.* **2014** 819324

[112] James M L and Gambhir S S 2012 A molecular imaging primer: modalities, imaging agents, and applications *Physiol. Rev.* **92** 897–965

[113] Weissleder R and Pittet M J 2008 Imaging in the era of molecular oncology *Nature* **452** 580–9

[114] Cheng X, Fan K, Wang L, Ying X, Sanders A J, Guo T and Ji J 2020 TfR1 binding with H-ferritin nanocarrier achieves prognostic diagnosis and enhances the therapeutic efficacy in clinical gastric cancer *Cell Death Dis.* **11** 92

[115] Yang F, Zheng Z, Zheng L, Qin J, Li H, Xue X and Fang G 2018 SATB1 siRNA-encapsulated immunoliposomes conjugated with CD44 antibodies target and eliminate gastric cancer-initiating cells *OncoTargets Ther.* **2018** 6811–25

[116] WangK R J, Qian Q, Song H, Bao C, Zhang X and Cui D 2011 BRCAA1 monoclonal antibody conjugated fluorescent magnetic nanoparticles for *in vivo* targeted magneto-fluorescent imaging of gastric cancer *J. Nanobiotechnol.* **9** 1–12

[117] Kitabatake S, Niwa Y, Miyahara R, Ohashi A, Matsuura T, Iguchi Y and Goto H 2006 Confocal endomicroscopy for the diagnosis of gastric cancer *in vivo Endoscopy* **38** 1110–4

[118] Gao H, Bao P, Dai S, Liu R, Ji S, Zeng S and Ding D 2019 Far-red/near-infrared emissive (1, 3-dimethyl) barbituric acid-based AIEgens for high-contrast detection of metastatic tumors in the lung *Chem. Asian J.* **14** 871–6

[119] Li R, Liu B and Gao J 2017 The application of nanoparticles in diagnosis and theranostics of gastric cancer *Cancer Lett.* **386** 123–30

[120] Zhang K, Du X, Yu K, Zhang K and Zhou Y 2018 Application of novel targeting nanoparticles contrast agent combined with contrast-enhanced computed tomography during screening for early-phase gastric carcinoma *Exp. Ther. Med.* **15** 47–54

[121] Davis M E, Chen Z and Shin D M 2008 Nanoparticle therapeutics: an emerging treatment modality for cancer *Nat. Rev. Drug Discov.* **7** 771–82

[122] Wu Q, Pan W, Wu G, Wu F, Guo Y and Zhang X 2023 CD40-targeting magnetic nanoparticles for MRI/optical dual-modality molecular imaging of vulnerable atherosclerotic plaques *Atherosclerosis* **369** 17–26

[123] Sack M, Alili L, Karaman E, Das S, Gupta A, Seal S and Brenneisen P 2014 Combination of conventional chemotherapeutics with redox-active cerium oxide nanoparticles—a novel aspect in cancer therapy *Mol. Cancer Ther.* **13** 1740–9

[124] Yang Q, Jones S W, Parker C L, Zamboni W C, Bear J E and Lai S K 2014 Evading immune cell uptake and clearance requires PEG grafting at densities substantially exceeding the minimum for brush conformation *Mol. Pharm.* **11** 1250–8

[125] Zeineldin R and Syoufjy J 2017 Cancer nanotechnology: opportunities for prevention, diagnosis, and therapy *Cancer Nanotechnology: Methods and Protocols* (Springer) pp 3–12

[126] Chouhan R S, Horvat M, Ahmed J, Alhokbany N, Alshehri S M and Gandhi S 2021 Magnetic nanoparticles—A multifunctional potential agent for diagnosis and therapy *Cancers* **13** 2213

[127] Widder K J, Senyei A E and Scarpelli D G 1978 Magnetic microspheres: a model system for site specific drug delivery *in vivo Proc. Soc. Exp. Biol. Med.* **158** 141–6

[128] Bulbake U, Doppalapudi S, Kommineni N and Khan W 2017 Liposomal formulations in clinical use: an updated review *Pharmaceutics* **9** 12

[129] Toub N, Bertrand J R, Tamaddon A, Elhamess H, Hillaireau H, Maksimenko A and … Couvreur P 2006 Efficacy of siRNA nanocapsules targeted against the EWS–Fli1 oncogene in Ewing sarcoma *Pharm. Res.* **23** 892–900

[130] Wang L Y, Li J H, Zhou X, Zheng Q C and Cheng X 2017 Clinical application of carbon nanoparticles in curative resection for colorectal carcinoma *OncoTargets Ther.* **2017** 5585–9

[131] Huang G, Liu Y and Chen L 2017 Chitosan and its derivatives as vehicles for drug delivery *Drug Deliv.* **24** 108–13

[132] Hu A, Chen C, Mantle M D, Wolf B, Gladden L F, Rajabi-Siahboomi A and Melia C D 2017 The properties of HPMC: PEO extended release hydrophilic matrices and their response to ionic environments *Pharm. Res.* **34** 941–56

[133] Alagaratnam S, Yang S Y, Loizidou M, Fuller B and Ramesh B 2019 Mechano-growth factor expression in colorectal cancer investigated with fluorescent gold nanoparticles *Anticancer Res.* **39** 1705–10

Chapter 8

Artificial intelligence in hepatitis and chronic liver disease

Akbar Hamid, Gira Sulabh and Vinod Kumar

Artificial Intelligence (AI) is a well-developing field of computer science that imitates human technical thinking to solve problems. The use of different AI models in hepatology is a recent development in the medical field for better diagnostics. Conventional diagnostic methods are being integrated with modern AI to enhance the performance of treatment. AI has the ability to mine the data in human parameters, and forecast the occurrence of hepatitis and other chronic liver diseases. Classifying the different stages of hepatitis, fatty liver disease and hemochromatosis are possible along with diagnosis and screening. Early disease prediction, complications and mortality can be studied using the algorithms such as regression models, since hepatitis early diagnosis is clinically limited in early stages. AI can predict the risk related to the vascular invasion of hepatocellular carcinoma and hepatitis related to cirrhosis. It also calculates the liver failure rate in hepatocellular carcinoma (HCC) patients. Ultimately AI will eventually help in reducing medical errors and managing the patient clinical output.

8.1 Introduction

AI has revolutionized numerous industries, and is considered to be one of the fastest-growing fields and its impact on healthcare is increasingly evident. Hepatology, particularly in the detection and treatment of hepatitis and other chronic liver diseases, is one area that has benefited from the revolutionary potential of AI. Medical conditions pose significant challenges to medical professionals due to their complexity, varied etiologies, and the need for accurate and timely interventions. With the advent of AI, there is newfound hope in addressing these challenges more effectively. This chapter examines the rising importance of AI in hepatitis and

doi:10.1088/978-0-7503-6134-7ch8

chronic liver disease, emphasizing its potential to improve patient outcomes, medication selection, diagnostic accuracy, and prognostic evaluation [1].

Liver diseases such as hepatitis and other chronic liver disease are considered to be a global health concern affecting millions of people worldwide every year. They encompass a wide range of medical conditions, including viral hepatitis (such as hepatitis B and C), non-alcoholic fatty liver disease (NAFLD), alcoholic liver disease, and HCC. These diseases can progress silently for years without causing any serious health issues, leading to liver fibrosis, cirrhosis, and hepatocellular carcinoma if left undetected and untreated, as can be seen in figure 8.1 [2]. The burden of liver-related consequences can be reduced and disease development can be stopped with early identification and prompt care. Traditionally, the diagnosis and management of hepatitis and chronic liver disease have relied on a combination of clinical evaluation, laboratory tests, medical imaging, and invasive procedures such as liver biopsies used for the detection of disease in patients. However, these methods have certain limitations [3]. For instance, liver biopsies, while considered the gold standard for fibrosis staging, are invasive, expensive, and prone to sampling errors. Moreover, interpreting the vast amounts of data generated from various diagnostic tests can be challenging for healthcare professionals, leading to potential human errors and delays in the diagnosis of the disease for the treatment which may lead to a much more serious condition of the patient [4]. As a result, artificial intelligence offers a viable answer to these problems by utilizing cutting-edge computational algorithms and machine learning techniques to quickly and accurately evaluate complicated data patterns. Large amounts of patient data, like test results, medical images, genetic profiles, clinical histories, and treatment outcomes, may be processed and integrated by AI algorithms [5]. By identifying patterns and associations that may not be immediately apparent to human clinicians, AI systems can provide valuable insights and support clinical decision-making [5].

Accurate diagnosis is one area where AI has been shown to have tremendous potential. The algorithms used for machine learning may be taught on massive datasets of liver disease cases, learning to recognize minute patterns and signals that might point to the presence of certain liver illnesses. For example, studies have shown that AI algorithms can accurately detect and classify liver lesions in medical

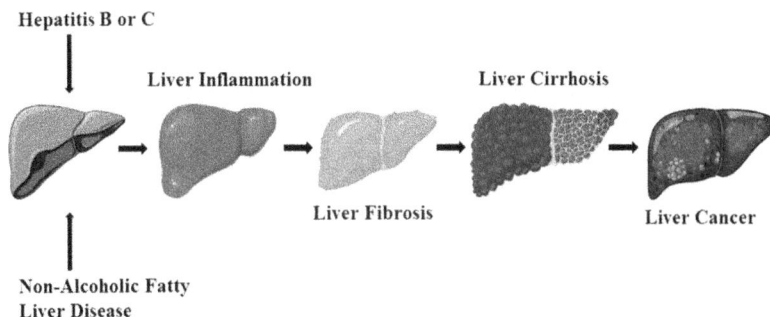

Figure 8.1. Different stages of liver damage once it is infected with either hepatitis virus or non-alcoholic fatty liver disease. Created via Biorender

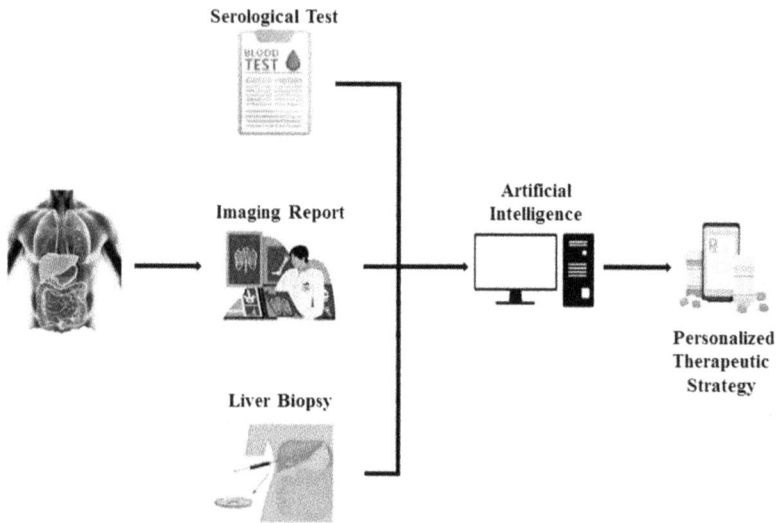

Figure 8.2. An overview of the diagnosis and therapy selection using AI in disease treatment. Created via Biorender

imaging, aiding in the early detection of hepatocellular carcinoma [6]. AI systems can also analyze laboratory results and clinical data to identify potential risk factors for liver disease, enabling earlier intervention and management. Furthermore, AI has the ability to enhance prognostic assessment in hepatitis and chronic liver disease [7]. By analyzing various patient factors and disease characteristics, AI algorithms can generate predictive models to estimate disease progression, treatment response, and overall patient outcomes, which can be understood with the help of figure 8.2. Clinical professionals may use this data to create personalized treatment plans, spot high-risk patients who can benefit from more frequent follow-up or early intervention, and maximize the use of healthcare resources.

AI has the potential to improve therapy choices and efficiency in addition to diagnosis and prognosis. AI systems may recognize trends in therapy response through data analysis and machine learning, assisting medical professionals in selecting the best suitable treatments based on specific patient profiles [8]. This can minimize trial-and-error approaches, reduce treatment costs, and improve patient outcomes. AI can also assist in monitoring treatment response over time, enabling timely adjustments and personalized interventions.

To fully utilize AI in hepatology, further research and partnerships between AI developers and medical practitioners are required as technology develops. We can significantly advance the treatment of liver illness and, eventually, decrease the impact of hepatitis and chronic liver disease worldwide by leveraging the potential of AI [9].

8.2 Artificial intelligence role in hepatitis disease

Hepatitis, a global public health concern, is an inflammation of the liver caused by viral infections (hepatitis A, B, C, D, and E), alcohol abuse, drug toxicity, autoimmune disorders, or metabolic diseases. Globally, it affects millions of individuals and can cause serious side effects such as liver cirrhosis and hepatocellular cancer. Once the patient develops liver cirrhosis they will experience several other health-related issues such as ascites, jaundice, red plams, etc. Figure 8.3 shows health issues caused by cirrhosis. The accurate and timely diagnosis of hepatitis, along with effective treatment strategies, is crucial for reducing its impact and improving patient outcomes. In recent years, AI has stepped up to this challenge, offering invaluable contributions across different stages of the disease continuum.

Hepatitis diagnosis and treatment is one of several significant domains where AI has had an important contribution. The identification of high-risk groups and the implementation of targeted treatments have been challenges for public health authorities and organizations globally [10]. AI algorithms, however, have the capability to analyze vast amounts of demographic, behavioural, and genetic data to pinpoint individuals at higher risk of contracting the virus. Health officials may now concentrate on preventative efforts like vaccination drives and awareness campaigns that can significantly lower the prevalence of hepatitis thanks to this knowledge [11].

Additionally, patient involvement and education are changing thanks to chatbots and virtual assistants driven by AI. These interactive systems can provide individualized information, respond to patient questions, and encourage commitment to medications. AI leads to better patient outcomes and an overall improvement in quality of life by allowing individuals to successfully manage their disease [12]. AI has a pivotal role in patient monitoring and disease management. Wearable devices and remote monitoring tools equipped with AI can track liver function, and other relevant parameters, providing real-time data to healthcare professionals. This continuous monitoring allows for early detection of disease exacerbation and prompt intervention, preventing disease progression and reducing hospitalizations. Moreover, by personalizing medicines for each patient, AI-driven personalized medicine is transforming the treatment of hepatitis. Hepatitis viruses can mutate

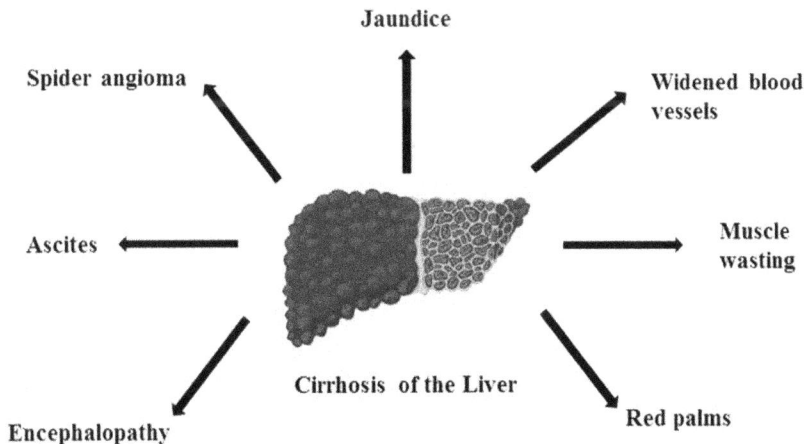

Figure 8.3. Health issues caused by cirrhosis of liver in patient. Created via Biorender

rapidly, leading to drug resistance and treatment failure. AI algorithms, however, can continuously analyze a patient's viral genetic data and treatment response, enabling real-time adjustments to medication regimens. This approach enhances treatment efficacy and minimizes adverse effects, optimizing patient outcomes and reducing the burden on healthcare systems [13, 14].

Nevertheless, despite these remarkable developments, integrating AI into hepatitis care doesn't come without difficulties. As AI systems depend on a significant quantity of sensitive medical data, maintaining patient data privacy and security as a top priority is necessary. To win over the public and ensure that AI technologies are widely used in healthcare, it is essential to strike a balance between utilizing the promise of AI and protecting patient privacy.

8.2.1 Limitations of the traditional method for the diagnosis and treatment of hepatitis disease

Although widely used for many years, conventional approaches for the diagnosis and treatment of hepatitis have certain major drawbacks that restrict their effectiveness and overall influence on patient outcomes. These flaws have motivated the investigation of novel strategies, including the use of AI and cutting-edge technology, to get over these obstacles and enhance hepatitis management.

Firstly, the sensitivity and specificity necessary for accurate and early detection are sometimes lacking in the usual diagnostic procedures for hepatitis, such as serological testing and liver biopsies [15]. Even though serological tests are frequently used to identify viral antigens and antibodies, they may result in false negatives when the virus is present but no antibodies have yet formed. Similar to blood tests, liver biopsies are intrusive, expensive, and risky, making them unsuitable for regular monitoring and follow-up. However, they are considered to be the gold standard for determining liver damage and staging hepatitis. These limitations can delay diagnosis and impede timely intervention, potentially allowing the disease to progress to more severe stages.

Moreover, antiviral drugs are the foundation of traditional hepatitis treatment methods, which can be helpful but also have side effects. These medications often target specific viral components, making them susceptible to drug resistance as the virus mutates over time. Also, the treatment plans are frequently uniform, making it difficult to adapt them to the special traits and treatment reactions of each patient. As a result, some patients may experience suboptimal treatment outcomes or develop complications due to the inability to adapt therapy based on their specific needs [16]. Another limitation lies in the monitoring and follow-up of patients with hepatitis. Periodic clinic visits and laboratory tests are commonly used for disease assessment, but they may not provide a real-time and continuous evaluation of a patient's condition. This kind of infrequent monitoring might overlook slight alterations in the course of the disease or the effectiveness of the treatment, delaying therapeutic modifications or obstructing possibilities for early intervention. Therefore, in order to ensure improved disease management, more dynamic and patient-centred monitoring methods are required [17].

The conventional approaches to diagnosing and treating hepatitis suffer from a lack of scalability and accessibility, especially in areas with few resources. Liver biopsies, as mentioned earlier, require specialized facilities and expertise, making them challenging to implement in certain regions [18]. In the same way, access to other common treatment options may be restricted in some places, depriving patients of the care they require [19]. These variations in access to healthcare can increase the burden of hepatitis globally and prevent successful attempts to manage the virus.

8.2.2 Artificial intelligence in hepatitis diagnosis

Accurate diagnosis is the cornerstone of effective disease management. The use of AI methods, in particular machine learning and deep learning algorithms, has shown considerable potential for improving hepatitis B and hepatitis C diagnosis. This has changed the way medical practitioners handle this important component of patient care. Medical image analysis is one of the main uses of AI in the diagnosis of hepatitis [30]. AI algorithms, particularly those based on deep learning and convolutional neural networks, seen in figure 8.4, have shown remarkable performance in interpreting liver imaging modalities such as ultrasound, computed tomography (CT), and magnetic resonance imaging (MRI). This assists radiologists and clinicians in making accurate and timely diagnoses [30]. These algorithms can automatically detect and segment liver lesions, assess liver texture and parenchymal changes, and identify signs of fibrosis and cirrhosis, which are common manifestations of chronic hepatitis. Early diagnosis of liver problems is made possible by AI's capacity to quickly and reliably assess huge quantities of imaging data, which enables prompt intervention and better patient outcomes. In addition to medical imaging, AI plays a pivotal role in interpreting laboratory test results used in hepatitis diagnosis. In order to determine the presence of viral infection and distinguish between various kinds of hepatitis, serological tests that look for viral antigens and antibodies are important [12]. AI algorithms can process vast databases of serological test results, along with clinical information from electronic health records, to identify patterns that signify hepatitis infection and assess disease severity. AI-powered diagnostic tools can offer medical practitioners insightful information and evidence-based suggestions for patient treatment by combining this data-driven methodology with domain-specific expertise.

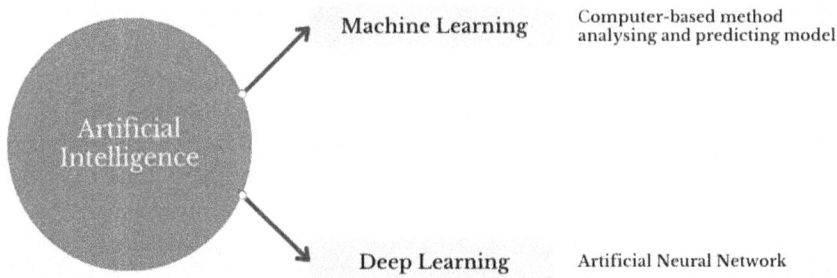

Figure 8.4. AI has been divided into two primary categories: machine learning and deep learning. Created via Biorender

Investigators have used artificial neural network (ANN), as artificial intelligence paradigms, to provide a reliable outcomes for clinical problems. An ANN is a mathematical model, which is inspired by the biological nervous system. Like in Nature, how a network functions is primarily determined by connections between its components. Through learning, ANNs may detect intricate patterns between inputs and outputs [20]. Also, AI has proven to have excellent abilities in predicting hepatitis growth and treatment response. Using machine learning algorithms, chronic patient data may be combined and evaluated, including laboratory results, imaging results, and clinical outcomes [21]. AI can help doctors create individualized treatment strategies for specific individuals by analyzing illness progression trends and factors affecting treatment success. This precision medicine approach optimizes therapeutic efficacy while minimizing adverse effects, thereby enhancing patient well-being and treatment adherence [21].

Risk prediction modelling is an important field where AI is effective in the diagnosis of hepatitis. By analyzing various risk factors, including demographic data, lifestyle habits, comorbidities, and genetic predispositions, AI algorithms can assess an individual's likelihood of developing hepatitis or experiencing disease progression. These risk prediction models allow for focused screening and early care for high-risk patients, decreasing the total impact of hepatitis on public health systems and averting disease consequences [22].

Hepatitis diagnosis is made even more simple by the incorporation of AI into electronic health record (EHR) systems, which aggregate and analyze huge amounts of patient data. Doctors may be alerted to probable hepatitis cases and assisted in making better decisions by AI-powered EHRs, which can automatically identify critical clinical markers and risk factors. The efficiency of the medical system is improved, diagnostic mistakes are decreased, and patients receive a higher level of treatment because of this thorough and data-driven approach [23].

The influence of AI technology on hepatitis detection is projected to increase as it develops and becomes more widely available, significantly advancing efforts to battle and manage this serious public health issue on a worldwide scale.

8.2.3 Treatment and management of hepatitis with artificial intelligence

The choice of the best possibilities for therapy is essential when hepatitis is identified. With the incorporation of AI, there has been a paradigm change in the treatment and management of hepatitis, providing creative solutions that optimize therapeutic approaches, improve patient outcomes, and expedite healthcare delivery [24]. A thorough and customized strategy is necessary to treat the various forms and varied disease regimens of hepatitis, a viral infection of the liver. Medical professionals may now offer individualized therapies, track patient progress, and forecast treatment outcomes with better accuracy and efficiency thanks to AI-driven technologies, which have emerged as potent tools in this field [24].

Drug research and development are some of the main implications of AI in the fight against hepatitis. AI has changed this field of research by speeding up the identification of prospective antiviral drugs, which was previously a time- and money-consuming procedure. AI algorithms can analyze libraries of molecular structures and predict the interaction between viral components and drug candidates with remarkable accuracy [25]. By simulating drug-receptor interactions, AI narrows down the list of potential drug candidates, accelerating the development of new antiviral therapies. This strategy makes it possible to investigate innovative therapy alternatives, address drug resistance, and increase the number of drugs accessible for the treatment of hepatitis. AI's potential extends beyond drug discovery to precision medicine, Because hepatitis viruses may change quickly, different individuals may respond differently to therapy [26]. In order to find trends that affect medicine effectiveness, AI can continually monitor patient data, including viral genetic data and treatment outcomes. AI systems that use machine learning can forecast the best treatment plans for specific patients by taking into account aspects like medication resistance, liver function, and allergies. This targeted strategy improves patient compliance and treatment outcomes while minimizing side effects and maximizing treatment effectiveness [26].

AI algorithms can find prognostic markers linked to disease development or remission by examining massive datasets of patient records, laboratory findings, and clinical outcomes. Thanks to these forecasting capabilities of AI, doctors may undertake early treatments and preventative measures, reducing illness complications and improving long-term results [27]. Additionally, AI has shown to be quite helpful in assisting medical professionals in making difficult treatment decisions. Clinical decision-support systems powered by AI combine patient data with the most recent scientific findings and clinical advice to provide real-time suggestions on possible treatments, dose modifications, and medication interactions. These decision-support tools improve medical judgment, lower the chance of mistakes, and encourage evidence-based practice [28].

AI has played an essential part in dealing with the management of hepatitis in public health in addition to treatment. An immense amount of demographic and illness data can potentially be analyzed by AI-powered epidemiological models to forecast disease outbreaks, estimate the impact of diseases, and guide public health initiatives. In order to manage and eradicate hepatitis as a hazard to the general population, the world is making efforts to do so. This forecasting skill helps with resource allocation, vaccine planning, and disease preventive activities [29]. AI has the potential to significantly improve hepatitis management and change medical procedures for the benefit of the millions of people who are impacted by this disease, provided that research is conducted and deployment is done responsibly.

Despite these amazing developments, integrating AI in the management and treatment of hepatitis does present some difficulties, such as establishing confidence in AI-driven healthcare solutions from the public.

8.2.4 Artificial intelligence-enabled hepatitis disease surveillance and prevention

AI has the potential to be extremely useful in disease surveillance and preventive initiatives in addition to diagnosis and treatment. AI systems can identify the latest developments and early warning indications of hepatitis outbreaks by analyzing vast amounts of information that come from EHRs, health department records, and social media. In order to slow the spread of the disease, public health officials can use this early diagnosis to assist them execute immediate actions and preventative measures, such as vaccination programs [21]. With the goal to identify early warning signs of future hepatitis outbreaks or vaccination reluctance, AI-driven systems can examine the language used in online conversations. Public health authorities may better focus programs and campaigns to increase awareness, encourage immunization, and dispel myths about hepatitis by using this relevant information [30].

AI plays a critical role in organizing vaccination activities for the prevention of disease. AI-powered algorithms are able to detect high-risk populations with low immunization rates by analyzing the population's demographics, illness frequency, and vaccine coverage rates [31]. These predictive models give healthcare systems the ability to spend resources proactively, create focused preventative plans, and forecast future healthcare requirements. Public health officials may use this information to specifically target outreach and vaccination initiatives, ensuring that hepatitis is prevented in susceptible groups [30].

AI-driven simulations can also forecast how the virus may change over time, enabling the creation of vaccinations that offer broader and more durable protection. AI may also monitor vaccination outcomes in real-time to evaluate the efficacy of currently available vaccines, enabling quick revisions to immunization plans as necessary [32]. AI-enabled surveillance is essential for tracking hepatitis-related complications and determining the severity of the condition. AI can uncover patterns of life-threatening cases and consequences by examining hospitalization data and clinical outcomes, leading focused interventions and treatment approaches. This thorough understanding of the disease's impact helps medical organizations to better manage resources and improve patient care [33].

Furthermore, contact tracing, a crucial part of disease prevention during outbreaks, is being transformed by AI. Machine learning AI-powered contact tracking systems can quickly find and alert people who may have been exposed to the virus, allowing for quick testing and action to stop future transmission [7]. AI simplifies the discovery of possible transmission chains by automating contact tracking procedures, effectively interrupting the cycle of illness.

8.3 Artificial intelligence role in non-alcoholic fatty liver disease

Millions of people worldwide are affected by Non-Alcoholic Fatty Liver Disease (NAFLD), which has become a serious global health problem. The term 'NAFLD' refers to a group of diseases where excessive amounts of fat build-up in the liver, causing inflammation and liver cell destruction as well as the possibility of developing into more severe stages including cirrhosis, hepatocellular carcinoma, and fibrosis [34]. Innovative methods are urgently needed in order to help with NAFLD's early detection, precise diagnosis, and personalized treatment due to its increasing frequency. AI, which has the potential to completely transform the healthcare industry, has recently emerged as a promising technology in the medical industry. With a focus on its uses, difficulties, and potential uses, AI is examined in this chapter's discussion of NAFLD [35].

The global obesity epidemic and the development of metabolic diseases like diabetes and dyslipidemia are the main causes for why NAFLD has become the most frequent cause of chronic liver disease globally. The burden of NAFLD extends beyond liver-related complications, as it is closely associated with an increased risk of cardiovascular disease, type 2 diabetes, and overall mortality. However, the early detection and accurate diagnosis of NAFLD remain challenging, hindering effective disease management and the prevention of disease progression [34].

The multidisciplinary discipline of computer science known as AI has shown incredible promise for use in medical fields. It entails the establishment of computer systems that are capable of carrying out operations like learning, analyzing situations, and coming up with solutions that would ordinarily need human intelligence [36]. Due to their capacity to analyze complicated data and extract useful information, machine learning and deep learning, the two subfields of AI, have become more popular. One of the key applications of AI in NAFLD lies in the early detection and diagnosis of the disease. Medical imaging techniques, such as ultrasound, CT, and MRI, play a crucial role in assessing liver fat content and distinguishing between simple steatosis and non-alcoholic steatohepatitis (NASH) [37]. Manually interpreting these photos, however, may be difficult and time-consuming. By precisely assessing and quantifying liver fat levels, AI algorithms have the ability to automate this procedure, resulting in quicker and more accurate diagnoses. Additionally, AI can help medical professionals in differentiating between NASH and simple steatosis, allowing them to identify individuals who are more likely to experience disease progression and develop specific therapies.

AI can assist in making use of NAFLD prediction models in addition to diagnostics. AI algorithms may find patterns and relationships in massive datasets of data from hospitals and laboratories that may not be obvious to human observers [38]. By calculating a person's probability of acquiring NAFLD and accompanying problems, these predictive models enable early intervention and preventative actions. Additionally, in order to offer targeted treatment suggestions, AI algorithms can incorporate patient-specific data, such as demographic, genetic, and lifestyle characteristics. The potential benefits of this personalized strategy include better patient care, better treatment results, and an eventual reduction in the overall condition of NAFLD [39].

Despite the positive potential of AI in NAFLD, there are still a number of obstacles to overcome. For the establishment of reliable AI models, high-quality, well-annotated data must be accessible. However, disparities in data completeness, uniformity, and quality among healthcare organizations and systems provide problems for data-driven projects. Moreover, rigorous validation studies and integration into existing clinical workflows are essential to evaluate the performance and effectiveness of AI algorithms in real-world settings.

8.3.1 Limitations of the traditional method for the diagnosis and treatment of non-alcoholic fatty liver disease

NAFLD is a complex liver disorder characterized by the accumulation of fat in the liver. It covers a broad spectrum of diseases, including simple steatosis, NASH, fibrosis, cirrhosis, and even hepatocellular cancer. Accurate diagnosis of NAFLD is essential for appropriate management and intervention. Traditional diagnostic techniques for NAFLD, however, have a number of drawbacks that reduce their efficacy and dependability.

Liver biopsy is a frequent yet expensive technique of NAFLD diagnosis. A tiny tissue sample from the liver is taken as part of this process for microscopic analysis. Although liver biopsy is regarded as the most reliable method for NAFLD diagnosis and staging, it has a number of limitations. First of all, it is an intrusive operation that has risks including bleeding, pain, and infection. This restricts its usage, especially in individuals who are hesitant to undergo an invasive operation or who have underlying medical issues. Because the medical condition may not be spread evenly throughout the liver, liver biopsy is also sensitive to sample hetero-geneity [40]. As a result, the diagnosis may be affected if the biopsy sample fails to properly represent the general status of the liver. Furthermore, liver biopsy is more difficult to access, particularly in areas with low resources, as it needs specialized facilities, trained workers, and expensive equipment. Imaging techniques, such as ultrasonography (US), CT scan, and MRI, are also utilized for the diagnosis of NAFLD [37]. Due to its low cost and non-invasive nature, ultrasonography is commonly utilized. However, it is not always reliable in distinguishing between mild and moderate hepatic steatosis. Furthermore, it might not be sensitive enough to spot early-stage fibrosis or inflammation, both of which are essential signs of NASH. In comparison to ultrasonography, a CT scan can reveal more specific information about the amount of fat and fibrosis in the liver [41]. However, it involves ionizing radiation and is relatively expensive. The associated radiation exposure risks limit its use for routine screening purposes. In determining the amount of liver fat present and distinguishing between steatosis and NASH, MRI, especially magnetic reso-nance spectroscopy (MRS), provides incredible precision. The extensive use of MRI for regular NAFLD screening and monitoring is nonetheless constrained by its high cost, restricted availability, and time-consuming nature [42].

Blood tests are frequently used to diagnose NAFLD, including those that measure liver enzymes and certain biomarkers. For the purpose of evaluating liver function, it is common practice to monitor liver enzymes such as alanine amino-transferase (ALT) and aspartate aminotransferase (AST). Although these enzymes lack specificity, many NAFLD patients, especially those with pure steatosis, may have levels that are within the normal range [41]. Because of this, depending just on liver enzymes may result in a missed or postponed diagnosis of NAFLD. Blood tests and biomarkers may not be able to offer a thorough evaluation of the severity of a disease, despite being advantageous for screening. Another strategy is to utilize composite scores, such as the Fatty Liver Index (FLI), which determines a score based on factors including body mass index, waist circumference, triglyceride levels, and gamma-glutamyl transferase (GGT). Although the FLI can assist in identifying those who are at risk for NAFLD, it is not a reliable diagnostic tool and cannot distinguish between various disease stages. Similar to this, non-invasive fibrosis biomarkers to calculate the degree of fibrosis have been established, such as the NAFLD Fibrosis Score (NFS) and Fibrosis-4 (FIB-4) index. These results, however, may need to be confirmed by further testing or imaging as they are not totally accurate. The diagnosis and treatment of NAFLD may be improved by techno-logical developments such as transient elastography, advanced MRI sequences, and new blood biomarkers [43].

8.3.2 Artificial intelligence in non-alcoholic fatty liver disease diagnosis

The field of medical diagnostics has seen the emergence of AI as a potent tool that is altering how diseases are identified and treated. The diagnosis of NAFLD, a medical condition marked by the build-up of fat in the liver of people who drink little to no alcohol, is one area where AI has shown substantial promise. A significant portion of the world's population now suffers from NAFLD, which must be diagnosed correctly and early in order to be effectively managed and prevented from progressing to more serious liver conditions including cirrhosis and hepatocellular carcinoma [44]. NAFLD is often diagnosed through invasive techniques like liver biopsies, which are not only costly and time-consuming but also run the risk of consequences. AI-based approaches use cutting-edge algorithms and machine learning to evaluate medical data and produce precise diagnoses. These methods are non-invasive and effective. The capability of AI to rapidly analyze vast amounts of data and discover patterns that human observers might miss is one of the major benefits of AI in NAFLD diagnosis [34].

Medical imaging plays a crucial role in the diagnosis of NAFLD, and AI has demonstrated its potential in this area. For instance, AI algorithms may examine ultrasound, CT, and MRI images to pinpoint certain markers connected to NAFLD, such as liver fat content, fibrosis, and inflammation. AI models may learn to detect these patterns with high accuracy by training on massive datasets of medical pictures, enabling radiologists to make more accurate diagnoses. By doing so, medical staff are freed up to concentrate on other important activities while simultaneously increasing the efficiency of diagnosis [45].

Medical imaging is only one sort of data that AI may use to improve NAFLD diagnosis; other categories include patient histories, test findings, and genetic data. AI models may create detailed patient profiles and produce unique risk evaluations for NAFLD by combining these data sources. This makes it possible to identify those who are at a high risk of contracting the disease early on, permitting suited therapies and lifestyle changes to stop its progression. Additionally, AI algorithms are capable of ongoing learning and adaptation based on actual patient outcomes, which helps them develop their diagnostic abilities over time and provide better patient care. Another area where AI has made significant contributions to NAFLD diagnosis is in the development of predictive models. AI systems can scan big datasets comprising a variety of patient data to identify risk factors and forecast the possibility of NAFLD onset or progression by utilizing machine learning techni-ques. These models can support doctors in making well-informed decisions about patient management and treatment plans, maximizing healthcare resources, and raising patient satisfaction [46].

Additionally, AI-driven decision-support systems can help medical professionals understand complicated data and navigate the enormous amount of NAFLD-related medical literature. These systems can provide evidence-based suggestions and help with the creation of individualized treatment plans by combining knowledge from a variety of sources, including clinical guidelines, research publications, and real-time patient data [47]. This not only improves the precision and effectiveness of diagnosis but also encourages standardization of treatment procedures and lowers clinical decision-making variability.

There are issues that need to be resolved despite the enormous promise of AI in the diagnosis of NAFLD. For the purpose of developing reliable AI models, it is essential to have access to a variety of high-quality datasets, and the absence of standardized data-collecting procedures and annotated datasets continues to be a major barrier

8.3.3 Treatment and management of non-alcoholic fatty liver disease with artificial intelligence

NAFLD is a prevalent and growing health concern worldwide. NAFLD has emerged as a major contributor to chronic liver disease due to the rising incidence of obesity and metabolic syndrome. A comprehensive strategy that emphasizes lifestyle changes, such as food and exercise, as well as pharmaceutical therapies is needed for the management and treatment of NAFLD. However, new developments in AI have demonstrated significant promise in terms of enhancing the diagnosis, prognosis, and customized management of NAFLD [48].

One of the key areas where AI can aid in the management of NAFLD is in the diagnosis and early detection of the disease. AI algorithms are now able to interpret medical imaging data from ultrasound, CT, and MRI to precisely detect and measure hepatic steatosis, a defining characteristic of NAFLD. This can enable healthcare providers to detect NAFLD at an early stage when interventions are most effective [49]. Furthermore, AI algorithms may examine a massive quantity of patient data, including medical history, test findings, and genetic data, to forecast the likelihood that the condition will worsen and that problems would arise in NAFLD patients. AI algorithms are able to create risk ratings and give individualized risk stratification for specific patients by fusing several data sources. The use of this data by healthcare professionals can improve patient outcomes by assisting them in prioritizing high-risk patients for additional assessment and intense management. In terms of treatment, AI can assist in the development of personalized therapeutic strategies for patients with NAFLD [50]. AI models can find patterns and correlations that might inform therapy choices by examining vast datasets of patient characteristics, treatment results, and medication reactions. For example, based on the features of the patient and genetic variables, AI algorithms can assist in predicting the reaction to particular drugs, such as vitamin E or pioglitazone. This personalized strategy can improve treatment results and lower the chance of negative consequences [51].

Additionally, patients with NAFLD can benefit from lifestyle therapies supported by AI-powered solutions. In order to offer real-time feedback and specific suggestions, these systems can evaluate food and exercise data obtained via wearable technology or smartphone applications. By monitoring the patient's adherence to a healthy diet and exercise regimen, AI algorithms can promote behaviour changes and help patients achieve their goals. This continuous support can improve patient compliance and long-term treatment outcomes [52].

Another promising application of AI in NAFLD management is the development of virtual patient models. These models, based on AI algorithms, can simulate the progression of NAFLD and assess the impact of different interventions on disease outcomes [52]. By integrating patient-specific data, such as liver function tests, imaging results, and lifestyle factors, these models can predict the long-term effects of interventions, such as weight loss or medication use. Virtual patient models can serve as valuable decision-support tools for healthcare providers, enabling them to make informed treatment decisions and evaluate the potential benefits and risks of different interventions.

8.3.4 Artificial intelligence-enabled non-alcoholic fatty liver disease surveillance and prevention

The issues related to NAFLD can be greatly improved with the use of AI, which has become an effective tool in disease surveillance and prevention. NAFLD is a disorder marked by the build-up of extra fat in the liver and is frequently associated with obesity, a poor diet, and sedentary lifestyles [35]. It has become a global health concern, affecting millions of people worldwide. AI-enabled approaches can revolutionize the management of NAFLD by improving early detection, risk prediction, personalized treatment plans, population-level surveillance, decision-support systems, and patient education and behaviour modification. One of the significant advantages of AI in NAFLD is early detection. AI algorithms are capable of quickly and accurately analyzing medical imaging data from CT scans, MRIs, and ultrasounds [53]. AI algorithms may assist medical professionals in starting effective therapies by identifying NAFLD symptoms at an early stage, such as liver fat accumulation and inflammation. Early detection is crucial because it allows for the implementation of lifestyle modifications, such as dietary changes and exercise, which can prevent disease progression and reduce the risk of complications, including liver cirrhosis and hepatocellular carcinoma. Moreover, AI can play a pivotal role in predicting the risk of NAFLD development. By analyzing a combination of genetic, environmental, and lifestyle factors, AI models can assess an individual's likelihood of developing NAFLD [54]. The capacity to forecast risk might assist healthcare workers in locating high-risk patients who can profit from specialized preventative actions. For example, individuals with a high genetic predisposition to NAFLD can be provided with personalized counselling on lifestyle modifications, including diet and exercise, to mitigate their risk [55].

AI can also contribute to the development of personalized treatment plans for NAFLD patients. AI algorithms can suggest customized treatment plans by integrating and examining diverse patient-specific data, such as medical history, genetic data, and lifestyle variables. These personalized treatment plans can optimize outcomes by considering individual characteristics and response patterns to different interventions. AI may also help in monitoring the effectiveness of the therapy and making necessary adjustments, ensuring that patients receive the best possible care. At a population level, AI can enable comprehensive surveillance of NAFLD. AI algorithms may find patterns, trends, and risk factors related to NAFLD by examining large-scale health data, such as EHRs and medical claims databases. Authorities in public health can use this information to better understand the prevalence and incidence of NAFLD in certain groups and geographical areas. With this knowledge, targeted prevention programs can be implemented to address the underlying causes of NAFLD, such as promoting healthier lifestyles and improving access to healthcare resources [56].

AI-powered decision-support systems have the potential to enhance clinical decision-making in NAFLD management. Such networks can offer real-time advice to doctors and nurses by fusing patient-specific data with the most recent findings, clinical recommendations, and professional expertise. These recommendations, which might include monitoring advice, treatment alternatives, and diagnostic ideas, guarantee that professionals have access to the most recent data when making crucial decisions regarding patient care. Better patient outcomes may result from increasing the precision and consistency of diagnosis and treatment regimens [55].

Furthermore, AI-enabled tools can empower patients to actively participate in the management of their NAFLD. Personalized instruction, medication adherence reminders, food advice, and lifestyle coaching may all be provided through mobile applications and virtual assistants. By providing patients with accessible and user-friendly tools, AI can support behaviour modification and encourage healthier choices. These tools can also facilitate remote monitoring and communication between patients and healthcare providers, enabling more efficient and proactive care management. In order to fully utilize AI in disease surveillance and prevention, collaboration between academics, healthcare professionals, policymakers, and technology developers is necessary. This will eventually improve outcomes for people with NAFLD and other related diseases.

8.4 Artificial intelligence role in hepatocellular carcinoma

AI has emerged as a powerful tool in the management of HCC, the most common type of liver cancer. Due to its ability to examine big datasets, identify patterns, and provide insights, AI has the potential to enhance a variety of HCC-related functions, including early detection, diagnosis, planning of treatments, and prognosis prediction. By applying machine learning algorithms, AI has the potential to revolutionize the way HCC is handled, hopefully resulting in improved patient outcomes and specific therapy [57]. One of the primary applications of AI in HCC is in the field of medical imaging. In order to assist in the timely detection and diagnosis of HCC, AI algorithms may evaluate radiological images such as CT scans, MRI, and ultrasound. These algorithms are able to spot minor signs of HCC such as nodularity, vascularity, and tumour size. AI is able to help radiologists and doctors in establishing cause and accurate diagnoses, enabling early intervention, and increasing patient survival rates by properly and quickly interpreting these pictures. Moreover, AI can aid in the risk stratification and prediction of HCC progression [58]. AI models can evaluate the risk of disease recurrence, metastasis, and therapy response in specific individuals by combining clinical, genetic, and histological data. In order to make sure that high-risk patients receive more extensive monitoring and immediate assistance, this information can assist doctors in creating individualized treatment regimens and surveillance techniques for HCC patients. Additionally, AI can help in the discovery of new prognostic markers or genetic signatures that can improve risk assessments and offer insightful information about patient outcomes [57].

Treatment planning is another area where AI can make a significant impact on HCC management. AI algorithms can suggest the best treatment plans for certain patients by examining patient-specific data, such as medical history, imaging results, and genetic profiles. This involves recommending suitable therapeutic methods, such as surgical resection, liver transplantation, radiofrequency ablation, or systemic medicines like targeted therapies or immunotherapies [59]. Additionally, AI can help anticipate therapy responses and track the evolution of the disease, allowing for prompt modifications to the treatment plan to enhance therapeutic efficacy. AI can also help forecast the prognosis and survival of individuals with HCC. AI algorithms may produce customized survival estimates for specific patients by evaluating large-scale datasets and taking into account a variety of prognostic variables. This can offer important insights into long-term results, assist both doctors and patients in making well-informed decisions about available treatments, and help set reasonable expectations. AI can also aid in identifying novel prognostic markers or genetic signatures that could further refine prognostic predictions in HCC [60].

Furthermore, AI has the potential to support precision medicine in HCC. AI algorithms can find possible therapy targets, biomarkers, and medication combinations that may be efficient in particular subgroups of HCC patients by examining comprehensive genomic and molecular data. This personalized approach to treatment can optimize therapy selection and improve treatment outcomes. By analyzing huge datasets and making predictions about treatment effectiveness based on molecular profiles, AI can also make it easier to find new drug candidates, possibly leading the way for the creation of suited medicines.

8.4.1 Limitations of the traditional method for the diagnosis and treatment of hepatocellular carcinoma

HCC is a kind of liver cancer that can be efficiently managed, but current approaches to detection and therapy have numerous drawbacks. These restrictions cover a wide range of topics, such as diagnosis, the degree of procedure invasiveness, accuracy, early identification, treatment alternatives, recurrence rates, and customized treatment plans. The late-stage diagnosis of HCC is one of the main drawbacks of the conventional method. Often, this type of cancer remains asymptomatic in its early stages, making it difficult to detect. As a result, HCC is frequently discovered in individuals after the tumour has already migrated to other regions of the liver or surrounding organs [61]. The likelihood of effective therapy and overall patient survival is greatly decreased by late-stage diagnosis. In addition to delayed detection, traditional diagnostic methods for HCC can be invasive and carry risks. Liver biopsy, a commonly used procedure for diagnosing HCC, involves extracting a small sample of liver tissue for examination. However, this procedure can be uncomfortable for patients and carries a risk of complications such as bleeding or infection. Moreover, the obtained sample may not fully represent the characteristics of the tumour due to tumour heterogeneity, leading to potential inaccuracies in diagnosis [62].

For the diagnosis of HCC, imaging methods MRI, CT, and ultrasound are also used. The ability to identify tiny tumours, distinguish HCC from other liver diseases, and precisely estimate the degree of tumour involvement are all limitations of these techniques. This lack of sensitivity and specificity can result in misdiagnosis or delayed diagnosis, further hindering effective treatment. The lack of trustworthy early detection markers for HCC is another major constraint. HCC lacks the distinct biomarkers that some other cancers do that can be used for early diagnosis. As a result, effective screening tests for early detection are limited or nonexistent. This limitation contributes to the late-stage diagnosis mentioned earlier, reducing treatment options and overall prognosis for patients [63].

Also, there are frequently few standard alternatives for treating HCC, particularly in advanced stages or for individuals who cannot have a surgical resection. Although chemotherapy and radiation treatment are frequently utilized, their efficacy may be restricted since HCC cells have a built-in resistance and there is a chance that they might harm nearby good liver tissue. These limitations necessitate the exploration of alternative and more targeted therapies to improve treatment outcomes. Recurrence rates are high in HCC, even after successful treatment. Traditional approaches, on the other hand, might not be able to monitor for recurring disease as efficiently, leading to delays in discovery and proper response. Close surveillance is crucial in HCC patients, but the limitations of traditional methods may hinder the timely identification of recurrent tumours [64].

Moreover, the traditional approach to HCC diagnosis and treatment lacks personalized strategies. Decisions regarding treatment are frequently made in accordance with broad standards, which may not take into account the unique variances in tumour features, patient comorbidities, or genetic variables. This restriction makes it difficult to create treatment regimens that are specifically catered to the needs of each patient, which may have an impact on the effectiveness and results of the therapy [65]. These limitations encompass late-stage diagnosis, invasive diagnostic procedures, limited sensitivity and specificity of imaging techniques, lack of early detection markers, limited treatment options for advanced stages, high recurrence rates, and the absence of personalized treatment strategies. However, ongoing advancements in medical research and technology offer hope for overcoming these limitations and improving the diagnosis, treatment, and overall management of HCC.

8.4.2 Artificial intelligence with hepatocellular carcinoma diagnosis

AI has emerged as a powerful tool in the diagnosis of HCC, the most common type of primary liver cancer. AI has the potential to increase the precision and effectiveness of HCC diagnosis, resulting in better patient outcomes. AI has the capacity to evaluate complicated medical data and identify patterns that may escape human observers. One of the primary applications of AI in HCC diagnosis is in the analysis of medical images [60]. The identification and characterization of HCC depend heavily on imaging methods including CT, MRI, and ultrasound. In order to identify patterns and traits indicating HCC, AI systems may be trained on huge collections of medical pictures. Radiologists may more easily discover and diagnose HCC at an early stage when treatment choices are more successful by using AI to apply these algorithms to fresh patient images [58]. Furthermore, AI can assist in the quantification and characterization of liver lesions. AI algorithms are able to estimate tumour size, evaluate vascular invasion, and find other significant aspects in radiological images that assist diagnose the stage and severity of HCC. This information is crucial for treatment planning and prognosis. By comparing patient photos to a sizable library of annotated images, AI-powered systems may also offer decision assistance, giving doctors insights and suggestions for more accurate diagnosis and treatment choices [66].

In addition to medical imaging, AI can leverage other sources of patient data to improve HCC diagnosis. A wide range of information is stored in EHRs, such as patient demographics, medical histories, test results, and pathology reports. These records may be searched through AI algorithms, which can then produce prediction models for the growth and progression of HCC. By considering a wide range of data points, AI can assist doctors in identifying high-risk individuals who may benefit from closer monitoring or earlier intervention. With the help of AI and biomarker, early or accurate diagnosis of the HCC can be acchived. Several potential biomarkers are listed in table 8.1. Moreover, AI has the potential to contribute to personalized medicine in HCC diagnosis [67]. AI systems can pinpoint certain biomarkers and genetic alterations linked to HCC by combining genetic and molecular data. Based on each patient's particular molecular profile, this information can help in customizing treatment approaches, such as targeted treatments or immunotherapies, for that patient. AI can also facilitate the prediction of treatment response and prognosis, enabling healthcare professionals to optimize therapeutic strategies and improve patient outcomes.

While AI shows great promise in HCC diagnosis, it is important to address certain challenges and considerations. One challenge is the need for high-quality, diverse, and well-annotated datasets to train AI algorithms effectively [68]. Collaborative efforts are required to collect and curate comprehensive datasets that reflect the heterogeneity of HCC, encompassing different stages, etiologies, and

Table 8.1. Some biomarkers used for the detection of HCC.

Marker	Application
AFP (alpha-fetoprotein)	Early diagnosis
TGF-β1 (transforming growth factor-β1)	Prognosis
VEGF (vascular endothelial growth factor)	Prognosis

demographic factors. AI can assist healthcare professionals in accurate diagnosis, prognostication, and treatment planning for HCC. While challenges exist, continued research, collaboration, and ethical considerations will pave the way for responsible and effective integration of AI in HCC care, ultimately improving patient outcomes and advancing our understanding of this complex disease.

8.4.3 Treatment and management of hepatocellular carcinoma with artificial intelligence

HCC is the most common type of primary liver cancer, and it poses a significant health challenge globally. It is essential to look into cutting-edge methods for the treatment and management of HCC because its incidence has been rising and its prognosis is still dismal. Personalized treatment plans, early identification, and monitoring of therapy response are just a few of the areas of cancer care that have been revolutionized by AI in recent years. The use of AI in the management and treatment of HCC has the potential to significantly improve patient outcomes and lessen the burden of this fatal condition [69]. Early detection of HCC is essential for effective therapy because it enables prompt intervention when the tumour activity is still confined and relatively mild. AI-based algorithms have demonstrated remarkable capabilities in interpreting medical images, such as CT scans, MRI, and ultrasound, with higher accuracy and efficiency than traditional methods. AI can help radiologists discover and characterize HCC abnormalities more precisely, lowering the possibility of a missed diagnosis and allowing quick referral to experts [70]. This is done by utilizing machine learning and deep learning approaches. Once HCC is diagnosed, treatment decisions become complex due to variations in tumour characteristics, patient factors, and available therapeutic options. Here, AI can play a pivotal role in assisting clinicians with personalized treatment recommendations. By analyzing vast amounts of patient data, including genomic profiles, clinical history, and treatment outcomes, AI models can identify patterns and correlations that may predict the most effective treatment strategies for individual patients. This may result in more specialized and focused therapy, perhaps improving the effectiveness of the latter while reducing unneeded adverse effects [71].

The common methods of treatment for early-stage HCC include surgical resection, liver transplantation, and ablation treatments. However, not all patients are suitable candidates for these procedures, and disease recurrence remains a significant concern. AI can help with risk stratification by estimating survival and recurrence probabilities based on a variety of clinical and biological variables [72]. The use of these prediction models can help doctors decide on the best course of therapy and post-treatment surveillance tactics. For patients with advanced HCC or those who are not eligible for curative therapies, systemic treatments like targeted therapies and immunotherapies offer potential benefits. AI can optimize the selection of these therapies by identifying biomarkers associated with treatment response or resistance. By analyzing diverse datasets from clinical trials and real-world patient data, AI models can uncover novel biomarkers and develop predictive models that guide treatment decisions, ultimately leading to improved outcomes and quality of life for patients [73].

Additionally, tracking the response to therapy is essential to determining its efficacy and making any required modifications in a timely manner. By analyzing changes in tumour features and circulating tumour DNA, AI-driven radiomics and liquid biopsy technologies can detect early disease progression or therapy response. These non-invasive techniques not only eliminate patient discomfort but also give doctors real-time data to modify treatment plans and improve therapeutic results [74].

AI has the potential to boost HCC research and treatment development in addition to enhancing individual patient care. Through AI-driven analysis of enormous genomic and molecular databases, the discovery of new therapeutic targets and the repurposing of current medications may be improved. Virtual screening of compounds against specific molecular targets can also expedite the drug discovery process, potentially leading to the development of more effective and less toxic treatments for HCC [75]. Continued research, collaboration between AI developers and healthcare professionals, and a strong commitment to ethical implementation are crucial to unlock the full potential of AI in the fight against HCC and other forms of cancer.

8.4.4 Artificial intelligence-enabled hepatocellular carcinoma disease surveillance and prevention

HCC, the most prevalent form of primary liver cancer, presents a major public health challenge worldwide. Early identification and prevention are essential for enhancing patient outcomes and lowering mortality because of their high incidence rates and few therapeutic choices. In recent years, the advent of AI has revolutionized the field of healthcare, offering unprecedented opportunities for disease surveillance and prevention in HCC [76]. Data collection and aggregation are the first steps towards AI-driven disease surveillance in HCC. Sophisticated AI algorithms are built using a large array of patient data, including medical records, imaging scans, genetic information, lifestyle variables, and environmental exposures. With the help of these potent algorithms, it is possible to analyze patterns and identify risk factors for the development of HCC. As a result, AI makes it easier to make more precise predictions, identify people who are at high risk of developing HCC early on, and implement timely treatments and individualized preventive plans while also boosting the efficiency of disease surveillance [75].

One of the primary applications of AI in HCC prevention is in the field of medical imaging analysis. Liver imaging, such as ultrasound, CT, and MRI, plays a crucial role in early detection and diagnosis. When trained on large datasets of imaging scans, AI systems can quickly and effectively interpret these pictures, finding even tiny abnormalities or early-stage malignancies that human observers would miss. AI-enabled image analysis helps diagnose the disease in its early stages, when treatment choices are most effective and the chance of survival is better, by improving the sensitivity and specificity of HCC diagnosis [77]. Another crucial element of HCC surveillance and prevention is AI-driven genomics. An individual's vulnerability to developing HCC is mostly influenced by hereditary factors; however, genetic markers linked to the disease that were previously unknown can now be found using AI algorithms. By analyzing vast genomic datasets, AI can identify genetic patterns and mutations that elevate the risk of HCC. This provides insightful information on the fundamental processes underlying the development of HCC and indicates prospective therapeutic targets for preventative strategies or cutting-edge therapy modalities [73].

In addition to genetics, environmental and lifestyle factors have a big impact on how HCC develops. AI can combine various facts to create detailed risk profiles for each individual. AI models can precisely forecast a person's probability of acquiring HCC by taking into account variables including alcohol intake, viral infections like hepatitis B and C, obesity, and other liver illnesses. Armed with this knowledge, healthcare professionals may give specific therapy and focused treatments to high-risk patients in an effort to assist them to change their behaviour and reduce their chance of developing HCC [74].

Moreover, AI is instrumental in analyzing real-time health data from various sources, particularly with the rise of wearable devices and health monitoring applications. Continuous tracking of individuals' health parameters can generate vast amounts of data that AI algorithms can process in real-time. AI can uncover early indicators of HCC or illness development by seeing abnormalities and finding departures from typical health trends. With fast intervention and appropriate medical care made possible by this real-time analysis, the condition may be stopped from progressing to more serious stages [78]. AI's impact on HCC prevention extends beyond the individual level to address population-level health challenges. AI may be used by public health authorities to predict and control the prevalence of HCC on more widespread levels. AI is able to pinpoint high-risk areas and develop specialized preventative plans by examining population patterns, geographic distribution, environmental variables, and other pertinent data. Implementing broad screening programs, planning hepatitis vaccination drives, or creating public health campaigns focused on encouraging better lives and lowering HCC risk factors are a few examples of these [79].

Through its applications in medical imaging, genomics, real-time health data analysis, and population-level forecasting, AI offers valuable tools to identify high-risk individuals, implement personalized interventions, and design targeted public health strategies. The influence of AI technology on HCC prevention holds tremendous potential for lowering the burden of this terrible disease on a worldwide scale as it develops and integrates with healthcare systems.

8.5 Conclusion

The utilization of AI in hepatitis and chronic liver diseases has exhibited promising results, fostering enhanced efficiency, accuracy, and patient outcomes. AI algorithms have demonstrated impressive capabilities in accurately diagnosing liver diseases from medical imaging, such as ultrasound, CT scans, and MRI, with a level of precision and speed that exceeds traditional methods. Early detection of these conditions is crucial for initiating timely interventions and preventing disease progression, and AI's ability to identify subtle anomalies in images has significantly contributed to this goal. Moreover, AI-driven decision-support systems have facilitated personalized treatment plans based on patient's individual characteristics, disease severity, and response to therapies. The vast amount of data generated in the field of hepatology can be effectively analyzed and interpreted by AI, aiding in prognostication and predicting treatment outcomes. This has led to the development of more efficient and targeted therapies, ultimately improving the overall quality of life for patients with hepatitis and chronic liver diseases. Additionally, AI algorithms can efficiently match donor organs with potential recipients, maximizing the chances of successful transplants and reducing waitlist times for patients in dire need of a liver transplant. This has the potential to save countless lives and alleviate the burden on healthcare systems.

Looking ahead, the future of AI in hepatitis and chronic liver diseases appears promising, with several exciting avenues for further exploration and advancement. One such aspect is the integration of AI with emerging technologies, such as genetic sequencing and omics data analysis, to unravel the genetic basis of liver diseases. AI can help identify novel genetic markers and pathways associated with disease susceptibility and progression, paving the way for more targeted therapies and personalized medicine approaches. Another future aspect lies in the realm of drug development. The use of AI-driven drug discovery platforms can accelerate the identification of potential therapeutic compounds, shortening the time and cost required to bring new treatments to the market. By simulating molecular inter-actions and predicting drug–target interactions, AI can revolutionize the pharma-ceutical industry and facilitate the discovery of novel treatments for hepatitis and chronic liver diseases.

However, to fully realize the potential of AI in hepatitis and chronic liver diseases, several challenges must be addressed. Data privacy and security concerns, ethical considerations, and the potential for bias in AI algorithms must be carefully managed to ensure patient safety and maintain public trust. Collaborative efforts between clinicians, researchers, and AI experts will be crucial in overcoming these challenges and ensuring that AI technologies are implemented responsibly and ethically. The integration of AI in hepatitis and chronic liver diseases has already yielded promising outcomes in diagnosis, treatment, and patient care. As technology continues to evolve, AI is expected to play an increasingly pivotal role in trans-forming hepatology and liver medicine. By harnessing the power of AI, we can aspire to a future where liver diseases are diagnosed early, treated effectively, and managed with precision, significantly improving the lives of millions of patients worldwide.

References

[1] Lee H W, Sung J J Y and Ahn S H 2021 Artificial intelligence in liver disease *J. Gastroenterol. Hepatol.* **36** 539–42
[2] Le Berre C, Sandborn W J, Aridhi S, Devignes M D, Fournier L, Smaïl-Tabbone M *et al* 2020 Application of artificial intelligence to gastroenterology and hepatology *Gastroenterology* **158** 76–94.e2

[3] Decharatanachart P, Chaiteerakij R, Tiyarattanachai T and Treeprasertsuk S 2021 Application of artificial intelligence in chronic liver diseases: a systematic review and meta-analysis *BMC Gastroenterol* **21** 1–16

[4] Asrani S K, Devarbhavi H, Eaton J and Kamath P S 2019 Burden of liver diseases in the world *J. Hepatol.* **70** 151–71

[5] Dana J, Venkatasamy A, Saviano A, Lupberger J, Hoshida Y, Vilgrain V *et al* 2022 Conventional and artificial intelligence-based imaging for biomarker discovery in chronic liver disease *Hepatol. Int.* **16** 509–22

[6] Nishida N and Kudo M 2023 Artificial intelligence models for the diagnosis and management of liver diseases *Ultrasonography* **42** 10

[7] Konerman M A, Beste L A, Van T, Liu B, Zhang X, Zhu J *et al* 2019 Machine learning models to predict disease progression among veterans with hepatitis C virus *PLoS One* **14** e0208141

[8] Yip T C-F, Ma A J, Wong V W-S, Tse Y-K, Chan H L-Y, Yuen P-C *et al* 2017 Laboratory parameter-based machine learning model for excluding non-alcoholic fatty liver disease (NAFLD) in the general population *Aliment. Pharmacol. Ther.* **46** 447–56

[9] Spann A, Yasodhara A, Kang J, Watt K, Wang B, Goldenberg A *et al* 2020 Applying machine learning in liver disease and transplantation: a comprehensive review *Hepatology* **71** 1093–105

[10] Liu W, Liu X, Peng M, Chen G Q, Liu P H, Cui X W *et al* 2021 Artificial intelligence for hepatitis evaluation *World J. Gastroenterol.* **27** 5715

[11] Doyle O, Leavitt N and Rigg J A 2020 Finding undiagnosed patients with hepatitis C infection: an application of artificial intelligence to patient claims data *Sci. Rep.* **10** 10521

[12] Panchal D and Shah S 2011 Artificial intelligence based expert system for hepatitis B diagnosis *Int. J. Model. Optim.* **1** 362–6

[13] Edeh M O, Dalal S, Dhaou I B, Agubosim C C, Umoke C C, Richard-Nnabu N E *et al* 2022 Artificial intelligence-based ensemble learning model for prediction of hepatitis C disease *Front. Public Health* **10** 892371

[14] Rashid J, Batool S, Kim J, Wasif Nisar M, Hussain A, Juneja S *et al* 2022 An augmented artificial intelligence approach for chronic diseases prediction *Front. Public Health* **10** 860396

[15] Oskam L, Slim E and Bührer-Sékula S 2003 Serology: recent developments, strengths, limitations and prospects: a state of the art overview *Lepr. Rev.* **74** 196–205

[16] Banerjee D and Reddy K R 2016 Review article: safety and tolerability of direct-acting anti-viral agents in the new era of hepatitis C therapy *Aliment. Pharmacol. Ther.* **43** 674–96

[17] Mendizabal M and Reddy K R 2017 Chronic hepatitis C and chronic kidney disease: advances, limitations and unchartered territories *J. Viral Hepat* **24** 442–53

[18] Perrillo R P 2005 Current treatment of chronic hepatitis B: benefits and limitations *Semin. Liver Dis.* **25** 20–8

[19] Sumida Y, Nakajima A and Itoh Y 2014 Limitations of liver biopsy and non-invasive diagnostic tests for the diagnosis of nonalcoholic fatty liver disease/nonalcoholic steatohepatitis *World J. Gastroenterol.* **20** 475–85

[20] Aval F, Behnaz N, Raoufy M and Monthly S A 2014 Predicting the outcomes of combination therapy in patients with chronic hepatitis C using artificial neural network *Hepat. Monthly* **6** e17028

[21] Metwally F, Khaled AbuSharekh E and Abu-Naser S S 2018 Diagnosis of hepatitis virus using artificial neural network *Int. J. Acad. Pedagogical Res.* **2** 1–7

[22] Sweidan S, El-Bakry H, El-Sappagh S *et al* 2006 Viral hepatitis diagnosis: a survey of artificial intelligent techniques *Int. J. Biol. Biomed.* **1** 106–16

[23] Obaido G, Ogbuokiri B, Swart T G, Ayawei N, Kasongo S M, Aruleba K *et al* 2022 An interpretable machine learning approach for hepatitis B diagnosis *Appl. Sci.* **12** 11127

[24] Butaru A E, Mămuleanu M, Streba C T, Doica I P, Diculescu M M, Gheonea D I *et al* 2022 Resource management through artificial intelligence in screening programs—key for the successful elimination of hepatitis C *Diagnostics* **12** 346

[25] Sarma D, Mittra T, Hoq M *et al* 2020 Artificial neural network model for hepatitis C stage detection *EDU J. Comput. Electr. Eng* **1** 11–16

[26] Jilani T A, Yasin H and Yasin M M 2011 PCA-ANN for classification of hepatitis C patients *Int. J. Comput. Appl.* **14** 1–6

[27] Huang J, Zhao C, Zhang X, Zhao Q *et al* 2022 Hepatitis B virus pathogenesis relevant immunosignals uncovering amino acids utilization related risk factors guide artificial intelligence-based precision medicine *Front. Pharmacol.* **13** 1079566

[28] Ahn J, Connell A, Simonetto D *et al* 2021 Application of artificial intelligence for the diagnosis and treatment of liver diseases *Hepatology* **73** 2546–63

[29] Yağanoğlu M 2022 Hepatitis C virus data analysis and prediction using machine learning *Data Knowl. Eng.* **142** 102087

[30] Peng J, Zou K, Zhou M, Teng Y, Zhu X, Zhang F *et al* 2021 An explainable artificial intelligence framework for the deterioration risk prediction of hepatitis patients *J. Med. Syst.* **45** 1–9

[31] Lin R H and Chuang C L 2010 A hybrid diagnosis model for determining the types of the liver disease *Comput. Biol. Med.* **40** 665–70

[32] Hashem S, Esmat G, Elakel W, Habashy S, Raouf S A, ElHefnawi M *et al* 2018 Comparison of machine learning approaches for prediction of advanced liver fibrosis in chronic hepatitis c patients *IEEE/ACM Trans. Comput. Biol. Bioinf.* **15** 861–8

[33] Chen Y *et al* 2017 Machine-learning-based classification of real-time tissue elastography for hepatic fibrosis in patients with chronic hepatitis B *Comput. Biol. Med.* **89** 18–23

[34] Li Y, Wang X, Zhang J, Zhang S and Jiao J 2022 Applications of artificial intelligence (AI) in researches on non-alcoholic fatty liver disease(NAFLD): a systematic review *Rev. Endocr. Metab. Disord.* **23** 387–400

[35] Wong G L H, Yuen P C, Ma A J, Chan A W H, Leung H H W and Wong V W S 2021 Artificial intelligence in prediction of non-alcoholic fatty liver disease and fibrosis *J. Gastroenterol. Hepatol.* **36** 543–50

[36] Zhang C and Yang M 2021 The emerging factors and treatment options for NAFLD-related hepatocellular carcinoma *Cancers* **13** 3740

[37] Lupsor-Platon M, Serban T, Silion A I, Tirpe G R, Tirpe A and Florea M 2021 Performance of ultrasound techniques and the potential of artificial intelligence in the evaluation of hepatocellular carcinoma and non-alcoholic fatty liver disease *Cancers* **13** 790

[38] Takahashi Y, Dungubat E *et al* 2023 Artificial intelligence and deep learning: new tools for histopathological diagnosis of nonalcoholic fatty liver disease/nonalcoholic steatohepatitis *Comput. Struct. Biotechnol. J.* **21** P2495–501

[39] Wong G, Yuen P *et al* 2021 Artificial intelligence in prediction of non-alcoholic fatty liver disease and fibrosis *J. Gastroenterol. Hepatol.* **36** 543–50

[40] Beaton M D 2012 Current treatment options for nonalcoholic fatty liver disease and nonalcoholic steatohepatitis *Can. J. Gastroenterol.* **26** 353

[41] Rinella M E, Loomba R, Caldwell S H, Kowdley K, Charlton M, Tetri B *et al* 2014 Controversies in the diagnosis and management of NAFLD and NASH *Gastroenterol. Hepatol.* **10** 219

[42] Pouwels S, Sakran N, Graham Y, Leal A, Pintar T, Yang W *et al* 2022 Non-alcoholic fatty liver disease (NAFLD): a review of pathophysiology, clinical management and effects of weight loss *BMC Endocr. Disord.* **22** 1–9

[43] Fedchuk L, Nascimbeni F, Pais R, Charlotte F, Housset C and Ratziu V 2014 Performance and limitations of steatosis biomarkers in patients with nonalcoholic fatty liver disease *Aliment. Pharmacol. Ther.* **40** 1209–22

[44] Dinani A M, Kowdley K V and Noureddin M 2021 Application of artificial intelligence for diagnosis and risk stratification in NAFLD and NASH: the state of the art *Hepatology* **74** 2233–40

[45] Aggarwal P and Alkhouri N 2021 Artificial intelligence in nonalcoholic fatty liver disease: a new frontier in diagnosis and treatment *Clin. Liver Dis.* **17** 392–7

[46] Okanoue T, Shima T, Mitsumoto Y, Umemura A, Yamaguchi K, Itoh Y *et al* 2021 Artificial intelligence/neural network system for the screening of nonalcoholic fatty liver disease and nonalcoholic steatohepatitis *Hepatol. Res.* **51** 554–69

[47] Zhang L and Mao Y 2022 Artificial intelligence in NAFLD: will liver biopsy still be necessary in the future? *Healthcare* **11** 117

[48] Ahn J C, Connell A, Simonetto D A, Hughes C and Shah V H 2021 Application of artificial intelligence for the diagnosis and treatment of liver diseases *Hepatology* **73** 2546–63

[49] Kröner P, Engels M *et al* 2021 Artificial intelligence in gastroenterology: a state-of-the-art review *World J. Gastroenterol.* **27** 6794–824

[50] Decharatanachart P, Chaiteerakij R, Tiyarattanachai T and Treeprasertsuk S 2021 Application of artificial intelligence in non-alcoholic fatty liver disease and liver fibrosis: a systematic review and meta-analysis *Ther. Adv. Gastroenterol.* **14** 1–17

[51] Li Y, Wang X, Zhang J, Zhang S and Jiao J 2022 Applications of artificial intelligence (AI) in researches on non-alcoholic fatty liver disease(NAFLD) : a systematic review *Rev. Endocr. Metab. Disord.* **23** 387–400

[52] Mahzari A 2022 Artificial intelligence in nonalcoholic fatty liver disease *Egypt Liver J.* **12** 69

[53] Wu C, Yeh W, Hsu W *et al* 2019 Prediction of fatty liver disease using machine learning algorithms *Comput. Methods Programs Biomed.* **170** 23–9

[54] Schmidt K A, Penrice D D and Simonetto D A 2022 Artificial intelligence in the assessment and management of nutrition and metabolism in liver disease *Curr. Hepatol. Rep.* **21** 120–30

[55] Subramanian M, Wojtusciszyn A, Favre L, Boughorbel S, Shan J, Letaief K B *et al* 2020 Precision medicine in the era of artificial intelligence: implications in chronic disease management *J. Transl. Med.* **18** 472

[56] Rau H, Hsu C, Lin Y, Atique S *et al* 2016 Development of a web-based liver cancer prediction model for type II diabetes patients by using an artificial neural network *Comput. Methods Programs Biomed.* **125** 58–65

[57] Pérez M and Grande R G 2020 Application of artificial intelligence in the diagnosis and treatment of hepatocellular carcinoma: a review *World J. Gastroenterol.* **26** 5617–28

[58] Pellat A, Barat M, Coriat R, Soyer P and Dohan A 2023 Artificial intelligence: a review of current applications in hepatocellular carcinoma imaging *Diagn. Interv. Imaging* **104** 24–36

[59] Spieler B, Sabottke C, Moawad A W, Gabr A M, Bashir M R, Do R K G *et al* 2021 Artificial intelligence in assessment of hepatocellular carcinoma treatment response *Abdom. Radiol.* **46** 3660–71

[60] Sato M, Tateishi R, Yatomi Y and Koike K 2021 Artificial intelligence in the diagnosis and management of hepatocellular carcinoma *J. Gastroenterol. Hepatol.* **36** 551–60

[61] Zhou J, Sun H, Wang Z, Cong W *et al* 2018 Guidelines for diagnosis and treatment of primary liver cancer in China (2017 Edition) *Liver Cancer* **7** 235–60

[62] Osho A, Rich N and Singal A G 2020 Role of imaging in management of hepatocellular carcinoma: surveillance, diagnosis, and treatment response *Hepatoma Res.* **6** 55

[63] Ballestri S, Romagnoli D *et al* 2015 Role of ultrasound in the diagnosis and treatment of nonalcoholic fatty liver disease and its complications *Expert Rev. Gastroenterol. Hepatol.* **9** 603–27

[64] Waghray A, Murali A and Menon K 2015 Hepatocellular carcinoma: from diagnosis to treatment *World J. Hepatol.* **7** 1020–9

[65] Wu Z, Wei C, Wang L and Li H 2021 Determining the traditional Chinese medicine (TCM) syndrome with the best prognosis of HBV-related HCC and exploring the related mechanism using *Evid. Based Complement. Alternat. Med.* **2021** 9991533

[66] Nakamura Y, Higaki T, Honda Y, Tatsugami F, Tani C, Fukumoto W *et al* 2021 Advanced CT techniques for assessing hepatocellular carcinoma *Radiol. Med.* **126** 925–35

[67] Castaldo A, De Lucia D R, Pontillo G, Gatti M, Cocozza S, Ugga L *et al* 2021 State of the art in artificial intelligence and radiomics in hepatocellular carcinoma *Diagnostics* **11** 1194

[68] Zhang J, Huang S, Xu Y and Wu J 2022 Diagnostic accuracy of artificial intelligence based on imaging data for preoperative prediction of microvascular invasion in hepatocellular carcinoma: a systematic review and meta-analysis *Front. Oncol.* **12** 763842

[69] Calderaro J, Seraphin T, Luedde T and Simon T 2022 Artificial intelligence for the prevention and clinical management of hepatocellular carcinoma *J. Hepatol.* **76** P1348–61

[70] Mansur A, Vrionis A, Charles J P, Hancel K, Panagides J C, Moloudi F *et al* 2023 The Role of artificial intelligence in the detection and implementation of biomarkers for hepatocellular carcinoma: outlook and opportunities *Cancers* **15** 2928

[71] Hsu P, Liang P, Chang W *et al* 2022 Artificial intelligence based on serum biomarkers predicts the efficacy of lenvatinib for unresectable hepatocellular carcinoma *Am. J. Cancer Res.* **12** 5576–88

[72] Mo A, Velten C, Jiang J M, Tang J, Ohri N, Kalnicki S *et al* 2022 Improving adjuvant liver-directed treatment recommendations for unresectable hepatocellular carcinoma: an artificial intelligence–based decision-making tool *JCO Clin. Cancer Inform.* **6** e22000024

[73] Kim H, Lampertico P, Nam J, Lee H *et al* 2022 An artificial intelligence model to predict hepatocellular carcinoma risk in Korean and Caucasian patients with chronic hepatitis B *J. Hepatol.* **76** P311–8

[74] Citone M, Fanelli F, Falcone G, Mondaini F, Cozzi D and Miele V 2020 A closer look to the new frontier of artificial intelligence in the percutaneous treatment of primary lesions of the liver *Med. Oncol.* **37** 55

[75] Adeoye J, Akinshipo A, Thomson P and Su Y X 2022 Artificial intelligence-based prediction for cancer-related outcomes in Africa: status and potential refinements *J. Glob. Health* **12** 03017

[76] Ataei A, Deng J and Muhammad W 2023 Liver cancer risk quantification through an artificial neural network based on personal health data *Clin. Oncol.* **62** 495–502

[77] Student B and Ahsan Z 2022 Artificial intelligence used for the diagnosis, treatment and surveillance of hepatocellular carcinoma: a systematic review *Undergraduate Res. Nat. Clin. Sci. Technol.* **6** 1–13

[78] Jujjavarapu S and Saurabh D 2018 Artificial neural network as a classifier for the identification of hepatocellular carcinoma through prognosticgene signatures *Curr. Genomics* **19** 483–90

[79] Cheng M *et al* 2020 Chinese expert consensus on multidisciplinary diagnosis and treatment of hepatocellular carcinoma with portal vein tumor thrombus *Liver Cancer* **9** 28–40

Chapter 9

Artificial intelligence applications for clinical decisions support

Bhaskar Sharma, Renu Negi, Anjali Yadav, Yogesh Sharma and Vivek K Chaturvedi

Clinical decision support (CDS) systems represent a groundbreaking advancement in healthcare, fundamentally changing how clinicians make critical decisions by offering evidence-based guidance and knowledge directly at the point of care. By seamlessly integrating with electronic health record (EHR) systems, these platforms harness extensive patient data, medical literature, and best practice guidelines, empowering clinicians with the insights needed for informed decision-making. Through sophisticated analysis of large datasets, CDS systems uncover nuanced patterns and insights that enable early intervention and optimize resource allocation, thereby enhancing patient care outcomes. Despite the transformative potential of CDS, concerns persist regarding algorithm bias, data privacy, and stakeholder engagement, necessitating careful consideration and ongoing refinement. Case studies underscore the tangible impact of CDS, demonstrating its ability to enhance adherence to clinical standards, reduce hospital readmissions, and elevate patient satisfaction levels. Furthermore, the integration of AI technologies bolsters the capabilities of CDS systems across various domains, including medical imaging analysis, virtual patient care, medication safety assurance, diagnostic support, medical research facilitation, and rehabilitation. Administrative applications of AI within CDS systems streamline essential tasks such as claims processing and clinical documentation, driving operational efficiency and alleviating administrative burdens on healthcare professionals. In summary, CDS systems play a pivotal role in revolutionizing healthcare delivery by equipping clinicians with actionable insights, improving clinical decision-making, and ultimately leading to better patient outcomes.

9.1 Introduction

A new age in healthcare has begun with CDS systems. These systems use data and technology to completely change the way clinicians make choices. These tools are meant to improve clinical reasoning by providing doctors with up-to-date, evidence-based advice and knowledge right at the point of care. Integrating with EHR systems and other clinical platforms gives CDS systems access to a huge amount of patient data, medical literature, and best practice standards. One of the best things about CDS systems is that they can look at large datasets and find patterns and trends that humans might not see right away. With the help of complex algorithms and machine learning (ML), CDS systems can sort through huge amounts of data to find patterns and insights that can help doctors make decisions. For instance, these systems can help doctors figure out which people are most likely to get certain illnesses or have bad things happen to them. This way, doctors can step in early and avoid problems before they happen.

CDS systems not only improve the specificity of diagnosis and treatment plans, but they also help healthcare settings make the best use of their resources and streamline their work processes. CDS systems free up doctors to work on more difficult and important parts of patient care by automating regular tasks and improving administrative processes. For example, these systems can automatically check all of a person's medications, flag possible drug combinations, and send real-time alerts for any odd test results. This lets doctors act quickly and avoids medical mistakes. However, using CDS systems also comes with problems and moral issues to think about. We need to talk about our worries about algorithm bias and unintended effects like relying too much on technology or losing the ability to use good professional sense. Also, keeping patient data private and safe is very important, especially since online dangers and data breaches are becoming more common. The effective implementation of CDS systems depends on the cooperation and involvement of many people, such as patients, clinicians, IT experts, and managers. Clinicians need to get the right training to use CDS tools correctly and make them work with their existing clinical processes. Involving patients in the creation and use of CDS systems also makes sure that these tools meet their needs and desires.

Case studies and real-life examples demonstrate the transformative impact of CDS on healthcare delivery and treatment outcomes. Research has demonstrated that CDS systems facilitate adherence to professional standards, reduce hospital readmissions, and enhance patient satisfaction. CDS systems empower physicians to deliver superior, more efficient, and patient-centric healthcare by providing them with access to current, evidence-based data and resources that facilitate informed decision-making. Currently, in the field of healthcare, CDS systems serve as a robust tool to enhance doctors' decision-making abilities and improve the quality of treatment provided. These methodologies have the potential to revolutionize the practices of medical professionals and pave the path for innovative healthcare delivery through the utilization of technology and data analytics. However, it is crucial to address the ethical, legal, and financial challenges that arise when adopting them. By allocating additional funding and introducing innovative concepts into CDS systems, it is possible to upgrade healthcare and enhance the well-being of individuals globally. This chapter will examine the benefits, challenges, and ethical concerns associated with the utilization of CDS systems in the healthcare industry.

The main objective is to highlight the crucial significance of CDS in modern medicine, as well as its potential to revolutionize healthcare practices and improve patient outcomes. Furthermore, the use of case studies and real-world illustrations will demonstrate the transformative impact of CDS on healthcare delivery.

9.2 Overview of clinical decision support

The CDS system encompasses a variety of computerized and non-computerized tools and interventions crafted to assist the clinician in their intricate decision-making procedures. It has played a vital role in healthcare by enhancing medical decisions with targeted clinical knowledge, patient information and other health information [1]. In this system, the attributes of the patient are matched with the computerized clinical knowledge base. Subsequently, the CDS provides the clinician with patient-specific assessments or recommendations, facilitating the decision-making process [2]. Currently, CDS is often employed through web applications or incorporated into EHR and computerized provider order entry (CPOE) systems. Users can access this system via desktop computers, tablets, smartphones, and various other devices, including biometric monitoring tools and wearable health technology. The data outputs from these devices may originate directly on the device or be linked to EHR databases [3].

9.2.1 Role of artificial intelligence (AI) in enhancing CDS

Incorporating AI into CDS is a game-changer, changing the way healthcare is provided and giving doctors the ability to make better, more evidence-based judgments. AI applications in CDS utilize advanced algorithms and ML techniques to analyze large volumes of patient data, medical literature, and clinical guidelines. This allows them to provide crucial insights and suggestions just when patients need them. Consider these important functions of AI in improving CDS.

9.2.2 Medical imaging and diagnostic services

AI serves a pivotal role in image analysis, currently employed by radiologists to diagnose the onset of diseases with precision. Additionally, it is an important asset for analyzing electrocardiogram (ECG) and electrocardiography, aiding in their decision-making. AI is enabled to diagnose the early stages of diseases, including breast and skin cancer, eye disease, and pneumonia, by analyzing body modalities and speech patterns in cases of psychotic and neurodegenerative diseases. In addition, Ultra Omics' next-generation electrocardiograph is utilized to scan the sense of heartbeat patterns and detect ischemic heart diseases. During the COVID-19 pandemic, AI significantly contributed through various tools such as x-ray, computed tomography (CT), ultrasound (USG), CT scans, x-rays, and MRI, aiding in early diagnosis. The results obtained from handcrafted feature learning (HCFL), deep neural networks (DNNs), and hybrid methods were able to predict COVID-19 cases. The transformer has been used to distinguish between COVID-19 and Pneumonia by analysing x-ray and CT images, thereby addressing the critical need for the rapid and effective management of COVID-19 cases. It is the tool used in medical image analysis including registration, detection, categorization, image-to-image translation, segmentation and video-based applications. Furthermore, the ImageNet-pretrained vision transformer (ViT)-B/32 network is another tool to detect COVID-19, using Patches of chest x-ray images. Wang *et al* introduced a novel hybrid approach using chest CT scans for automatic COVID-19 detection. This technique relies on computer vision and incorporates wavelet Renyi entropy (WRE) alongside a proposed three-segment biography-grounded optimization (3SBBO) algorithm. Compared to kernel-based extreme learning machines, extreme learning machines with bat algorithms, and radial basis function neural networks, this method demonstrated superior performance in COVID-19 detection. Furthermore, AI encompasses the use of deep learning methods such as generative adversarial networks (GNAs), or artificial networks, which have an impact on radiology. Additionally, ChatGPT comes into the picture and has been used by the public for medical advice that substitutes professional medical bits of advice. It has been used for possible diagnosis and treatment suggestions based on clinical features [4].

9.2.3 Virtual patient care

The potential application of AI, ML algorithm and advancement in wearable technology in healthcare has been explored. Therefore, patient care, monitoring and management by using sensible wearable technology has become part of standard care. In addition, AI has played a vital role in monitoring chronic diseases such as diabetes mellitus, hypertension, sleep apnea, and chronic bronchitis asthma by using wearable, non-invasive sensors. These sensors track physiological parameters including respiratory rate, pulse rate, breathing patterns, waveform, blood pressure, and ECG. The acquired data is stored in the cloud and subsequently analyzed for applications in elderly care [5]. The COVID pandemic has prompted advancement in wearable technology. These devices were used to monitor physiological changes in biometrics and enable real-time patient monitoring through online connectivity [6]. Bogu and Snyder proposed the utilization of wearable sensor data as a means to predict COVID-19 attributes at early stages [7]. Through ongoing real-time research involving wearable technology in COVID-19 cases, this approach not only enhances our understanding of the disease but also reveals clinical characteristics that may have been overlooked by individuals and later substantiated through laboratory investigations. Remote patient monitoring (RPM) is a subset of telehealth that allows patients to get healthcare at a distance. RPM enhances the efficacy of medical intervention by leveraging sensor or communication technology. It makes it possible to examine health data and patient medical conditions [8].

9.2.4 Patient safety

Medication errors like drug–drug interaction (DDI) are documented as common, with up to 65% of inpatients being exposed to one or more potentially harmful combinations. The CDS system plays a vital role in reducing medication errors [9]. Computer provider order entry (CPOE) incorporates drug safety software, featuring protective measures for dosage, therapy duplication and checks DDI [10]. The types of alerts generated by these systems are among the most widely disseminated forms of decision support. However, studies have revealed considerable variability in how alerts for DDIs are displayed, prioritization, and the algorithms employed for identifying DDIs [10, 11]. Other systems that focus on enhancing patient safety encompass electronic drug dispensing systems (EDDS) and bar-code point-of-care (BPOC) medication administration systems. These are frequently integrated to establish a 'closed loop,' wherein every stage of the process (prescribing, transcribing, dispensing, and administering) is automated and takes place within an interconnected system. In general, CDS systems focusing on patient safety, particularly through computerized physician order entry (CPOE) and related systems, have demonstrated success in mitigating prescribing and dosing errors. They achieve this through features like automated warnings for contraindications, drug-event monitoring, and other functionalities. Patient safety emerges as a secondary objective or inherent requirement in nearly all categories of CDS systems, irrespective of their primary implementation purpose.

9.2.5 Diagnostic support

CDS systems, also referred to as diagnostic decision support systems (DDSSs), are a crucial tool in the clinical field, adding in diagnosis. These systems facilitate computerized consultation where they receive data or user input and subsequently generate a roster of potential diagnoses [12]. A DDSS employs uncertain logic to diagnose peripheral neuropathy [13, 14]. The system comprises 24 input fields, encompassing symptoms and diagnostic test results. This system achieved a 93% accuracy rate for identifying motor, sensory, mixed neuropathies, or normal cases. Its value is particularly pronounced in countries where access to clinical expertise is limited [15]. In addition, DXplain is an electronic-based DDSS that provides clinical-based diagnostic manifestations. In a randomized controlled trial with 87 family medicine residents, participants assigned to utilize the system exhibited notably improved accuracy [15].

9.2.6 Medical research and drug discovery

AI plays a vital role in the domain of medical research and drug discovery. It helps to analyse the intriguing data utilized in medical research and drug discovery. It is employed to seek scientific research work, integrates various types of data and supports drug innovation [16]. Pharmaceutical agencies are increasingly prioritizing the integration of AI to streamline the drug development process. Researchers leverage predictive analytics to identify appropriate candidates for clinical trials and develop accurate models of biological mechanisms [17]. ML plays a vital role in drug development by facilitating the pre-clinical stages. It assists in cohort selection, participant organization, data collection and analysis. It enhances the chances to achieve patient-oriented view, generalizability, efficacy and achievement of clinical trials. Furthermore, ChatGPT serves as an AI tool for clinical trials, aiding in data collection and furnishing information regarding clinical trials. It facilitates the summarization of pertinent publications and identification of crucial discoveries, enabling medical researchers to proficiently navigate extensive online evidence [18]. Additionally, ChatGPT assists in translating medical terminology for medical students [19]. Using an AI workbench platform, Toronto-based Deep Genomics developed a novel genetic target and respective oligonucleotide drug candidate, DG12P1, to target a rare inherited variant of Wilson's disease [20]. AI can detect the lead compounds and expedite the validation of drug targets [21, 22]. AI plays a critical role in drug repurposing by predicting interactions between drugs and targets that evade polypharmacology [21]. Within drug discovery, AI technologies such as bioinformatics and cheminformatics models significantly reduce the high costs and time required for drug discovery [20, 23].

9.2.7 Rehabilitation

AI has played a crucial role in the field of rehabilitation, encompassing both physical (robotics) and virtual domains (informatics). ML, a subset of AI, is used for perioperative medicine, brain–computer interface technology, myoelectric control, and symbiotic neuroprosthetics. ML techniques are increasingly utilized in the musculoskeletal domain, encompassing tasks such as patient data assessment, CDS, and diagnostic imaging. Moreover, in the domain of therapy, an artificial cognitive system was employed to facilitate rehabilitation exercises by analyzing signals from machinery [24]. These advancements in technology, AI, and robotics are reshaping conventional approaches.

9.2.8 Administrative applications

AI plays a vital role in administrative applications in the healthcare system. In the field of administrative applications, AI is less revolutionary than observed in patient care; nevertheless, it holds the capacity to yield significant efficiencies. Administrative applications are essential since 25% of the work time for nurses is dedicated to administrative tasks [25]. Robotic process automation (RPA) stands out as the most dependable technology to address this challenge, offering versatile applications in healthcare such as claims processing, clinical documentation, revenue cycle management, and medical record administration [26]. The integral role of CDS in the healthcare system involves the management of administrative functions and offering assistance in diagnostic coding, procedure ordering, and the triage of patients for testing. A CDS system was designed to solve the inconsistencies associated with emergency department (ED) admission and categorization of illnesses, and standardized codes were used to represent diseases and diagnoses [27]. It contributes to improving the quality of clinical documentation. The obstetric CDSS integrated an enhanced prompting system, resulting in a significant improvement in documenting indications for labour induction and estimated fetal weight compared to a control hospital [28].

9.3 Types of AI algorithms in CDS

9.3.1 Machine learning algorithms

ML algorithms have revolutionized healthcare by enabling accurate pattern recognition and disease prediction. The evaluation of large datasets is where ML approaches shine, which is why they are ideal for healthcare data analysis.

Everything from genetic information to medical pictures to patient data falls under this category. A significant use of ML algorithms in healthcare is the detection and prediction of disease trends [29]. Logistic regression is a popular ML method for binary classification applications like disease prevalence prediction. A patient's probability of having a given ailment is determined using data inputs such as demographics, medical history, and clinical test results. Support vector machines (SVMs) are a powerful tool for both classification and regression. When the distance between the classes is rather considerable, this technique performs admirably [30]. It is possible to employ SVMs for disease identification using characteristics derived from genetic data, medical imaging, and other patient data sources. Random forest is an example of an ensemble learning technique that uses several decisions to improve prediction accuracy. Its most prevalent applications in medical research include disease categorization, patient outcome prediction, and risk factor identification utilizing a range of input parameters. Neural networks, and more specifically deep learning architectures such as convolutional neural networks (CNNs) and recurrent neural networks (RNNs), are experts at dealing with complex and high-dimensional data, such as time-series data and medical images. Tasks like medical image identification (e.g., tumour detection in MRI or CT scans) and sickness progression prediction are made possible by combining CNNs with RNNs, which permit sequential data analysis. Decision trees offer a simple and understandable ML method for categorization jobs. One typical use of these algorithms is medical decision trees, which take patient information and utilize it to steer a chain of yes/no decisions that ultimately lead to a diagnosis and treatment strategy. K-Nearest Neighbors (k-NN) is a non-parametric method that has been widely used for regression and classification. For patient categorization, it employs the feature space's majority class and k-nearest neighbours. Disease identification and patient risk categorization are only two of the many medical sectors where k-NN has proven useful.

9.3.2 Bayesian Gaussian regression

The premise upon which the Naive Bayes approach rests is the independence of attributes. Gaussian Naive Bayes is extensively used in medical diagnosis issues requiring continuous features due to its efficacy with high-dimensional data. Long Short-Term Memory (LSTM) RNNs excel in detecting patterns of interdependence in sequential data that span several time periods. They are utilized in a time-series analysis of patient data, which is employed to predict the progression of a disease or the effectiveness of a treatment. These ML algorithms, when combined with other state-of-the-art approaches, aid in the development of reliable CDS systems and predictive models for use in illness diagnosis, prognosis, and treatment planning. Their dynamic application in healthcare is opening up new avenues for improved patient care and more streamlined medical processes [31].

9.4 Supervised learning

Supervised AI learning is a powerful approach for diagnosis and treatment prediction in healthcare. It involves training AI models on labelled data, where the input features represent patient information, and the corresponding output labels indicate the diagnosis or treatment outcomes. The trained AI models can then generalize patterns from the labelled data to make predictions on new, unseen patient cases. Here's how supervised AI learning is applied in diagnosis and treatment prediction.

9.4.1 Diagnosis and treatment prediction

Data collection, pertinent patient data, such as demographics, medical history, clinical test findings, imaging [32] and other diagnostic information, is gathered and associated with the respective diagnosis. Feature engineering involves preprocessing and trans-forming acquired data in a manner appropriate for training AI models. Feature engineering is the process of choosing and extracting the most pertinent traits to assist in precise diagnosis [33]. Model training involves using labelled data to train a supervised AI model, such as logistic regression, SVMs, random forest, or neural networks. The model is trained to correlate input characteristics with an accurate diagnosis using labelled examples. In model evaluation, the trained model is assessed for performance using a distinct set of data (validation or test set). Metrics such as accuracy, precision, recall, and F1-score are employed to assess the model's diagnostic perform-ance. Once the model is shown to be accurate and dependable, it may be used to make diagnoses on new patient data. The model uses the patient's input characteristics to estimate the diagnosis and treatment. Clinical decision-making might be greatly improved by supervised AI learning for diagnosis and therapy prediction. These AI models can analyse large volumes of patient data and learn from past instances to help doctors make better diagnoses and more tailored treatment plans. If we want accurate and trustworthy predictions in the actual world of healthcare, we need to train our models on high-quality data that is representative of the community of patients.

9.5 Unsupervised learning

The use of unlabelled data in unsupervised AI learning allows for the efficient identification of patterns and the gathering of patient data. While supervised learning entails labelling examples for the AI model to learn from, unsupervised learning seeks to discover structures, similarities, and patterns in the data on its own. With the use of unsupervised AI learning, patterns may be discovered and patient records can be organized. A lot of different kinds of information can be collected and set up to be used in data preparation. This includes personal information about patients, health records, test results, and details about their treatments. We can be sure that the data is ready for unsupervised learning after doing this. As part of data preparation, you may have to deal with missing numbers, scale features, and get rid of noise. We could use a number of unsupervised AI methods, like GMM, Hierarchical Clustering, K-means, and Density-Based Spatial Clustering of Applications with Noise (DBSCAN), to put together patient data [34]. The algorithm to use is based on the qualities of the data and the goals of the study. When the chosen unstructured AI model is run on the patient data, it groups patients who have similar traits. It is made up of patients whose data shows trends or traits that are similar to those in other clusters. Once the groups have been made, the next step is to look through them and see if there are any trends. The process involves looking for patterns and differences between the patients in each cluster by looking at their traits and characteristics. Patterns and observations can be found by breaking down the types of patients in each group. These patterns might help us figure out how diseases start, how treatments work, or how certain risk factors impact different groups of patients. There are many ways that these trends can be used to help people. Clustering data can be used by healthcare workers for many things, including risk stratification, finding the right people for a clinical study, customizing medication plans, and spotting early signs of sickness progression. Visualization tools like scatter plots, heatmaps, and dimensionality reduction methods (such as t-SNE) can help people understand the structure of the patient data better by showing the groups visually.

9.6 Deep learning and neural networks

Unsupervised AI learning is effective when data doesn't have clear titles or when data structure is needed to address an issue. This technology helps clinicians make fact-based judgments by detecting patterns and relationships that are hard to find by hand. It enhances patient care too. Be careful when reviewing and adding to the data to ensure the grouping appropriately reveals essential and clinically relevant patterns. Deep learning, the most advanced AI technology, can find patterns in enormous datasets. This makes it beneficial for patient and illness research and analysis. Because they can organize raw data into representations and features, deep learning models, especially deep learning neural networks, can operate with large, multidimensional datasets. Deep AI learning can help identify essential information in complex patient and sickness data.

Deep learning can handle medical photos, genetic data, EHRs, and time-series data like vital signs. DNNs can handle various dimensions and modalities of raw data. CNNs can excel at looking at pictures [35]. They immediately learn hierarchical elements like edges, textures, and forms from medical photos. This allows them to split images, recognize objects, and categorize illnesses (such as MRI scans for cancers). Autoencoders are uncontrolled deep learning models used to decrease dimensionality and extract features. They may be able to simplify patient data without losing critical information if they learn to shorten it. Training deep learning models requires a lot of labelled data, which healthcare organizations often lack. Transfer learning can enhance trained models using ImageNet. Medical jobs that require a lot of unlabelled data benefit from this. This model training method is quicker and more effective.

Multimodal data fusion teaches deep learning models to manage many patient data types. Genetic data, medical images, and EHRs are examples. Multimodal data fusion might illuminate complicated data relationships, providing a better view of individuals' ailments and features [36]. Since deep learning models are difficult, researchers are still trying to explain how they work. To feel more secure and seek treatment aid, folks must simplify models. Deep AI learning can enhance diagnosis, uncover novel biomarkers, and personalize drugs in healthcare. Data privacy, model interpretability, and morality must be considered while using deep AI learning in healthcare. This research might aid patients by assessing their conditions and creating individualized treatment strategies.

9.7 Natural language processing (NLP) techniques

Neural networks, specifically CNNs for image processing and RNNs for signal processing, have emerged as powerful tools in healthcare. These deep learning architectures have revolutionized medical image analysis and signal-processing tasks, contributing to improved diagnostics, disease detection, and patient care. Here's how neural networks are applied in image and signal processing in healthcare.

9.7.1 Convolutional neural networks (CNNs) for medical image analysis

CNNs are specifically designed for processing images and have shown remarkable success in various medical imaging tasks:

Image segmentation: CNNs can segment medical images, such as MRI or CT scans, to identify and delineate regions of interest. This is crucial for tumour detection, organ segmentation, and treatment planning [35].

Disease classification: CNNs can classify medical images into different disease categories, such as classifying skin lesions for melanoma detection or diagnosing various lung diseases from chest x-rays.

Object detection: CNNs can detect and localize specific objects or abnormalities within medical images, such as identifying retinal lesions in fundus images for diabetic retinopathy screening.

Image super-resolution: CNNs can enhance the resolution of medical images, enabling more precise diagnoses and treatment planning.

9.7.2 Recurrent neural networks (RNNs) for signal processing

RNNs are specialized for processing sequential data, making them ideal for analyzing time-series signals in healthcare:

Vital signs monitoring: RNNs can process continuous physiological signals, such as heart rate, blood pressure, and ECGs, to monitor patient health and detect anomalies or arrhythmias.

Disease progression prediction: RNNs can analyze time-series patient data to predict disease progression and patient outcomes, aiding in treatment planning and decision-making.

Natural language processing (NLP) for medical reports: RNNs, particularly LSTM networks, can process medical reports, clinical notes, and EHRs to extract valuable information and insights.

Multimodal data fusion: In some cases, neural networks can be designed to handle both image and signal data simultaneously, known as multimodal data fusion.

Combining medical imaging and vital signs: Multimodal neural networks can integrate medical imaging data with time-series vital signs data for a more comprehensive patient analysis.

Multimodal disease diagnosis: Combining data from different modalities (e.g., imaging, genomics, clinical data) can enhance disease diagnosis and treatment prediction, particularly in complex diseases.

Neural networks in image and signal processing have the potential to significantly impact healthcare, facilitating early disease detection, improving diagnostics accuracy, and enabling personalized treatment strategies. However, the successful application of neural networks requires high-quality and large datasets, collaboration between medical experts and data scientists, and robust model validation and interpretation to ensure the reliable and responsible use of these technologies in clinical settings. As research in this field progresses, we can expect continued advancements in medical image and signal processing, leading to better patient care and outcomes, such AI based implementations are listed in table 9.1 representing the AI tools used in healthcare.

Table 9.1. Representing several AI-based implementations in the field of healthcare.

Sl. No.	Current AI-based clinical data support systems	Application in clinical trial	References
1.	AI-PRS (AI-Polygenic risk scores)	Optimum dose estimation and combinations of drugs to be used for HIV treatment	[37]
2.	Bayesian network (BN)	Predict PPIs (protein–protein Interactions)	[38]
3.	EHR data	Detection, acquisition, and maintenance of patients	[39]
4.	AI-aided colonoscopy	Detection of colorectal neoplasia	[40]
5.	Genome-based cardiovascular medicine. Used to stratify baseline BP	Cardiovascular diseases	[41]
6.	SDQ (smart data quality)	AI in vaccine research	[42]
7.	SVM algorithm	Common variable immunodeficiency (CVID)	[43]
8.	Clinical trial simulation (CTS) tool Alzheimer's disease assessment Scale-cognitive sub-scale (ADAS-Cog) scores	Mild-to-moderate Alzheimer's disease	[44]
9.	IDx-DR diagnostic system	Detect diabetic retinopathy	[45]
10	WISENSE system	Esophagogastroduodenoscopy (EGD) automatically generate photo documentation during EGD	[46]
11.	Extreme gradient boosting (XGB), logistic regression (LR), random forest (RF), and Naive Bayes model (NB)	Clear cell renal cell carcinoma (ccRCC) with bone metastasis	[47]
12.	Automated EHR phenotyping (AEP)	Accurately identifies patients with epilepsy	[48]

(Continued)

Table 9.1. (*Continued*)

Sl. No.	Current AI-based clinical data support systems	Application in clinical trial	References
13.	Robot-assisted radical cystectomy (RARC)	Bladder cancer	[49]
14.	Variant combinations pathogenicity predictor (VarCoPP)	Identifies pathogenic variant combinations in gene pairs (for genetic understanding of rare diseases)	[50]
15.	Telemonitoring	Collect the telephonic recorded speech collected under acoustically non-controlled conditions utilizing different statistical machine learning techniques and strategies. Used in Parkinson's disease	[51]
16.	ANNs and DNNs	Predict the Parkinson's using the deep learning algorithm	[52]
17.	Inflammatory bowel disease (IBD)	AI is to identify patients for clinical trials via an automated endoscopic screening process known as AI-recruitment (AI-R).	[53]
18.	Colonoscopy	Reduce miss rates during colonoscopy	[54]
19.	Depression	Early detection of depression using a conversational AI bot	[55]
20	Schizophrenia	AI approach to patient selection for a clinical trial by identifying a subgroup of schizophrenia with an improved treatment effect	[56]
21.	Asthma	Asthma-guidance and prediction system (A-GPS), an Artificial intelligence (AI)-assisted CDS tool, in optimizing asthma management through a randomized clinical trial (RCT).	[57]
22.	Heart disease	Identify heart diseases by auscultation	[58]
23.	Laparoscopic cholecystectomy	Smart endoscopic surgery (SES), is a surgical system that uses artificial intelligence (AI) to detect the anatomical landmarks that expert surgeons base on to perform certain surgical maneuvers	[59]
24.	Suspected cardiac chest pain	RAPIDx AI used for diagnostic and prognostic assessment of suspected cardiac chest pain	[60]

9.8 Current AI-based clinical data support system

9.9 Challenges and considerations

9.9.1 Current AI-based CDS systems

Several AI-based CDS systems have been successfully implemented and used in real-world healthcare settings. These systems leverage AI technologies to assist healthcare professionals in making informed and evidence-based decisions. Some notable examples include the following.

IBM Watson for Oncology: IBM Watson for Oncology is an AI-powered CDS system that provides treatment recommendations for cancer patients. It analyzes large volumes of medical literature, clinical trial data, and patient records to offer personalized treatment options based on the patient's specific condition and genetic profile.

Google DeepMind's Streams: Streams is a mobile app developed by Google DeepMind in collaboration with the National Health Service (NHS) in the UK. It uses AI to help clinicians detect acute kidney injury by analyzing patient data and providing real-time alerts for early intervention.

Aidoc: Aidoc is an AI-powered radiology platform that assists radiologists in detecting and prioritizing critical findings in medical imaging studies, such as CT scans and x-rays. The system uses deep learning algorithms to highlight abnormalities and potential pathologies.

IDx-DR: IDx-DR is an AI-based diagnostic system that detects diabetic retinopathy from retinal images. It received US Food and Drug Administration (FDA) approval as the first autonomous AI system to make a clinical decision without requiring additional physician interpretation.

CLEW: CLEW is an AI-powered critical care platform that uses predictive analytics to identify patients at risk of clinical deterioration in the intensive care unit (ICU). The system continuously monitors vital signs and provides early warning alerts to healthcare providers.

Tempus: Tempus is an AI-driven healthcare platform that uses ML to analyze clinical and molecular data to inform cancer treatment decisions. It assists oncologists in tailoring treatments based on patients' molecular profiles and responses to therapies.

Zebra Medical Vision: Zebra Medical Vision offers a suite of AI algorithms that analyze medical imaging data for various conditions, including liver diseases, lung diseases, and cardiovascular risks. It provides radiologists with additional insights and improves diagnostic accuracy.

Medtronic's insulin pump with auto mode: Medtronic's AI-powered insulin pump system automatically adjusts insulin delivery based on real-time glucose readings, reducing the need for manual adjustments and offering better glucose control for diabetes patients.

These examples demonstrate the growing adoption of AI-based CDS systems across different areas of healthcare, including radiology, pathology, oncology, critical care, and chronic disease management. As AI technology continues to evolve and more research is conducted, we can expect even more innovative and impactful AI-driven CDS solutions to emerge in real-world healthcare settings.

9.10 Regulatory and ethical issues (HIPAA, GDPR, etc)

AI-driven healthcare presents several ethical considerations and regulatory aspects that must be carefully addressed to ensure patient safety, privacy, and equitable access to healthcare. Some of the key ethical considerations and regulatory aspects are as follows.

Data privacy and security: AI in healthcare requires access to sensitive patient data, raising concerns about data privacy and security. Healthcare organizations must implement robust security measures to protect patient data from unauthorized access, breaches, and misuse.

Informed consent: Patients must be adequately informed about the use of AI in their healthcare and provide informed consent for their data to be used for AI-driven decision-making.

Transparency and explainability: AI algorithms can be complex and difficult to interpret. Healthcare professionals need to understand the rationale behind AI-driven recommendations to trust and utilize them effectively. Transparent and explainable AI models are essential to build trust between clinicians and AI systems.

Algorithm bias: AI models trained on biased data can perpetuate healthcare disparities and lead to inequitable treatment recommendations for certain patient groups. Ensuring fairness and minimizing bias in AI algorithms is crucial for equitable patient care.

Autonomy and human oversight: AI should complement, not replace, the expertise and judgment of healthcare professionals. Maintaining human oversight is essential to ensure that AI-driven recommendations align with patient preferences and values.

Accountability and liability: Determining responsibility and liability in cases of AI-driven errors or adverse outcomes can be challenging. Clear guidelines and protocols are needed to assign responsibility and address legal considerations.

Generalizability and bias in AI models: AI models trained on specific populations may not generalize well to other groups or regions. Efforts should be made to ensure that AI models are diverse and representative to avoid perpetuating bias and disparities.

Regulatory approval and validation: AI-based medical devices and CDS systems require regulatory approvals, such as FDA clearance. Rigorous validation and testing are essential to ensure the safety and efficacy of AI-driven healthcare applications.

Resource allocation and accessibility: AI-driven healthcare technologies should be accessible to all patient populations, including underserved communities. Ensuring equitable access to AI-driven healthcare is crucial to avoid exacerbating existing healthcare disparities.

Over-reliance on AI: Over-reliance on AI-generated recommendations without clinical validation or human oversight may lead to suboptimal patient care.

Healthcare professionals should use AI as a tool to enhance decision-making, not as a substitute for clinical judgment.

Addressing these ethical considerations and regulatory aspects requires collaboration among healthcare organizations, AI developers, policymakers, and ethicists. Implementing responsible AI practices and adhering to established ethical guidelines can help maximize the benefits of AI-driven healthcare while mitigating potential risks and challenges. Striking the right balance between innovation and ethical principles is crucial for the successful and sustainable integration of AI in healthcare.

9.11 Challenges for clinical translation

The recent spate of articles and datasets demonstrates the impressive progress made by oncologic AI. There is a significant chasm, however, between proof of AI success and proof of therapeutic efficacy. According to a recent meta-analysis, the use of deep learning in medical imaging has only been tested in two published randomized clinical studies, with just nine planned trials in total. Deep learning algorithms have been the subject of hundreds of published researches on their effectiveness [61]. An absence of both high-quality and massive volumes of data may be a major obstacle to the development of clinical AI applications in cancer and healthcare generally. Varoquaux and Cheplygina [62] and Thompson [63] are only two of many sources that discuss the issues surrounding data collecting, transparency, bias, and reliability. The difficulty of AI models in comprehending, believing, replicating, and applying to different contexts has also received much attention [64]. Even though these issues are critical to the advancement of AI, we will now discuss certain concepts unique to the clinical translation of models that have proven effective throughout their early phases of development and assessment. These include practicality, usability, and clinical validity. Although these considerations are often overlooked during model building and evaluation, they are crucial for taking clinical AI beyond the lab and into the treatment of cancer patients. According to Park *et al*, the standard procedure for demonstrating a model's clinical validity involves doing internal validation, external validation, prospective testing, and finally, local testing in the target population [65]. To ensure that the study can be replicated and done correctly, one must adhere to new guidelines like FAIR data, CONSORT/ SPIRTAI, and the (still in development) TRIPOD-AI checklists [64]. With these guidelines, we can finally standardize the processes used to create AI models and have a yardstick by which to evaluate the quality of AI research. The majority of published AI research makes use of a blinded test set conducted internally. According to Kim *et al*, only a tiny fraction of models includes future testing or standard comparisons with human experts, and even fewer employ an external validation set [66]. Since the majority of AI models do not rely on hypotheses when selecting features, real-world outcomes might vary greatly depending on how the test data distribution differs from the training data [67]. This highlights the need to use several external assessment sets. Edge cases, or scenarios not well represented in the training data, might thus make predicting the model's performance challenging [68]. In oncology, finding uncommon outcomes is crucial for safe cancer treatment, hence they must be included while proving a model's clinical validity. Preliminary testing in 'silent' conditions can help ensure the model's viability in production settings [69]. Even while there is some proof that a model is safe to employ during run-in, it could be difficult to predict how well it would perform in really unusual scenarios. You need to prove clinical validity before you can prove clinical value. This differs from performance validation in that it incorporates the assessment of clinically significant metrics. Achieving good results on widely used endpoints like sensitivity, specificity, or area under the receiver operating characteristic curve may be sufficient for certain diagnostic applications. However, clinical outcomes must be verified at every stage of the treatment pathway for their influence to be felt in the real world. This translates to better quality of life, less healthcare resource use, a higher likelihood of survival, better management of the illness, and decreased risk of adverse effects in cancer. Randomized research is the best way to evaluate these hypotheses. The most effective method would be to randomly assign patients to the AI technique and then directly compare the clinical outcomes. Research in this area has been conducted on occasion. The accuracy of colonoscopy polyp detection rates is one such example [70]. The rate of tumour detection was the primary outcome of this research. More study is required to determine how AI systems might enhance the quality of life or living in the long term, although they were proven to be superior. A second approach to AI clinical trials is to employ randomized therapies once a verified model has classified all patients' risks. One research that attempted this and succeeded used EHR data to identify radiation patients at risk of ED visits [71]. The next step was to randomly assign high-risk individuals to either routine treatment or additional checkups to ensure their health. Both the number of visits to the emergency department and the length of hospital stays were significantly reduced in the randomized high-risk individuals who received additional visits compared to the low-risk patients who did not get such treatment. Although this research design is not sufficient for clinical benefit evidence, it is perfect for AI-based risk-prediction models—a significant portion of AI models that are currently in development. It usually takes a lot of time and effort to conduct a randomized clinical trial. AI interventions are already challenging, and their unique characteristics further make things worse. With the addition of fresh data, AI models can improve with time. What would the protocol be for including this in a typical randomized trial? There has to be a re-evaluation of the conventional randomized clinical trial if AI is to be demonstrated to have therapeutic utility through randomized trials [70]. To identify issues and enhance the experience, the platform should provide a means for users to provide feedback [71]. Systems must be able to communicate with one another at the point of care, inside and across facilities for operations to operate smoothly [72]. Additionally, each dataset under consideration has its own distinct set of usability issues. There are several challenges associated with the new data streams, such as mobile health data and wearable activity trackers [73]. Ensuring the AI software is straightforward to comprehend is a crucial aspect of producing anything functional. The increasing complexity of data streams makes it more difficult to attribute algorithmic predictions to underlying biological or clinical factors. While this 'black box' effect might work in other consumer goods industries, it would be extremely challenging to apply it to healthcare decisions due to the gravity of the matter and the potential influence of legislation [74, 75]. Fortunately, studies investigating interpretability concerns are becoming increasinly common. Some aspects of AI prediction can be illuminated by methods such as feature visualizations, variable significance metrics, hidden-states analysis, and saliency maps [76, 77]. Clinically validated approaches can be more easily implemented if one is aware of the developments in human factors research and collaborates with competent experts. Finally, clinical institutions and departments may need to allocate funds for robust IT support services to transform algorithms into solutions that are effective in the clinic.

Another crucial concept in clinical usefulness is addressing issues that arise from the simultaneous or sequential deployment of numerous AI models at various touchpoints. These events are likely to occur more frequently and require careful orchestration based on end-user responsibilities, communication, access, and training. Many different healthcare providers interact with cancer patients in some way throughout treatment, and some of these providers may be heavy users of an AI app (figure 9.1). These individuals may primarily focus on diagnosis or treatment, or perhaps both. On the one hand, cancer is mostly diagnosed by pathologists and radiologists; on the other hand, medical, radiation, and surgical specialists are the ones who typically treat the disease. There are opportunities to bring together and coordinate various AI applications at points along the route where multiple areas converge, such as tumour boards. A particular AI software might find its way into the hands of many different types of healthcare professionals, including physicians,

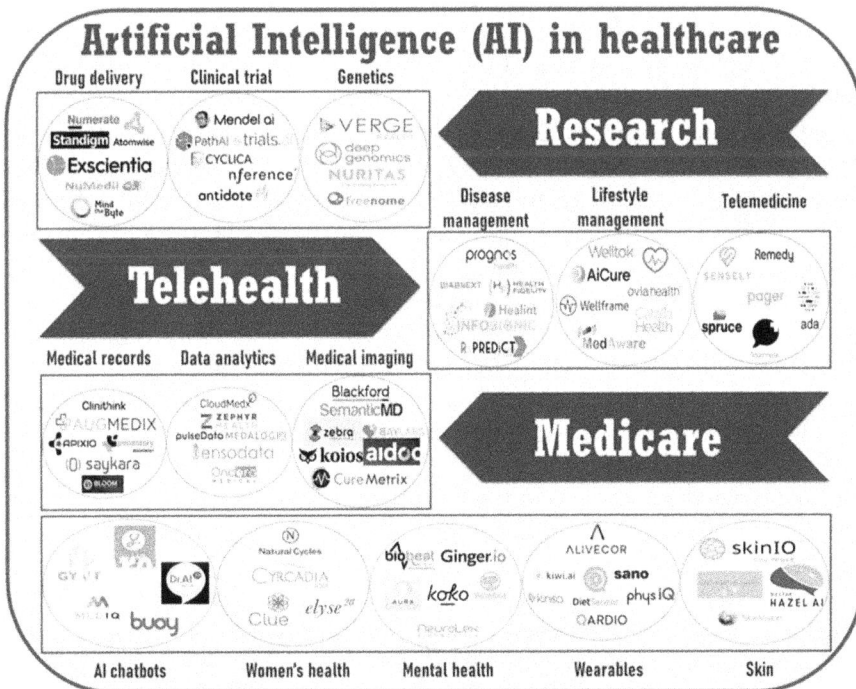

Figure 9.1. Illustration depicting several implementations of AI in the field of healthcare.

nurses, PAs, therapists, social workers, and even medical students. Who exactly is the 'designated user' whose job it is to make use of and share such data in this scenario? For instance, what if a patient's CT scan includes an AI-generated cancer diagnosis? What if this prediction is subsequently inputted into another algorithm that suggests surgery as a treatment? Who is liable for decisions taken following the plan is another concern that arises. For the time being, we do not have concrete solutions to these issues, and we expect that they will arise individually, case by case. To assist medical AI developers and cancer care professionals in navigating these complex issues, further funding, research, and direction are required for this clinical orchestration of AI models. Although there are currently very few AI applications for oncologic indications that have been authorized by the FDA, there are many more in the works. As a result, there is a lot of interest in finding ways to streamline the process from development to clinical translation. So, the FDA is now working on prescribing AI and ML-specific protocols for clinical usage. The most current plan of action takes into account the aforementioned clinical principles and lays the groundwork for adding more details to a framework for the safe clinical translation of AI [80].

9.12 Obstacles, restrictions, and missing knowledge

Additionally, the poll revealed a few restrictions and difficulties. To start with, it is not fair to rely just on accuracy as a measure to assess the effectiveness of a model when evaluating ML in some publications. The ML algorithm cannot be objectively evaluated using a single statistic. Second, there was no assurance of data quality, and the datasets used for medical AI applications were tiny in size. Consequently, the worse quality of the input data and the relatively short amount of the dataset may restrict the AI model's performance. Overfitting was anticipated to occur since the AI model was trained and validated using just a tiny dataset. Unfortunately, the model's generalizability proved poor. Thirdly, there are currently no universally approved AI assessment methodologies among researchers in the field. Due to the continued reliance on human cognition in evaluation, AI models can only be assessed qualitatively. Having said that, the majority of the publications included in this study only detailed the AI approaches and did not assess them in any way. Medical experts evaluated AIs in just a small number of studies. Lastly, a lot of the research relied only on pre-existing ML or AI techniques. Medical AI applications may not address doctors' real clinical demands because of a lack of creativity and prior knowledge of these AI techniques that were developed without the involvement of medical specialists.

After surveying the medical AI literature, we also identified two areas where more study is needed. To begin, deep learning techniques such as MLP, CNNs, RNNs, and transformers have been the subject of the vast bulk of research in the multidisciplinary area of AI and medicine. Models like transformers that rely on deep learning have millions of parameters and are notoriously difficult to understand. But AI, not state-of-the-art deep learning models, should be the emphasis of data scientists and AI specialists working in the multidisciplinary area of AI and healthcare. Second, only doctors should assess the usefulness of medical AI applications. Unfortunately, neither AI nor medical expert evaluations are present in the majority of medical AI applications. Good human–computer interaction (HCI) and logical explanations for medical professionals should characterize medical AI solutions.

9.13 Future trends

We anticipate that AI will play a significant role in many surgical procedures and diagnostics in the years to come. AI's ability to boost these models' openness and win over doctors' trust makes it an indispensable tool. We propose that to tackle the aforementioned problems, it would be preferable to evaluate ML using a variety of measures, including specificity and sensitivity, in addition to accuracy. Additionally, cross-validation is the way to go for validating the learned model. To further enhance the generalizability of the ML model, it would be wise to gather and construct the dataset from a variety of sources in the future, including other hospitals. Furthermore, federated ML might be utilized to safeguard identifying medical records. Few-shot learning [56], data augmentation [54], and transfer learning [55] are some more strategies that might be explored to handle the problem of small dataset sizes. Thirdly, there is no genuine agreement on how to evaluate AI. There is a lack of a standardized, objective measure for evaluation. Some researchers have suggested an evaluation method for generic AI assessments. One such method is the system causability scale (SCS), which was introduced by Holzinger *et al* [53] and offers a fresh perspective on quality explanation. It was able to swiftly determine if the explainable model was suitable for its intended purpose by using the Likert scale approach. Nevertheless, we contend that human-centred evaluation needs to underpin medical AI evaluation. To be more precise, it has to be reviewed by specialists in both medicine and AI. If we want to make sure that medical AI applications can generate explainable clinical inferences, for instance, we can ask medical specialists to test the methods using relevant clinical tasks. Experts in AI, on the other hand, may assess the AI apps' robustness and generalizability. Lastly, it would be beneficial for medical experts to be involved in the planning and execution of future research on medical AI applications. Collaborating across disciplines is essential for the successful implementation of medical AI. In particular, medical professionals should contribute their extensive medical expertise; their critiques and recommendations will enhance the development of AI systems. It is the responsibility of data scientists and AI specialists to guarantee that medical AI apps can aid doctors in reaching an explicable clinical conclusion. As a result, we anticipate that the medical field will warm up to medical AI models. A potential strategy for accomplishing this goal is to enhance HCIs. Through the use of an intelligently crafted HCI medical app, collaboration between medical professionals and AI specialists will be within reach.

9.14 Future trends and developments

9.14.1 Advancements in AI algorithms

AI algorithms analyse vast amounts of patient data, outperforming traditional tools like the Modified Early Warning Score (MEWS) in assisting medical professionals in making informed decisions about patient care [81]. This advancement is crucial for improving patient outcomes and enhancing the efficiency of healthcare delivery. The integration of CDS systems with EHRs and other healthcare IT systems is crucial for ensuring seamless data exchange and continuity of care. The Kidney Failure Risk equation (KFRE) and the Statin Choice Decision Aid are two such examples [82]. NLP technologies enable CDS systems to extract valuable insights from unstructured clinical notes, research articles, and other textual sources providing relevant information in a timely manner, enhancing the capability of decision-making, and improving the quality of care [83]. In diagnostics, AI has shown significant potential, especially in imaging. AI-based assistance for lung nodule detection on CT scans and other areas has led to nearly 400 FDA approvals of AI algorithms for the radiology field [84, 85]. This capability to process and analyse structured and unstructured data has the potential to transform diagnostic accuracy and efficiency. With over 48% of hospital CEOs and strategy executives confident that health systems will have the infrastructure to utilize AI to augment clinical decision-making by 2028, the implementation of AI in routine clinical care represents a substantial opportunity. AI algorithms are analysing patient data to customize treatments, with wearables and mobile health devices enhancing CDS in cardiovascular disease prevention. This personalized medicine offers effective, targeted therapies with improved outcomes and reduced side effects. The COVID-19 pandemic has accelerated the use of remote monitoring and telemedicine technologies, utilizing AI for data analysis and decision support, enhancing patient care in remote locations. Staff members of a nursing call centre provide guidance for at-home treatment via question-and-answer sessions using AI-algorithmic tools [86]. As the technology continues to evolve, it is essential for healthcare providers to build the necessary infrastructure to support AI technology, ensuring that its benefits are fully realized.

9.15 Expansion to point-of-care devices

The healthcare industry is integrating CDS systems into point-of-care devices, including handheld and wearable sensors that deliver decision support capabilities directly to the bedside, providing real-time data-driven insights to improve patient care. The US FDA has released revised guidance documents, including the Final CDS Guidance, which emphasizes the importance of CDS software intended for healthcare professionals (HCPs) as devices [87]. This shift reflects the growing recognition of CDS systems' potential to improve healthcare delivery by leveraging clinical knowledge, patient data, and other health information to support medical decisions. Point-of-care devices that can be integrated with CDS systems include for example, CDS Hooks: these are specifications that allow health systems to embed near real-time functionality within EHRs, enabling interoperability among different stakeholders, collecting specific data elements when a clinician performs a set event. Order Sets Tools tailored to specific patients with specific conditions, providing prompts, reminders, insights, and cautions, enhance workflow efficiency by saving clinicians time for data analysis. The future of CDS systems is likely to be shaped by advancements in AI and ML, which can process vast amounts of data to provide evidence-based recommendations for diagnosis, treatment, and follow-up [88]. These technologies can integrate data from multiple sources, including imaging, clinical, pathology, and genomics, to offer predictive analysis and recommended treatment pathways. The integration of AI in imaging interpretation and reporting processes is expected to reduce diagnostic errors and improve workflow efficiencies, particularly for junior radiologists [84]. Moreover, CDS applications are crucial for managing the rising cost of care by optimizing the use of medical imaging. By selecting the most appropriate imaging based on a patient's unique clinical condition and current evidence-based guidelines, CDS systems can help reduce unnecessary radiation exposure and costs [89]. As healthcare continues to digitalize and implement sustainable systems, the future of CDS appears promising, with the potential to significantly improve patient outcomes and healthcare delivery.

9.16 AI-driven drug discovery

AI is transforming the pharmaceutical industry, particularly in drug discovery and development. AI algorithms, such as DNNs, are accelerating the drug discovery process by analysing vast datasets to identify potential drug candidates and predict their effectiveness [90]. This advancement not only reduces the time and cost associated with traditional drug development but also enhances the accuracy of drug discovery, leading to better-quality products. AI is revolutionizing virtual screening and drug design by analysing protein structure, predicting drug interactions, and designing drugs with higher potency and specificity [20]. AI's role in CDS extends beyond drug discovery. It aids in the optimization of drug dosages, ensuring batch-to-batch consistency, and facilitating quick decision-making in clinical trials [91]. Moreover, AI can contribute to the safety and efficacy assessment of drugs, ensuring proper market positioning and costing through comprehensive market analysis. Despite the promising advancements, AI-driven drug discovery faces challenges like high-quality, reliable data, ethical and regulatory considerations, and patient privacy and data security, despite advancements in AI algorithms [92]. However, the future of AI in drug discovery and CDS looks bright, with the potential to significantly improve patient outcomes and healthcare delivery.

9.17 AI in public health and epidemiology

AI is significantly advancing public health and epidemiology, particularly through its application in CDS. AI chatbots, for instance, are instrumental in generating predictive models of public health outcomes by analyzing data from patient records, social media, and other sources like AiCure that coaches patients to manage their condition and adhere to instructions, offering personalized care and support. Watson for Oncology examines data from records and medical notes to generate an evidence-based treatment plan for oncologists, enhancing the precision of treatment planning [93]. This technology enables healthcare professionals to make informed decisions with greater accuracy and speed, aiding in the early identification of disease trends and the development of personalized treatment plans [94]. AI's role extends to simulating public health policy decisions, providing interactive advice on public health issues, and offering detailed information on the potential impact of policies. This capability allows for a more informed decision-making process in public health management and policy-making [95]. Moreover, AI's ability to automate the summarization of public health data through NLP techniques enhances the understanding of public health trends and patterns, informing decision-making and policy-making for improved health outcomes [96]. AI-driven systems like EPIWATCH provide early signals of epidemics before official detection by health authorities, demonstrating the potential for rapid epidemic intelligence and open-source data to improve public health security [97]. This early detection capability is crucial for mitigating the health and economic impacts of serious epidemics and pandemics, allowing for more timely and effective responses. AI integration in public health enhances data-driven decision-making, identifies threats, and monitors health trends, improving service efficiency and reducing health disparities.

9.18 Conclusion

AI in clinics may enhance patient outcomes and treatment strategies. It cannot be fully used in clinical practice until other difficulties have been addressed. AI in clinical oncology is now used for certain cancer treatment activities. Effective cancer care models require huge, well-labelled datasets. Clinical validity, usefulness, and usability should be prioritized as AI algorithms advance. This should be done to develop and assess needs-based models. EHRs are transforming into critical healthcare data sources and enormous databases for AI research and forecasting. ML and deep learning networks can combine risks to enhance patient outcomes. AI will assist physicians in balancing complex goals and risks, allowing for multi-outcome optimization when healthcare systems integrate AI. Doctors must understand AI prediction models in order to adapt to this new area and must examine biases. Additional training and professional development are required for healthcare staff. When providing patients with AI-generated knowledge, medical students want a revamped curriculum that prioritizes emotional intelligence and comprehension. Explaining anything is critical when developing and implementing AI-powered CDS systems. Because medicine is so complicated, developers, policymakers, and healthcare practitioners find it difficult to establish explainability. Clear standards and criteria are required to make AI-powered CDS systems visible. No AI explainability language may be dangerous for manufacturers and impede regulatory clearance. A global conference and 'explainability white paper' might help standardize language, boosting scientific research, law, and AI-powered medical device CDSSs. To fully investigate and evaluate AI-powered CDS systems, researchers from different fields must work together. To summarize, AI can enhance clinical therapy and outcomes. To use AI in clinical practice, we must first address questions of clinical validity, usefulness, and explainability.

References

[1] Patrício L, Sangiorgi D, Mahr D, Čaić M, Kalantari S and Sundar S 2020 Leveraging service design for healthcare transformation: toward people-centered, integrated, and technology-enabled healthcare systems *J. Service Manag.* **31** 889–909

[2] Velickovski F *et al* 2014 Clinical Decision Support Systems (CDSS) for preventive management of COPD patients *J. Transl. Med.* **12 Suppl 2** S9

[3] Butcher C J and Hussain W J F 2022 Digital healthcare: the future *Future Healthcare J.* **9** 113

[4] Ray P P and Majumder P J 2023 The potential of ChatGPT to transform healthcare and address ethical challenges in artificial intelligence-driven medicine *J. Clin. Neurol.* **19** 509

[5] Monteriù A, Prist M R, Frontoni E, Longhi S, Pietroni F, Casaccia S *et al* 2018 A smart sensing architecture for domestic monitoring: methodological approach and experimental validation *Sensors* **18** 2310

[6] Natarajan A, Su H-W and Heneghan C J N 2020 Assessment of physiological signs associated with COVID-19 measured using wearable devices *npj Digital Med.* **3** 156

[7] Bogu G K and Snyder M P J M 2021 Deep learning-based detection of COVID-19 using wearables data *MedRxiv* 2021.01.08.21249474

[8] Tantray J, Kosey S, Prajapati J B and Prajapati B 2024 The future of the healthcare system: a meta-analysis of remote patient monitoring *Handbook on Augmenting Telehealth Services* (Boca Raton, FL: CRC Press) pp 105–26

[9] Javaid M, Haleem A, Singh R P, Suman R and Rab S 2022 Significance of machine learning in healthcare: features, pillars and applications *Int. J. Intell. Netw.* **3** 58–73

[10] Nayyar A, Gadhavi L, Zaman N and Healthcare t I M T 2021 Machine learning in healthcare: review, opportunities and challenges *Machine Learning and the Internet of Medical Things in Healthcare* (Elsevier) pp 23–45

[11] Sadiku M N, Zhou Y and Musa S M 2018 Natural language processing *Int. J. Adv. Sci. Res. Eng.* **4** 68–70

[12] Ghosh P 2018 AI early diagnosis could save heart and cancer patients (BBC) https://www.bbc.co.uk/news/health-42357257

[13] Kunhimangalam R, Ovallath S and Joseph P K 2013 A novel fuzzy expert system for the identification of severity of carpal tunnel syndrome *BioMed Res. Int.* **2013** 846780

[14] Kunhimangalam R, Ovallath S and Joseph P K 2014 A clinical decision support system with an integrated EMR for diagnosis of peripheral neuropathy *J. Med. Syst.* **38** 1–14

[15] Wang D, Khosla A, Gargeya R, Irshad H and Beck A H 2016 Deep learning for identifying metastatic breast cancer arXiv:1606.05718

[16] O'Mara-Eves A, Thomas J, McNaught J, Miwa M and Ananiadou S 2015 Using text mining for study identification in systematic reviews: a systematic review of current approaches *Syst. Rev.* **4** 1–22

[17] Shelmerdine S C, Martin H, Shirodkar K, Shamshuddin S and Weir-McCall J R 2022 Can artificial intelligence pass the Fellowship of the Royal College of Radiologists examination? Multi-reader diagnostic accuracy study *BMJ* **379** e072826

[18] Khan R A, Jawaid M, Khan A R and Sajjad M 2023 ChatGPT-reshaping medical education and clinical management *Pakistan J. Med. Sci.* **39** 605

[19] Javaid M, Haleem A and Singh R PStandards, Evaluations 2023 ChatGPT for healthcare services: an emerging stage for an innovative perspective *BenchCouncil Trans. Benchm. Stand. Eval.* **3** 100105

[20] Vora L K, Gholap A D, Jetha K, Thakur R R S, Solanki H K and Chavda V P 2023 Artificial intelligence in pharmaceutical technology and drug delivery design *Pharmaceutics* **15** 1916

[21] Mak K-K and Pichika M R 2019 Artificial intelligence in drug development: present status and future prospects *Drug Discov. Today* **24** 773–80

[22] Paul D, Sanap G, Shenoy S, Kalyane D, Kalia K and Tekade R K 2021 Artificial intelligence in drug discovery and development *Drug Discov. Today* **26** 80

[23] Son W S 2018 Drug discovery enhanced by artificial intelligence *Biomed. J. Sci. Tech. Res.* **12** 8936–8

[24] Anderson D 2019 Rehabilitation. Artificial intelligence and applications in PM&R *Am. J. Phys. Med. Rehabil.* **98** e128–9

[25] Iroju O G, Olaleke J O J I J I T and Science C 2015 A systematic review of natural language processing in healthcare *Int. J. Inform. Technol. Comput. Sci.* **7** 44–50

[26] Trunfio M and Rossi S 2022 Advances in metaverse investigation: streams of research and future agenda *Virtual Worlds* **1** 103–29

[27] Orth M, Averina M, Chatzipanagiotou S, Faure G, Haushofer A, Kusec V *et al* 2019 Opinion: redefining the role of the physician in laboratory medicine in the context of emerging technologies, personalised medicine and patient autonomy ('4P medicine') *J. Clin. Pathol.* **72** 191–7

[28] Organization W H 2022 Regional strategy for fostering digital health in the Eastern Mediterranean Region (2023–2027)World Health Organization. Regional Office for the Eastern Mediterranean https://www.emro.who.int/about-who/rc69-presentations/regional-strategy-for-fostering-digital-health-in-the-eastern-mediterranean-region.html

[29] Alpaydin E 2020 *Introduction to Machine Learning* (Cambridge, MA: MIT Press)

[30] Kamiński B, Jakubczyk M and Szufel P 2018 A framework for sensitivity analysis of decision trees *Central Eur. J. Oper. Res.* **26** 135–59

[31] Liu J, Zhang Z and Razavian N 2018 Deep EHR: chronic disease prediction using medical notes *Proc. 3rd Machine Learning for Healthcare Conf.* vol 85 (PMLR) 440–64

[32] Patel M J, Andreescu C, Price J C, Edelman K L, Reynolds III CF and Aizenstein H J 2015 Machine learning approaches for integrating clinical and imaging features in late-life depression classification and response prediction *Int. J. Geriatric Psych.* **30** 1056–67

[33] Liang Z, Zhang G, Huang J X and Hu Q V 2014 Deep learning for healthcare decision making with EMRs *2014 IEEE Int. Conf. on Bioinformatics and Biomedicine (BIBM)* (Piscataway, NJ: IEEE)

[34] Alloghani M, Al-Jumeily D, Mustafina J, Hussain A, Aljaaf A J and science ulfd 2020 A systematic review on supervised and unsupervised machine learning algorithms for data science *Supervised and Unsupervised Learning for Data Science* (Springer) pp 3–21

[35] Leijnen S and van Veen F 2020 The neural network zoo *Proceedings* **47** 9

[36] Rao S R, DesRoches C M, Donelan K, Campbell E G, Miralles P D and Jha A K 2011 Electronic health records in small physician practices: availability, use, and perceived benefits *J. Am. Med. Inform. Assoc.* **18** 271–5

[37] Shen Y, Liu T, Chen J, Li X, Liu L, Shen J *et al* 2020 Harnessing artificial intelligence to optimize long-term maintenance dosing for antiretroviral-naive adults with HIV-1 infection *Adv. Therapeut.* **3** 1900114

[38] Gao S and Wang X J B 2011 Quantitative utilization of prior biological knowledge in the Bayesian network modeling of gene expression data *BMC Bioinform.* **12** 13

[39] O'Brien E C, Raman S R, Ellis A, Hammill B G, Berdan L G, Rorick T *et al* 2021 The use of electronic health records for recruitment in clinical trials: a mixed methods analysis of the harmony outcomes electronic health record ancillary study *Trials* **22** 8

[40] Lou S, Du F, Song W, Xia Y, Yue X, Yang D *et al* 2023 Artificial intelligence for colorectal neoplasia detection during colonoscopy: a systematic review and meta-analysis of randomized clinical trials *eClin. Med.* **66** 102341

[41] Krittanawong C, Johnson K W and Tang WH W 2019 How artificial intelligence could redefine clinical trials in cardiovascular medicine: lessons learned from oncology *Future Med.* **16** 87–92

[42] Sharma A, Virmani T, Pathak V, Sharma A, Pathak K, Kumar G *et al* 2022 Artificial intelligence-based data-driven strategy to accelerate research, development, and clinical trials of COVID vaccine *BioMed Res. Int.* **2022** 7205241

[43] Orange J S, Glessner J T, Resnick E, Sullivan K E, Lucas M, Ferry B *et al* 2011 Genome-wide association identifies diverse causes of common variable immunodeficiency *J. Allerg. Clin. Immunol.* **127** 1360–76

[44] Romero K, Ito K, Rogers J, Polhamus D, Qiu R, Stephenson D *et al* 2015 The future is now: model-based clinical trial design for Alzheimer's disease *Clin. Pharmacol. Therap.* **97** 210–4

[45] Abràmoff M D, Lavin P T, Birch M, Shah N and Folk J C 2018 Pivotal trial of an autonomous AI-based diagnostic system for detection of diabetic retinopathy in primary care offices *npj Dig. Med.* **1** 39

[46] Wu L, Zhang J, Zhou W, An P, Shen L, Liu J *et al* 2019 Randomised controlled trial of WISENSE, a real-time quality improving system for monitoring blind spots during esophagogastroduodenoscopy *Gut* **68** 2161–9

[47] Le Y, Xu W and Guo W 2023 Treatment. The construction and validation of a new predictive model for overall survival of clear cell renal cell carcinoma patients with bone metastasis based on machine learning algorithm *Technol. Cancer Res. Treat.* **22** 15330338231165131

[48] Fernandes M, Cardall A, Jing J, Ge W, Moura L M, Jacobs C *et al* 2023 Identification of patients with epilepsy using automated electronic health records phenotyping *Epilepsia* **64** 1472–81

[49] Khetrapal P, Wong J K L, Tan W P, Rupasinghe T, Tan W S, Williams S B *et al* 2023 Robot-assisted radical cystectomy versus open radical cystectomy: a systematic review and meta-analysis of perioperative, oncological, and quality of life outcomes using randomized controlled trials *Eur. Urol.* **84** 393–405

[50] Papadimitriou S, Gazzo A, Versbraegen N, Nachtegael C, Aerts J, Moreau Y *et al* 2019 Predicting disease-causing variant combinations *PNAS* **116** 11878–87

[51] Arora S and Tsanas A 2021 Assessing Parkinson's disease at scale using telephone-recorded speech: insights from the Parkinson's voice initiative *Diagnostics* **11** 1892

[52] Umar kamil M A, Rahman M, Waseem A, Ali M D and Khursheed M T 2023 Utilizing machine learning techniques for timely diagnosis of Parkinson's disease *Int. Res. J. Eng. Technol.* **10** 444–51

[53] Holzinger A, Carrington A and Müller H 2020 Measuring the quality of explanations: the system causability scale (SCS). Comparing human and machine explanations *Künstl Intell.* **34** 193–8

[54] Wei M T, Shankar U, Parvin R, Abbas S H, Chaudhary S, Friedlander Y *et al* 2022 Evaluation of computer aided detection during colonoscopy in the community (AI-SEE): a multicenter randomized clinical trial *Am. J. Gastroenterol.* **118** 1841–7

[55] Kaywan P, Ahmed K, Ibaida A, Miao Y and Gu B J P 2023 Early detection of depression using a conversational AI bot: a non-clinical trial *PLOS One* **18** e0279743

[56] Mellem M S, Kollada M, Tiller J and Lauritzen T 2021 Explainable AI enables clinical trial patient selection to retrospectively improve treatment effects in schizophrenia *BMC Med. Inform. Decision Making* **21** 162

[57] Seol H Y, Shrestha P, Muth J F, Wi C-I, Sohn S, Ryu E *et al* 2021 Artificial intelligence-assisted clinical decision support for childhood asthma management: a randomized clinical trial *PLOS One* **16** e0255261

[58] Thompson W R, Reinisch A J, Unterberger M J and Schriefl A J 2019 Artificial intelligence-assisted auscultation of heart murmurs: validation by virtual clinical trial *Pediatric Cardiol.* **40** 623–9

[59] Nakanuma H, Endo Y, Fujinaga A, Kawamura M, Kawasaki T, Masuda T *et al* 2023 An intraoperative artificial intelligence system identifying anatomical landmarks for laparoscopic cholecystectomy: a prospective clinical feasibility trial (J-SUMMIT-C-01) *Surg. Endosc.* **37** 1933–42

[60] Khan E, Lambrakis K, Briffa T, Cullen L, Karnon J, Papendick C *et al* 2022 Re-Engineering the clinical approach to suspected cardiac chest pain assessment in the emergency department by expediting research evidence to practice using artificial intelligence (RAPIDx AI)—a cluster randomised clinical trial design *Heart Lung Circ.* **31** S224–S5

[61] Chen M M, Terzic A, Becker A S, Johnson J M, Wu C C, Wintermark M *et al* 2022 Artificial intelligence in oncologic imaging *Eur. J. Radiol. Open* **9** 100441

[62] Varoquaux G and Cheplygina V J 2021 How I failed machine learning in medical imaging—shortcomings and recommendations arXiv:2103.10292

[63] Thompson M 2018 *Cultural Theory* (Milton Park: Routledge)

[64] Rozenfeld Y, Beam J, Maier H, Haggerson W, Boudreau K, Carlson J *et al* 2020 A model of disparities: risk factors associated with COVID-19 infection *Int. J. Equity Health* **19** 126

[65] Park S H *et al* 2021 Key principles of clinical validation, device approval, and insurance coverage decisions of artificial intelligence *Kor. J. Radiol.* **22** 442–53

[66] Kim D W *et al* 2020 Inconsistency in the use of the term "validation" in studies reporting the performance of deep learning algorithms in providing diagnosis from medical imaging *PLoS One* **15** e0238908

[67] Moreno-Torres J G, Raeder T, Alaiz-Rodríguez R, Chawla N V and Herrera F 2012 A unifying view on dataset shift in classification *Pattern Recog.* **45** 521–30

[68] Liu X, Rivera S C, Moher D, Calvert M J, Denniston A K, Ashrafian H *et al* 2020 Reporting guidelines for clinical trial reports for interventions involving artificial intelligence: the CONSORT-AI extension *BMJ* **2020** 3164

[69] Sebastian A M and Peter D J L 1991 Artificial intelligence in cancer research: trends, challenges and future directions *Life (Basel)* **12** 1991

[70] Wang Y, Yin W and Zeng J 2019 Global convergence of ADMM in nonconvex nonsmooth optimization *J. Sci. Comput.* **78** 29–63

[71] da Silva H E C *et al* 2023 The use of artificial intelligence tools in cancer detection compared to the traditional diagnostic imaging methods: An overview of the systematic reviews *PLoS One* **18** e0292063

[72] Kelly C J, Karthikesalingam A, Suleyman M, Corrado G and King D 2019 Key challenges for delivering clinical impact with artificial intelligence *BMC Med.* **17** 195

[73] Cutillo C M, Sharma K R, Foschini L, Kundu S, Mackintosh M, Mandl K D *et al* 2020 Machine intelligence in healthcare—perspectives on trustworthiness, explainability, usability, and transparency *npj Dig. Med.* **3** 47

[74] Kim S, Chen J, Cheng T, Gindulyte A, He J, He S *et al* 2019 PubChem 2019 update: improved access to chemical data *Nucl. Acids Res.* **47** D1102–D9

[75] Beg S, Ragunath K, Wyman A, Banks M, Trudgill N, Pritchard M D *et al* 2017 Quality standards in upper gastrointestinal endoscopy: a position statement of the British Society of Gastroenterology (BSG) and Association of Upper Gastrointestinal Surgeons of Great Britain and Ireland (AUGIS) *Gut* **66** 1886–99

[76] Doshi-Velez F and Kim B 2017 Towards a rigorous science of interpretable machine learning arXiv:1702.08608

[77] Zhao S, Lin Q, Ran J, Musa S S, Yang G, Wang W *et al* 2020 Preliminary estimation of the basic reproduction number of novel coronavirus (2019-nCoV) in China, from 2019 to 2020: a data-driven analysis in the early phase of the outbreak *Int. J. Infect. Diseas.* **92** 214–7

[78] Guo Z, Zhang Y and Lu W J 2019 Attention guided graph convolutional networks for relation extraction *Proc. of the 57th Annual Meeting of the Association for Computational Linguistics* 241–51

[79] Olah C, Satyanarayan A, Johnson I, Carter S, Schubert L, Ye K *et al* 2018 The building blocks of interpretability *Distill* **3** e10

[80] US FDA Artificial Intelligence & Medical Products: How CBER, CDER, CDRH, and OCP are Working Together? https://www.fda.gov/media/177030/download

[81] Gardner-Thorpe J, Love N, Wrightson J, Walsh S and Keeling N 2006 The value of Modified Early Warning Score (MEWS) in surgical in-patients: a prospective observational study *Ann. R. Coll. Surg. Eng.* **88** 571–5

[82] Alexiuk M and Tangri N 2024 Prediction models for earlier stages of chronic kidney disease *Curr. Opin. Nephrol. Hyperten.* **33** 325–30

[83] Sikkema L, Ramírez-Suástegui C, Strobl D C, Gillett T E, Zappia L, Madissoon E *et al* 2023 An integrated cell atlas of the lung in health and disease *Nat. Med.* **29** 1563–77

[84] Hosny A, Parmar C, Quackenbush J, Schwartz L H and Aerts H J W L 2018 Artificial intelligence in radiology *Nat. Rev.* **18** 500–10

[85] Lee H, Poncé S, Bushick K, Hajinazar S, Lafuente-Bartolome J, Leveillee J *et al* 2023 Electron–phonon physics from first principles using the EPW code *npj Comput. Mater.* **9** 156

[86] Haleem A, Javaid M, Singh R P and Suman R 2021 Telemedicine for healthcare: capabilities, features, barriers, and applications *Sens. Int.* **2** 100117

[87] US FDA 2022 Clinical Decision Support Software Guidance for Industry and Food and Drug Administration Staff https://www.fda.gov/regulatory-information/search-fda-guid-ance-documents/clinical-decision-support-software

[88] Mahadevaiah G, Rv P, Bermejo I, Jaffray D, Dekker A and Wee L 2020 Artificial intelligence-based clinical decision support in modern medical physics: selection, acceptance, commissioning, and quality assurance *Med. Phys.* **47** e228–e35

[89] Broder J S, Halabi S S *et al* 2014 Improving the application of imaging clinical decision support tools: making the complex simple *J. Am. Coll. Radiol* **11** 257–61

[90] Dara S, Dhamercherla S, Jadav S S, Babu C M and Ahsan M J 2022 Machine learning in drug discovery: a review *Artif. Intell. Rev.* **55** 1947–99

[91] Paul J, Lim W M, O'Cass A, Hao A W and Bresciani S 2021 Scientific procedures and rationales for systematic literature reviews (SPAR-4-SLR) *Int. J. Consum. Stud.* **45** O1–O16

[92] Blanco-Gonzalez A, Cabezon A, Seco-Gonzalez A, Conde-Torres D, Antelo-Riveiro P, Pineiro A *et al* 2023 The role of ai in drug discovery: challenges, opportunities, and strategies *Pharmaceuticals* **16** 891

[93] Shi C, Luo S, Xu M and Tang J (eds) 2021 Learning gradient fields for molecular conformation generation *Proceedings of the 38th International Conference on Machine Learning* (PMLR)

[94] Chatterjee S, Bhattacharya M, Nag S, Dhama K and Chakraborty C 2023 A detailed overview of SARS-CoV-2 omicron: its sub-variants, mutations and pathophysiology, clinical characteristics, immunological landscape, immune escape, and therapies *Viruses* **15** 167

[95] Jungwirth D and Haluza D 2023 Artificial intelligence and public health: an exploratory study *Int. J. Environ. Res. Public Health* **20** 4541

[96] Olawade D B, Wada O J and Ling J 2023 Using artificial intelligence to improve public health: a narrative review *Front. Public Health* **11** 1196397

[97] MacIntyre C R, Lim S and Quigley A 1997 Preventing the next pandemic: use of artificial intelligence for epidemic monitoring and alerts *Cell Rep. Med.* **3** 100867

IOP Publishing

Nanobiotechnology and Artificial Intelligence in
Gastrointestinal Diseases

Vivek K Chaturvedi, Anurag Kumar Singh, Jay Singh and Dawesh P Yadav

Chapter 10

Role of artificial intelligence in an early diagnosis and prediction of gastric cancer as an advanced therapeutic technique

Juhi Singh and Vinod Kumar Dixit

One of the most prevalent malignant tumors with a high fatality rate is gastric cancer (GC). Human professionals' meticulous assessments of medical pictures are crucial for making accurate diagnoses and treatment choices for GC. This ailment has historically proven difficult to diagnose. Furthermore, the imaging settings, limited expertise, objective criteria, and inter-observer inconsistencies impede the development of accuracy. Healthcare research has advanced thanks to artificial intelligence (AI). Applications that help with cancer diagnosis and prognosis have been developed as a result of the accessibility of open-source healthcare statistics. Accurate evaluation, diagnosis, and treatment of stomach malignant growth and *Helicobacter pylori* bacteria can be achieved with AI-assisted image analysis; links between these subfields can give more information than traditional analysis. AI-assisted categorization of genomic, epigenetic, and metagenomic data may lead to improved personalized therapy recommendations for gastrointestinal malignancies. In a number of therapeutic settings, including GC, researchers are looking at the extensive uses of AI. With endoscopic inspection and pathologic evidence during GC screening, AI can identify precancerous conditions and help with early cancer identification. AI can help tumor, nodes, and metastases (TNM) staging and subtype categorization in the diagnosis of GC. AI can assist with prognosis prediction and surgical margin estimation for treatment options. Here, we include some AI methods for early stomach cancer prediction. Even though several methods advocated in various texts have shown excellent prediction outcomes, cancer mortality has not decreased. As a result, further in-depth study is needed in the field of cancer prediction in relation to AI that may be applied as a therapy.

10.1 Introduction

GC is the fifth most common malignant tumor and the fourth leading cause of cancer-related death. In 2020, over one million fresh cases of cancer and 769 000 casualties (that is in every 13 patients 1 death) were reported. Men experience mortality and incidence rates twice as high as women do, with Eastern Asia having the highest rates overall. Advanced stomach cancer has a terrible prognosis, with a less than 30% 5-year survival rate. However, early stomach cancer can have a 90% chance of survival, but because of its vague symptoms, it is difficult to find [1, 2]. The most frequent procedure for early detection is endoscopic inspection, and a biopsy is required for a conclusive diagnosis [3]. The subtypes and stages of the tumor can be identified using pathology and computed tomography (CT) imaging, which can be used to guide treatment choices and forecast prognoses. Radical resection is recommended for patients with the initial stages of stomach cancer, whereas advanced cases may necessitate a triage approach that includes surgery, chemotherapy, and radiotherapy [4, 5]. Excellent prognoses for particular forms of stomach cancer have been demonstrated by immunotherapy and molecularly targeted medications [6]. In the realm of stomach cancer, AI technology has been extensively used for image analysis, prognosis, and diagnosis. Limited experience, objective standards, and inter-observer differences can all be addressed by AI [7]. Traditional ML methods rely on handcrafted features, while deep learning (DL) has achieved great success in medical image processing. DL models are currently effectively used in medical image processing using massive datasets and better methods. This chapter aims to contribute a comprehensive overview of AI, its condition and role in diagnosis, and recommendations for future research in related domains to medical professionals engaged in the detection of stomach cancer [8–10].

In recent years, there has been an abundance of biomedical data available in the medical field, leading to the emergence of the big data era [11]. Physicians now face the challenge of effectively analyzing this data rather than just collecting it. AI refers to a machine's ability to learn and display intelligence [12]. In the age of personalized medicine, AI can assist in more effectively converting massive data into useful insights, minimizing errors, enhancing diagnostic precision, offering real-time forecasts, and even providing advice after discharge. Cancer management is being revolutionized and reshaped by AI, which has seen increased application in recent years. Interpreting images is one example of how AI is used to manage cancer [13], surgical interventions [14], drug discovery, surgical skills training and assessment [15], hospital-wide data analysis [16], and personalized treatment [17]. AI is largely utilized for prognosis prediction, therapy advice, and early identification of stomach cancer. The methodical investigation of AI-assisted techniques is covered in this chapter, along with AI's potential drawbacks and potential future applications. Based on four factors, we have presented the state of AI in GC in this review: (1) Clinical big data analysis and prognosis prediction; (2) precise sampling from early diagnosis (endoscopy); (3) digital pathological diagnosis; (4) molecules and genes (figure 10.1).

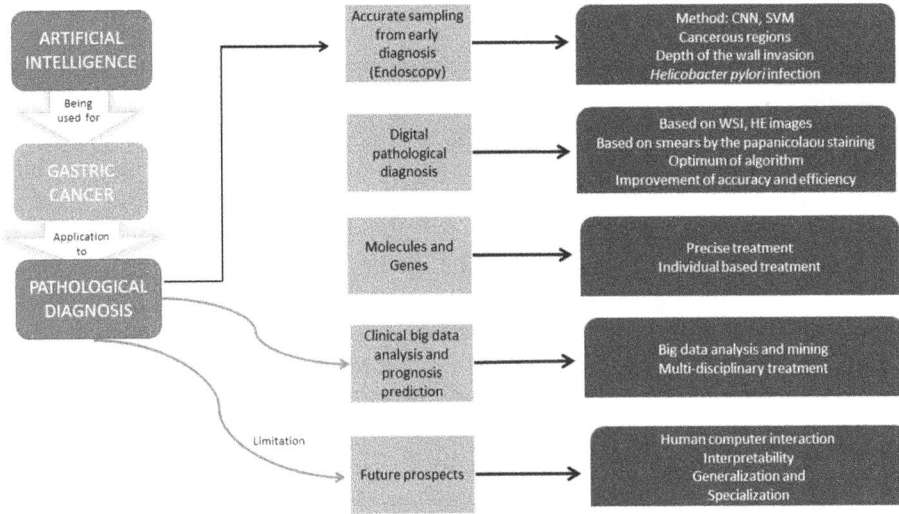

Figure 10.1. The alignment diagram of this chapter.

10.2 Developing history of AI

In stomach cancer research, treatment and prevention has increasingly relied on advanced technologies, including AI. The development of AI has revolutionized the way that stomach cancer is treated, as it allows for advanced screening, diagnosis, and prognosis prediction. AI, on the other hand, refers to the intelligence exhibited by machines. The term 'cognitive machines,' which was first used in 1956, describes devices or computers that mimic human cognitive processes like learning and problem-solving [18]. Machine learning (ML) is a subset of AI that utilizes computer algorithms to improve through experience [19]. Radiology, neurology, orthopedics, pathology, ophthalmology, and gastroenterology are just a few of the medical specialties where ML methods like random forest, support vector machines (SVM), and artificial neural networks (ANNs) have been used to develop models based on training data. In many ongoing projects as of 2020, DL has taken the lead. In order to gradually extract higher-level features from the initial input, it employs many layers. In a nutshell, DL is used to implement (ML, which is an important field of AI. Several AI models have emerged in the field of stomach cancer thanks to recent improvements in hardware and computational capability [20–27]. While studies concentrated on recurrence, metastasis, and forecasting survival for prognosis [32–34], the usage of AI-assisted diagnostics primarily comprises blood reports, medical imaging such as computed tomography (CT) and endoscopy [26–29]. The use of AI in medicine has been eagerly investigated, and DL technology has quickly attracted attention as the best ML technique. DL has been utilized extensively in medicine [25–27], particularly for tumors including skin [28], breast [29], and stomach [30, 31] cancers.

10.3 AI's role in the early detection of GC

Due to the vague and generic signs of GC, it is sometimes not discovered until it has progressed to an advanced stage, which has a bad prognosis. However, the five-year survival rate for stomach cancer can be greatly raised by up to 90% with early and correct identification.[35, 36] However, the capacity to diagnose early stomach cancer is constrained by the availability of skilled imaging specialists, and diagnostic efficacy greatly depends on their clinical background. All false diagnoses and missed diagnoses happen, even to the most qualified professionals. AI techniques are able to process and analyze vast volumes of data, mimicking human cognitive function, and help gastroenterologists make diagnoses and decisions. Endoscopy, pathology, and CT imaging are just a few of the medical imaging domains where AI has already been put to use. Extraction of picture features [37, 38], early detection of stomach cancer [39–43], early diagnosis of precancerous conditions [40], narrow-band imaging for magnifying endoscopic optimization, and use of Raman endoscopy are all steps in AI-assisted endoscopic diagnosis[44, 45]. Automatic GC identification [46], detection of GC using whole slide imaging (WSI) [47–50], automatic identification of tumor-infiltrating lymphocytes (TILs) [51], and segmentation of lesion areas [52–54] are all components of AI-assisted pathologic diagnosis. Preoperative peritoneal metastasis detection [54], perigastric metastatic lymph node detection [55], and the utilization of two more innovative imaging approaches [56] are the main goals of AI-assisted CT diagnosis. The diagnostic performance of these AI models is on a level with human experts in some situations. Detecting GC and precancerous lesions early on is crucial for improving survival rates. Although endoscopy is widely used for GC screenings, diagnosing early gastric cancer (EGC) through image analysis can be challenging and subjective due to cognitive and technical factors. Fortunately, there are effective methods to improve diagnostic accuracy such as use of image enhanced endoscopy, as well as narrow-band imaging (NBI) and blue-laser imaging (BLI), which are more efficient than traditional white light imaging. To increase diagnosis accuracy and prevent pointless biopsies, AI-assisted evaluation enables a more objective evaluation strategy. Recently, the detection of EGC has been the topic of numerous investigations.

Convolutional neural network (CNN) algorithms have been found to reliably detect EGC in pictures taken using standard and magnifying endoscopy in recent research [13]. The ability of this technique to distinguish EGC from normal tissue or gastritis in real-time utilizing video images has been demonstrated to be extremely successful [57, 58]. Results have revealed that CNN systems perform similarly to expert systems and outperform non-expert systems in accurately identifying EGC. Additionally, the use of AI significantly speeds up the detection process compared to endoscopists [60]. Deep convolutional neural networks (DCNNs) have been used in a unique system created by Wu *et al* that can identify EGC and stomach regions without blind spots [61]. Various devices can cooperate in real time to make sure the endoscope can see the whole gastric mucosa, which is necessary to detect early neoplastic changes. A trial with randomized controlled experiment including 324 patients compared the 'WISENSE system—which stands for smart and sense—to traditional endoscopy'. When compared to the controls, WISENSE dramatically reduced the percentage of blind spots (5.9% versus 22.4%, p 0.001) [57]. One more tool is developed that involved 1 million images of endoscopy of more than 80 000 patients. It is called 'GRAIDS' (Gastrointestinal Artificial Intelligence Diagnostic System). With accuracy equivalent to professional endoscopists and superior to non-expert endoscopists, the device may identify upper GI cancer in real time [59]. It is possible to determine the level of invasion using a computer-aided detection system based on CNNs. According to research, this approach is more precise and exacting than those carried out by skilled endoscopists. 'ENDOANGEL' which is an AI system that provides real-time information and can also carry out a number of functions in EGC diagnosis, such as white light endoscopy detection, enlarging narrow-band imaging, and predicting invasion depth. Although its sensitivity and negative predictive value were only slightly higher, ENDOANGEL's specificity, accuracy, and positive predictive value (93.22%, 91%, and 90%, respectively) were noticeably superior to those of endoscopists (72.33%, 76.19%, and 70.56%, respectively). These studies have contributed to the development of AI for clinical use, despite some limitations. For example, validation with unaltered images and videos is necessary for accurate results. With further improvements, the performance of AI in clinical settings is expected to improve [61].

10.3.1 Screening of GC by AI

The research into applying AI to detect gastric carcinoma (GC) is both highly anticipated and well-liked. Atrophic gastritis (AG), which is caused by *H. pylori* (HP), is the first step in the development of GC. This is followed by gastric intestinal metaplasia (GIM), dysplasia, and eventually malignancy [62, 63]. To reduce the incidence of GC, it is important to identify these precancerous gastric diseases and screen high-risk individuals [64]. Unfortunately, due to modest morphological alterations, GC is frequently detected in an advanced stage, leading to a five-year survival probability of only 30%. A substantially greater survival percentage of 91.5% can be achieved, however, for those who receive a diagnosis at an early stage [65]. Therefore, early detection of GC is crucial. The common method for GC screening is through endoscopic examination, which unfortunately has reported miss rates ranging from 4.6% to 25.8% by endoscopists in previous studies [65–68]. Improved techniques in endoscopy with enhanced image capabilities can potentially aid in detecting GC [69], but their widespread use is limited by the need for specialized training and expertise. Visually analyzing 'whole slide imaging' (WSI), medical images achieve after biopsy or resection is crucial for the accurate diagnosis of GC [70]. Nevertheless, pathologists must concentrate for extended periods of time and carry out a lot of work to find stomach cancer because of the size variations in malignant regions and the enormous scale of WSI. To solve these problems, AI might offer automated, accurate, and quick histo-pathological analysis and endoscopic detection. Even endoscopic pictures have been used to try to detect the presence of *H. pylori* infection [71–75].

Yan *et al* [72] talked about a three-category categorization method that incorporates the eliminated state in their investigation. An accuracy rate of above 0.8 was attained by all researchers, which is comparable to that of experienced endoscopists. In comparison to predicting HP infection, researchers found that detecting AG and GIM had a greater accuracy prevalence of 0.9 [76–78]. However, they struggled to accurately identify a variety of precancerous conditions and stomach neoplasms [79–81]. Researchers investigated conventional ML techniques [82, 83] and used DL models [84, 86, 89] to identify GC in endoscopic pictures. To increase detection precision, they additionally used self-designed network topologies [87, 88] and sophisticated image-enhanced endoscopy [43, 49]. Researchers have also concentrated on finding GC in disease pictures [89].

10.3.2 Accuracy of sampling from early endoscopic diagnosis

To accomplish endoscopic diagnosis of stomach cancer, magnifying endoscopy is usually used in combination with narrow spectrum imaging technologies such as narrow-band imaging [61], flexible spectral imaging colour enhancement, and BLI. However, this method requires well-trained medical professionals to perform the diagnostic examinations [63–65]. Unfortunately, endoscopy may miss roughly 10% of cases of upper gastrointestinal tract cancer, particularly GC [65]. Researchers are looking at using AI to help in the detection of stomach cancer during endoscopy to address this problem. The aim is to reduce the instances of missed diagnoses caused by inexperience or fatigue among endoscopic doctors. CNN, a widely used AI model, has demonstrated efficacy in identifying malignant and non-cancerous areas during endoscopy. These AI techniques are as accurate as or more accurate than skilled endoscopists, with an accuracy range of 86%–92.5% [67]. This shows that using AI approaches to aid in decision-making can be quite helpful. The rate at which detection is achieved is on the same level with that of the most expert endoscopists because of the great sensitivity of AI approaches, which may reach 100% [69]. SVM is a further AI model that is frequently utilized in the detection of stomach cancer. Images from a magnifying endoscopy might be used by a system based on SVM analysis to quantitatively detect stomach cancer. In comparison to other regions, the tumor region's SVM output value was noticeably different [71]. Endoscopists used a computer-aided diagnostic (CAD) system based on SVM to diagnose early GC with a diagnostic accuracy of 96.3%, a positive prognostic value of 98.3%, a precision of 96.7%, and a level of specificity of 95% [71]. AI can be useful for both detection and characterization when using endoscopic pictures to diagnose stomach cancer. The computer-aided pattern recognition system [72] and the CNN computer-aided detection (CNN-CAD) system [73] were used to determine the depth of wall invasion of GC.

10.3.3 Digital pathological diagnosis

Digital versions of the glass slides used for pathological investigation are known as WSIs. For tumor classification [46] depth of invasion discrimination [90] micro-satellite instability prediction, and minimizing the lack of sufficient well-annotated training data [91], stomach cancer has been studied using AI approaches, such as DL-based neural networks. However, further improvements are necessary. WSI, a virtual equivalent of glass slides, is comparable to optical microscopy in diagnosing GCs. AI applications in pathological diagnosis emerged with advances in WSI. By providing two deep CNN-based techniques, Leon *et al* [47] evaluated the use of deep CNN in the automated identification of stomach cancer pathological pictures. Using all of the photos, one did morphological feature analysis, while the other separately looked into the local distinctive features. According to Sharma *et al* [46] the CNN architecture could accurately classify cancer with an accuracy of 0.6990 and detect necrosis with an accuracy of 0.8144 in pathological image analysis. According to the experiment results, the proposed model demonstrated excellent performance in detecting GCs with an average accuracy of 89.72%. In order to differentiate between stomach cancer, adenoma, and non-neoplastic tissue, Iizuka *et al* [48] used CNNs and recurrent neural networks. However, the automatic segmentation of lesion zones proved an issue in the AI-assisted pathological identification of stomach malignancy. To address the absence of thoroughly annotated pathological imaging data, Liang *et al* [28] proposed a new neural network architecture and approach called overlapping area prediction. The DL approach was used for the first time to segment disease pictures in order to find stomach tumors. The model achieved an intersection over union coefficient (IOU) of 88.3% and 91.1% accuracy, which went above what was expected for supervised learning. Qu *et al* [91] developed a novel intermediate dataset and a stepwise fine-tuning-based strategy to improve the classification performance of deep neural networks.

The efficiency of the suggested DL model for medical picture segmentation was proved by Sun *et al* [92] with a mean accuracy of 91.60% and a mean IoU of 82.65%. The Mask R-CNN model is a useful tool for medical picture segmentation, according to different research [93]. In the field of genetic pathology, DL data interpretation has the potential to yield valuable insights into understanding and treating stomach cancer: the importance of genes, biomarkers, and their interpretation [93]. Liang *et al* identified certain genes and their functions in carcinogenesis by analyzing numerous transcription datasets and tabulating genomic data from stomach cancer patients and healthy persons [51]. Datasets were analyzed and ranked using Rank Prod and INMEX. Gene expression data was obtained from the Gene Expression Omnibus database and combined with literature analysis and bioinformatics data to identify promising genes to increase comprehension, Geno Ontology and route analysis were employed. Progastricism (PGC) and collagen type VI alpha 3 chains (COL6A3) were two of the 1153 differentially expressed genes that remained after elimination, which can serve as biomarkers for GC [79]. AI-assisted applications have enormous potential benefits for detecting GC and improving image segmentation efficiency and diagnostic time.

AI analysis is utilized in the area of digital pathology to identify cancer, segment it, classify mutations, forecast clinical outcomes, and discover new drugs. The unification of pathology and oncology is becoming more crucial with the emergence of precision oncology. Limiting radiation exposure and performing numerous computations have advantages, but AI can also aid patients and medical staff [63, 93].

To ascertain the advantages of AI in patient care, Vollmer *et al* offer 20 implementation, statistical methodology, and repeatability-related issues [94]. Patients and healthcare systems may benefit from a practical framework that uses a common technical vocabulary and relies on empirical research. AI may also take human and emotional judgment out of computer-aided diagnosis decision-making.

10.4 Role of AI from endoscopic diagnosis to treatment

A guide for using ML in clinical endoscopy to diagnose gastrointestinal diseases accurately is an idea that Van Der Sommen *et al* [95] have put forth. Each medical professional must have a good technical foundation in order to adequately comprehend the influence of ML on gastrointestinal diagnosis [95]. In terms of anatomy, the stomach is different from other gastrointestinal organs such the colon and esophagus [96]. Clinicians need several in-depth searches to prevent any omissions due to the broader bent lumen of the device, which may necessitate more tedious observations [96].

Infection with *H. pylori* is another factor which masks the early signs of EGC [96], leading to variation in endoscopic diagnosis [9, 97]. As a result, adopting AI from colon cancer to abdominal cancer may be inadvisable. Endoscopy, such as EMR (endoscopic mucosal excision for EGC), is another alternative for treating tumors in the stomach [98]. EMR is renowned in Japan and the West due to its low risk of metastasis lymph node cancer [98–100]. However, local lesions greater than 15 mm may increase difficulty in assessing tumor depth and recurrence. ESD (endoscopic submucosal dissection) is a formidable opponent to open/laparoscopic surgery for treating EGC [98].

To improve endoscopic resection in clinical practice, Zhu *et al* developed a highly accurate and specific CNN-CAD system [101]. However, AI's specific role in endoscopic resection procedures remains limited. While AI-based detection systems can predict the depth of tumor invasion and reduce unnecessary gastrectomy, they are unable to manage the resection procedure or activate alarms for high-risk consequences including bleeding, perforation, and peritonitis. ESD-related complications remain a very difficult problem in GC, with a 3.5% rate [102]. The creation and training of AI-based approaches, particularly those comprising ML or DL that require adequate data training, should be assigned to hospitals with significant patient volumes. In a clinical guide on the use of AI in endoscopy [101], Namikawa *et al* gathered its applications in stomach-related disciplines such as clinical detection, classification, and blind spot monitoring. Additionally, they expected that in the future, AI might be fully taught to differentiate between stomach neoplastic and non-plastic tumors, contributing more significantly [96]. However, the use of AI in the management of stomach cancer is still in its infancy. In contrast to endoscopic diagnosis of GC, which is mostly based on image interpretation, AI in chemo radiotherapy could require multimodal data interpretation, such as genetic characterization, immuno-histochemistry results, mutation analysis, or insensitivity prediction. DeepIC50, a 1D CNN model, was created by Joo *et al* that reliably predicts drug responsiveness in GC patients and cell lines [95].

10.5 Artificial intelligence in surgery

AI's application in surgery will involve computer-assisted improvements to human performance [103]. Proper surgical education and evaluation are essential components of the medical field. Fard *et al* utilized ML techniques to evaluate robotic surgery skills, and a future date [15], AI is anticipated to be employed throughout and after surgical operations [14]. A patient-specific surgical risk assessment and postoperative results may be established using AI analysis of preoperative clinical data. In order to forecast postoperative problems in patients with stomach cancer, Chien *et al* employed artificial neural networks (ANNs) [18]. During surgery, EMR data can be an integrating operational data for real-time direction and adverse event prevention. Autonomous robots capable of performing surgical procedures under human supervision might be developed in the future. To improve cancer care, postoperative data might be combined with hospitalization data [18].

10.6 Molecules and genes

The usage of molecular and genetic approaches is growing to diagnose and predict tumors. Early intervention may be possible if high-risk stomach cancer patients are identified. For localized GC patients receiving treatment, detecting circulating tumor DNA may aid in the facilitation of tailored neo-adjuvant treatment to increase survival in patients at high risk of resurgence [104]. To maximize efficacy and avoid overtreatment, comprehensive molecular signatures can be exploited to personalize therapy to each patient [105]. In this field, AI is frequently applied (table 10.1). In order to direct medical care and forecast prognosis, a classifier can discriminate between the gene expression patterns of different subtypes of GC [106]. Various algorithms may be utilized to develop a comprehensive data mining model for the aim of detecting biomarkers based on gene expression data and biological aspects of stomach cancer based on gene characteristics from the prediction model [107]. Due to the intricacy of cancer, current targeted therapies are built on ideas that have undergone experimental verification and explain one potential mechanism of carcinogenesis while neglecting other disease-related facts [5, 6]. Patients may have severe adverse effects as well as unintended effects on healthy tissues [7, 8].

Table 10.1. The use of AI in genetics.

Authors	Year	Disease	Algorithm	Identifying object	No. of cases	Results
Yan *et al* [107]	2013	GC	DM and ML	Feature genes	216	Sn,>90%; Sp,>90%
Ishii *et al* [106]	2013	GC (2 subtypes)	Bayesian network	The pattern of expression of genes classifier,100%	46	Accuracy of the

Interactome data can be used to better understand the molecular causes of cancer, which can be represented as network structures with components representing biological entities (e.g. genes, proteins, mRNAs, and metabolites) and edges representing their associations/interactions (e.g. gene co-expression, signaling transduction, gene regulation, and physical interaction between proteins) [9–14]. AI algorithms can effectively process biological network data for classification [15], clustering, and prediction tasks, improving our understanding of carcinogenesis and exploring new cancer-fighting targets [16]. We have witnessed rapid progress during the last few decades regarding biology analysis algorithms. On the one hand, network-based biology analysis algorithms offer a number of different network methodologies for identifying cancer targets. Furthermore, distinct network-based biology analysis algorithms may look at network data from different angles, they can compensate for each other to produce accurate biological explanations [108]. High-performance, diverse, and complicated molecular data may be handled using ML-based biology analysis in an effective manner, and biological networks can be mined for features or relationships. Increasing the number of algorithms will enable more accurate target identification and cancer medication development [108–110].

In recent years, two of the most important parts of AI biological analysis have been to uncover potential oncology targets [114–116] and the fast development of cancer-associated techniques [111–113]. These technologies are divided into five categories in figure 10.2 epigenetic, genomics, proteomics, metabolomics, and multiomics integration analysis. Epigenetics is the study of DNA and DNA-related protein alterations that modify gene expression without altering DNA sequence (figure 10.2) [54]. AI is essential for investigating epigenetic data and designing targeted therapeutics. As an illustration, regulatory networks relating to histone lysine demethylation may be studied using transcriptome and epigenetic data [116].

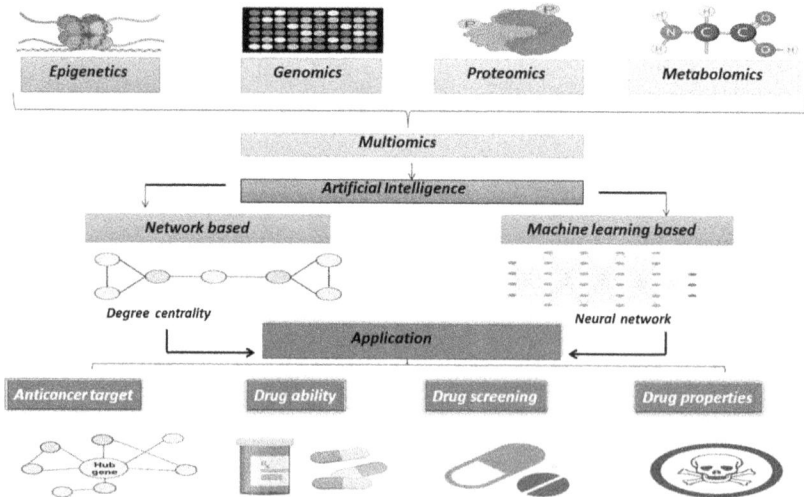

Figure 10.2. The discovery of cancer treatment targets using AI to combine multiomics data (such as epigenetics, genomics, proteomics and metabolomics).

They established the importance of epigenetic regulators such as KDM1A, KDM3A, EZH2, and DOT1L in oncogenesis and drug resistance, emphasizing their importance in mitogenic control and therapeutic potential [114].

Genome-scale experiments, such as sequencing, are used in genomics to investigate the function of every genetic component in an organism [107]. Applications include mapping genomic areas with high biochemical activity, discovering biomarkers for patient classification, predicting gene function, and establishing genotype–phenotype relationships. In order to identify cancer subtypes and therapeutic targets, comparative genomics analysis of molecular datasets has been greatly enhanced by recent network-based biology analysis approaches [109]. Medi *et al* [117], for example, incorporated gene expression patterns into genome-scale molecular associations to find therapeutic targets for cervical cancer, comprising receptors, micro RNAs, transcription factors, proteins (such as CRYAB, CDK1, PARP1, WNK1, and KAT2B), and metabolites (arachidonic acids). Cantini *et al* [118] used a network-based biology analysis methodology to merge several genomic layers into a biological network to uncover cancer driver genes such as F11R, HDGF, PRCC, ATF3, BTG2, and CD46 as oncogenes and potential indicators for pancreatic cancer. Following that, they implemented a consensus clustering approach.

Proteomics is the study of proteins. Proteomic investigations are carried out to mark up and compare genomic patterns, estimate protein abundance, find modifications after translation, and discover protein–protein interactions (PPIs) [119]. PPIs are often employed for the processing of proteomics data [120] and serve key roles in organizing and modulating biological processes. Vinayagam *et al* [114], for example, used control theory to examine the human PPI interaction network in order to discover essential proteins that impact the network's controllability [121]. By varying the number of driver nodes in the network in response to the removal of that protein, the hub may be classed as 'indispensable,' 'neutral,' or 'dispensable,' which correlates with increasing, no impact, or reducing the number of driver nodes in the network in response to the removal of the key protein. The findings show that these critical proteins are the primary targets of drugs, viruses, and disease-causing mutations. In addition, intelligent network controllability analysis of data from 1547 discovered 46 additional cancer-associated genes in addition to 56 essential genes across nine malignancies. According to a network-based biological evaluation framework, there are significant changes in gene expression for disorders whose proteins are close to phenolic targets but not for those whose proteins are distant to polyphenol targets [120]. This network link offers a way to determine how polyphenols affect illnesses as well as a foundation for finding new anticancer targets.

By analyzing the metabolites present in bodily fluids, cells, and tissues, the study of metabolism is frequently employed to identify biomarkers [122]. The sensitivity of biotechnology allows for the detection of subtle changes in metabolic pathways, providing understanding of the processes behind cancer and diverse physiological states. In order to do metabolomic studies and give systems-level knowledge of the function of metabolites in cancer, researchers are currently using biological networks

[122]. To analyze flow control and find driver responses in metabolic networks, for instance, Basler *et al* [123] suggested a network-based paradigm. *Escherichia coli* driver responses were shown to be subject to intricate cellular regulation, pointing to their crucial function in aiding cellular control. According to correlation data, the driven response is a viable therapeutic target since it slows cancer development.

The handling of integrated omics information and the intricacy of tumor–host relationships are necessary for multiomics integration analysis [124]. Multiomics data offers researchers related molecular profiles to analyse carcinogenesis in comparison to single omics investigations [124]. In order to properly understand the intricate interlayer regulatory connections in cancer progression, integrated multiomics information in a hierarchical design to AI biology study has become an effective tool. With the use of this strategy, we may take advantage of earlier data that can be condensed and displayed as networks, giving us insights into the process of carcinogenesis as a whole [125]. Gov *et al* [126] undertook a comparative study of transcriptome data to uncover biomolecules such as genes, receptors, membrane proteins, TFs, and miRNAs. They then used the links between these molecules to build a tissue-specific network for ovarian cancer, and identified GATA2 and miR-124–3p as potential biomarkers.

10.7 AI models' function in prognosis prediction

GC patients are divided into several risk categories using the TNM staging method. Patients having a similar TNM stage, however, might have varying chances of surviving. The accepted technique for determining risk variables for prognosis is the Cox proportional hazard (CPH) model. The prognostic parameters which were previously shown to have been more accurate for predicting survival have been corroborated by a nomogram based on CPH. However, the nomogram technique's predictive power has its own constraints when taking linear analysis into account. The complexity of the human body includes several nonlinear elements that may affect survival. As illustrated in table 10.2, nonlinear statistical models that use ANN have proven to be more accurate at forecasting patients' chances of surviving stomach cancer. Biglarian *et al* predicted the survival of stomach cancer patients by comparing an ANN to the CPH model [127]. When Amiri *et al* evaluated the weights in the ANN using a variety of hidden nodes [128], they observed that five nodes provided the best accuracy.

Nilsaz-Dezfouli *et al* developed the system [129] using a single-time-point ANN model and the ability to handle filtered input. ANNs were surpassed by Bayesian neural networks, according to Korhani Kangi and Bahrampour in terms of predicting survival [130]. TNM staging was not as effective as the survival recurrent network (SRN) [130]. Prior to surgery, it offered a trustworthy prognosis for long-term survival of GC that was statistically superior to cTNM and pTNM, or clinical and pathological TNM, respectively [129]. Unquestionably, much more data is needed to continue improving ANN models. Jiang *et al*'s [131] prognostic classifier was created by applying SVM to survival analysis. The findings showed that overall survival and disease-free survival could be predicted with greater accuracy than the

Table 10.2. Utilisation of AI in stomach cancer prognosis based on several research populations.

Authors	Year	Country/region	Number of cases	Study population	Methods	Results
Jiang et al [131]	2018	China	786 cases	Hospital	SVM classifier	AUCs (up to 0.834)
Lu et al [132]	2017	China	939 patients	Hospital	MMHG	Accuracy (69.28%)
Korhani Kangi and Bahrampour [130]	2018	Iran	339 patients	Hospital	ANN, BNN	Sensitivity (88.2% for ANN, 90.3% for BNN), specificity (95.4% for ANN, 90.9% for BNN)
Zhang et al [133]	2020	China	669 cases	Hospital	ML	AUCs (up to 0.831)
Bollschweiler et al [135]	2004	Germany Japan	135 cases	Cancer centre	ANN	Accuracy (93%)
Jagric et al [136]	2010	Slovenia	213 cases	Cancer centre	Vertex quantification neural network developingnet works	Sensitivity (71%), specificity (96.1%)
Liu et al [134]	2018	China	432 GC tissue Samples	Hospital	SVM classifier	Accuracy (up to 94.19%)
Hensler et al [42]	2005	Germany Japan	4302 cases	Cancer centre	QUEEN technique	Accuracy (72.73%)

American Joint Committee on Cancer's tumor-node-metastasis staging classification. Additionally, the suggested SVM classification of stomach cancer was utilized to forecast the efficacy of adjuvant chemotherapy, enabling the treatment of stomach cancer on an individual basis. One of the major reasons for mortality was recurrence for people with stomach cancer, Therefore, in the course of routine therapeutic activity, a precise estimate of the risk of recurrence was crucial. Recent findings state that the AI-assisted recurrence prediction method outperformed conventional statistical techniques. The radiomic fingerprints of advanced stomach cancer in 669 people in a row were extracted from CT scans using ML techniques by Zhang et al [133]. They subsequently developed a CT-based radiomic model to predict the recurrence of advanced stomach cancer. The SVM classifier was created by Liu et al [134] with the intent to predict resurgence in patients with stomach cancer.

Lymph node metastases from stomach cancer are a highly reliable indicator [64]. The use of AI-assisted prediction tools has made it possible to more accurately assess the metastasis risk due to the absence of reliable ways to forecast the metastasis of GC. ANNs were shown to significantly improve the lymph node metastasis prediction accuracy by Bollschweiler et al [41]. Hensler et al [42] described a unique ANN approach for detecting lymph node metastases before surgery. The proposed model surpassed the Maruyama Diagnostic System established at the National Cancer Centre in Tokyo in terms of accuracy and dependability. Using the expression of gene profiling dataset GSE26253, they discovered that a variety of characteristic genes, including PLCG1, PRKACA, and TGFBR1, may be linked to the reappearance of GC [63]. Using the GSE26253 gene expression profile dataset, a collection of feature genes, including PLCG1, PRKACA, and TGFBR1, were discovered to possibly be associated with GC relapse. GC lymph node metastases were a major predictive factor. The use of AI-assisted prediction tools has made it possible to more accurately assess the metastasis risk due to the absence of reliable ways to forecast the spread of GC. Bollschweiler et al [135] introduced a novel ANN technique for the preoperative evaluation of lymph node metastasis and demonstrated how ANNs may considerably increase the prognostic accuracy of lymph node metastasis. When compared to the Maruyama Diagnostic System developed at the National Cancer Centre in Tokyo, the proposed model displayed improved accuracy and reliability. It was also demonstrated that the possibility of liver metastases could significantly reduce a patient's long-term prognosis for stomach cancer. Jagric et al [136] developed a learning vector quantization network to predict postoperative liver metastases in patients with GC, and it produced a remarkably high predictive value.

10.7.1 Metastasis and staging prediction

The capacity to anticipate lymph node metastases (LNMs) is crucial for clinical decision-making, that might involve endoscopic mucosa excision, neo-adjuvant chemotherapy, or major surgery. Currently, the lymph nodes' dimensions, contours, and densities serve as the primary determinants of the imaging diagnosis of LNMs.

The N status pre-treatment screening was frequently insufficient. Recent studies have shown that ANNs can predict LNM with a markedly higher degree of accuracy [135]. Furthermore, neural network-based liver metastasis prediction has been shown to have a strong negative predictive value and a respectably high sensitivity [136]. The early diagnosis of peritoneal metastases was enhanced by DL method for ascites cytopathology evaluation [137].

An ANN model that included clinical, pathological, and genetic polymorphism data correctly predicted the preoperative stage of GC 81.82% of the time [138] (table 10.3). To increase the predicted accuracy of the ANN models, it will be important to combine clinical, pathological, and biological data with biological markers.

10.7.2 AI aided treatment decisions

Advanced GC (AGC) patients have been recommended to have adjuvant chemotherapy and targeted molecular treatment; resection is the preferred curative treatment for EGC. Additionally, adjuvant immunotherapy has been included in preoperative treatment regimens. Some of the uses of AI in the management of GC are compiled in table 10.4. Several researches [139–146] investigated the use of AI approaches in resection surgery, chemotherapy, and molecular drug decision-making, while other studies employed clinico-pathologic characteristics, CT, immuno-histochemical stain, and lymph-node WSIs to assess the outcome of treatment. These applications showed how AI may be used in various GC therapy modalities.

10.7.3 Clinical massive data analysis and prognostic prediction

AI is often employed in clinical big data analysis and prognosis prediction, similar to how patient history, clinical nursing data, pathology, and imaging data have been integrated and used for data analysis and mining (table 10.5). Complex conditions should be treated using multidisciplinary methods that combine gastrointestinal, radiology, pathology, medicine, surgery, and radiation oncology [147]. For instance, AI has been used to predict complications after gastrectomy to significantly lower postoperative mortality and morbidity [135], reinforce early detection and screening to enhance the long-term survival and standard of life of EGC patients, predict the preoperative staging of tumors through the use of clinico-pathological datasets and genetic susceptibility tests, and predict tumor recurrence in patients with carcinoma of the stomach to develop [147].

10.8 Survival analysis

The prognosis determines the malignancy of the tumor and forecasts patient survival. A major prognostic factor for GC is TNM staging. It is nonetheless constrained because people with different stages may have varying survival rates. The typical model for survival analysis is Cox regression. Age, sex, histology, depth of the tumor, the number of metastatic and examined lymph nodes, the presence of distant metastases, and the amount of the resection were the eight criteria included

Table 10.3. For individuals with stomach cancer, a method for predicting metastases.

Authors	Goal	Prediction	Variables	Patient count for validation	Results
Bollschweiler *et al* (2004) [135]	LNM	The maruyama computer programme (MCP) and the ANN	Tumor dimensions, position, and Borrmann classification, T category	135	Accuracy: ANN, 64% to 93%; MCP, 42% to 70%
Gao *et al* (2019) [54]	LNM	Using ANN, a CT scan may detect perigastric metastatic lymph nodes.	CT images	100	mAP, 0.7801; AUC, 0.9541
Hensler *et al* (2005) [42]	LNM	The maruyama diagnostic system (MDS) and QUEEN	Age, gender, tumor type, invasive depth, Borrmann classification, tumor size, transverse and concentric locations, and tumor size	34	QUEEN, 72.73% accuracy, about 10% greater sensitivity, and approximately 18% better specificity over MDS
Jagric *et al* (2010) [136]	Liver metastasis	DL vector quantization neural networks, forecast liver metastases	Size of the tumor, Lauren histological type, adjuvant chemotherapy and radiation treatment, TNM N position, UICC stage, number of positive lymph nodes, and percentage of positive nodes among all nodes removed	73	Sensitivity for a developing sample is 71%; specificity is 96.1%. The sensitivity of the test sample is 66.7%; the specificity is 97.1%
Lai *et al* (2008) [138]	Staging	staging before surgery using ANN	Diagnostic data, pathological information, and genetic variations	121	Accuracy: 81.82%

CT: computed tomography, ANN: artificial neural network; QUEEN: quality assured efficient engineering of feed forward neural networks with supervised learning.

Table 10.4. AI's use in making treatment decisions for GC.

Authors	Aim	Data	Method	Result
An et al (2020) [139]	Delineate resection 1 margin for EGC	1244 images and ESD videos	U-Net þþ	IoU: 67.6% (image), 70.4% (video); Sen.: 81.7% (image), 89.5% (video)
Wang et al (2021) [140]	Prognosis prediction	1164 patients; lymph node pathological images	U-net, Res Net	Hazard ratio: 2.04 (univariable), C-index: 0.694
Jiang et al (2021) [141]	Prognosis prediction	1615 patients; CT	S-net	C-index: 0.719 (DFS), 0.724 (OS)
Ling et al (2020) [142]	Delineate resection margin for EGC	1670 images and ESD videos	U-Net þ þ	Acc: 82.7% (differentiated), 88.1% (undifferentiated)
Meier et al (2020) [143]	Prognosis prediction	248 patients; IHC-stained TMAs	Google Net	Hazard ratio: 1.273 (Cox), 1.234 (Uno), 1.149 (Log rank)
Zhang et al (2020) [144]	Prognosis prediction	640 patients; CT	Res Net	C-index: 0.78 (OS)
Hyung et al (2017) [145]	Prognosis prediction	1549 patients; clinico-pathologic factors	Five-layer neural network	AUC: 0.844–0.852 (five-year survival)
Joo et al (2019) [95]	Predict molecular drug response	GDSC, CCLE, TGGA dataset	DeepIC50	
Tan et al (2020) [146]	Predict chemotherapy response	116 patients	Delta radiomics	Acc: 0.728–0.828

Acc, accuracy Area under the receiver-operating characteristic curve is known as AUC; concordance index is known as C-index; and computed tomography is known as CT. The term 'disease-free survival' ESD, or endoscopic sub-mucosal dissection, stands for early stomach cancer. The term immuno-histochemistry; IoU stands for Intersection over Union. The total survival rate; Sen., sensibility the distinctiveness of; the tissue microarray.

Table 10.5. The use of AI to forecast prognosis.

Authors	Year	Disease	Algorithm	Prognosis forecast	No. of cases	Results
Chien et al [18]	2008	GC	ANN, DT, LR	An after-surgery problem	521	ANN was a more effective approach than DT and LR
Lai et al [138]	2008	Primary GC	ANN	Tumor stage predicted before surgery	121	Accuracy,81.82%
Jagric et al [136]	2010	GC	LVQNN	Liver metastases following a tumor removal operation	213	Sn, 71%; Sp96.1%
Liu et al [134]	2018	EGC	data analysis	Invasive-free screening	618	Accuracy, 77.84%; AI can efficiently analyze the threat of EGC and help doctors in strengthening the diagnosis and assessment of EGC

EGC is for early gastric cancer; DT stands for decision tree; LR stands for logistic regression; and LVQNN stands for learning vector quantization neural networks; ANN stands for artificial neural network.

in the proposed five-year survival prediction model. The proposed approach beat the Cox regression model with a precision of 83.5%. A ResNet-based model was put forth to forecast the individuals with AGC's highest overall survival rate [133].

Additionally, based on preoperative CT images, A DL-based imaging signature (DeLIS) was created by Jiang et al [131] to predict survival without disease and prolonged survival for GC patients. In a multicenter investigation, the suggested DeLIS demonstrated independent predictive value from conventional clinico-pathologic variables. With a C-index of 0.792–0.802 and a net re-categorization increase of 10.1%–28.3%, the integrated model improved performance by combining imaging signals and clinical criteria. They also found that adjuvant therapy would be more beneficial for those with higher DeLIS scores. Additionally, researchers looked at AI-based digital pathology prognosis.

Pathologists often assess positive cells for prognosis by counting them in certain perspectives. Subjectivity and inter-observer heterogeneity, however, compromised its accuracy. Based on tissue microarrays stained with immuno-histochemistry, a DL model without hypotheses was created to predict risk. The revised Google Net was subjected to the application of loss functions (Cox loss, Uno loss, and Log-rank loss) to account for the time-to-event element of survival information. A group of proliferative markers (Ki67) and immune cell markers (CD8, CD20, and CD68) were also included in their investigation of the tumor microenvironment. Bollschweiler et al found that the immune-related CNN score generated can add to prognosis prediction utilizing qualitative analysis [135].

Additionally, N staging is an important prognostic marker, and pathologists must laboriously examine and count metastatic lymph nodes (MLNs) in order to accurately determine it. As a DL framework to examine the lymph-node WSI, the overall tumor-area-to-MLN-area ratio (T/MLN), which was discovered to be a self-sufficient prognostic predictor, was presented. The system employs U-net for segmentation, ResNet for categorization, and T/MLN for computation. Using just N phases, tests using multicenter data sets show that T/MLN is an effective predictive measure with a hazard ratio of 2.05 and a greater C-index of 0.694 above 0.646 [146].

10.9 Conclusion and future prospects

In 1955, John McCarthy was the first to use the phrase AI. The ability of machines to learn and solve problems is the basis for the notion of AI. AI is divided into five primary subfields: ANNs, DL, vision in computers, natural language processing (NLP), and ML. Figure 10.3 illustrates the relationship between ML, AI, and DL. While DL is built on the intricate ANN designs, ML creates algorithms to analyse data. NLP is a field that gives computers the ability to extract meaningful data from content, like digital health records, allowing in-depth research (figure 10.3). ANNs simulate the way the nervous system functions in humans, which has multiple layers and can recognize subtle or complicated patterns. For saved photos or live videos, computer vision does machine recognition. There are numerous uses for computer vision, such as image-guided surgery, digital pathology

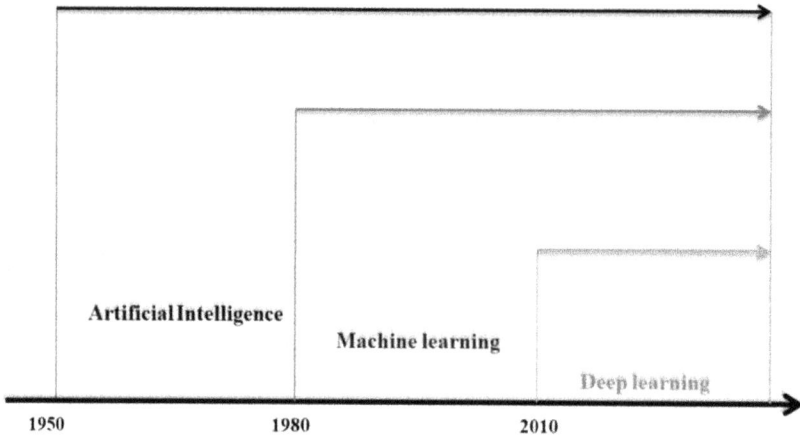

Figure 10.3. AI concept.

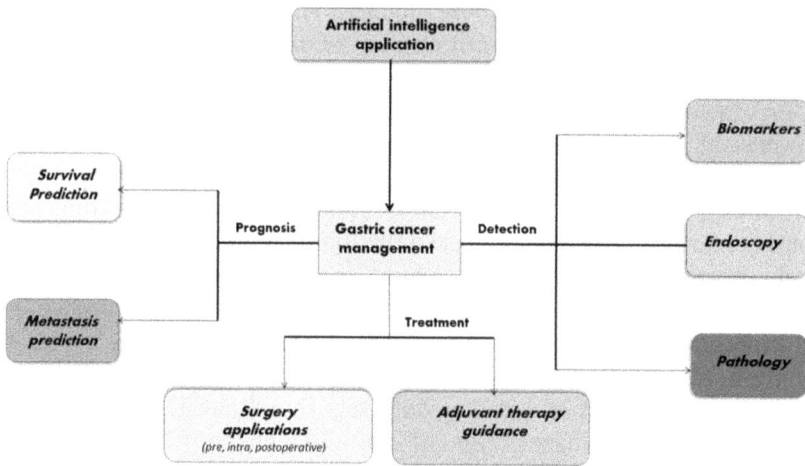

Figure 10.4. AI applications in the treatment of cancer of the stomach.

interpretation, and computer-assisted endoscopic diagnostics. Recent investigations have shown that it has great potential for use in the treatment of stomach cancer. AI can help with early detection, treatment planning, and prognosis forecasting in cases of stomach cancer. The primary uses of AI in stomach cancer are illustrated in (figures 10.4 and 10.5).

Future clinical practice in the era of precision medicine will require the integration of omics data with clinical information. The workload of doctors could be significantly reduced with the help of AI technology. In recent years, AI-assisted endoscopic diagnosis for stomach cancer has significantly improved thanks to picture recognition. These researches mainly concentrate on four areas: identifying HP infection, identifying CAG, detecting EGC and estimating the degree of invasion. High detection rate and processing speed were shown by an AI-assisted system. Additionally, when used

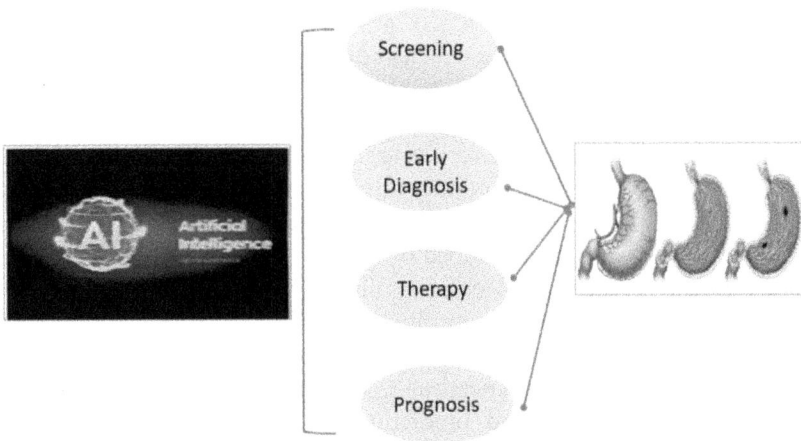

Figure 10.5. AI implementation in GC.

for video images, real-time identification together with endoscopic inspection were evaluated, although further study is required before it can be implemented in clinical practice in the future. Additionally, it is utilized to develop models that predict surgical complications and lymph node metastasis, therapeutic prognosis and the reaction. In addition, a different study found that an ANN model outperformed a decision tree model at predicting hospital charges [135].

The use of AI approaches does have some restrictions, though. First, there aren't many high-quality instruction and approval datasets available. Second, most AI algorithms are 'black boxes,' meaning that no one has a complete grasp of how they operate. The use of AI upon patient permission and identification of the misdiagnosis's perpetrator or inappropriate course of therapy are two additional ethical and safety concerns. AI is also unable to establish causal connections. Physicians must rigorously assess and interpret AI-generated predictions in ways that have therapeutic relevance [125]. Additionally, most modern systems use supervised learning, which is based on carefully human-labeled data. However, given the dearth of domain experts, it is challenging to collect a sizable volume of high-quality labeled data for medical activities, while more unlabeled data remain untapped. To make use of the underutilized unlabeled data, numerous strategies for self- and semi-supervised learning have lately been introduced. These methods might be applied in GC AI to address the problem of sparsely tagged data [130].

In the early identification, diagnosis, and treatment of disease, many diagnostic imaging techniques can play special and unique roles in decision-making processes related to GC. While pathologic investigation must be used to confirm GC, its preliminary diagnosis is acceptable for endoscopic investigation. Additionally, AGC may be identified using CT scanning, hence it cannot be utilized to make the diagnosis. The use of a single modality to inform decisions could result in incorrect diagnosis. Building multi-modality algorithms is advantageous in order to reach more thorough diagnostic conclusions. Additionally, large-scale imaging data can be gathered more affordably than expensive molecular data. In order to understand the connection between disease-related gene expression patterns and imaging characteristics, a new research field called radio genomics has arisen [114].

For glioblastoma [109], carcinoma of the breast [110], and malignancies of the lungs [111], it has drawn a lot of attention and it may be able to help with better treatment selection, prognosis forecasting, and cancer knowledge in general. Researchers working across cancers may advance our knowledge of tumor-related chemicals given that pan-cancer compounds are present in a variety of tumor types. The Database of Pan-Cancer, developed by TGGA, for forms of human carcinoma is reclassified based on their molecular similarity [112]. Knowledge from cancers with similar characteristics may be applied to the study of GC. Additionally, the majority of previous research has concentrated on a small number of modeling issues, such as diagnosing precancerous conditions or tumors, categorizing the phases or cancer subgroups, and predicting treatment effectiveness or survival outcomes. These duties are, nevertheless, inevitably related. In order to create a more reliable GC diagnosis, multi-task learning algorithms may be able to take advantage of useful information by learning several related tasks at once [113]. The tumor's growth is also an unpredictable process that takes place over time.

The evolution of pictures over time may be crucial in determining the prognosis and responsiveness to treatment. Building time-dependent modeling based on image information from different patient phases, such as initial detection, pre-therapy, post therapy, etc, may therefore be beneficial. It might aid in our understanding of the dynamic process through which cancer develops. Additionally, given that different modalities are used at various stages of GC, combining multi-modality and multi-task algorithms may enhance prediction accuracy.

Epigenetic, genomes, proteomics, metabolomics, and other fields fall under the purview of using AI to find novel targets for cancer therapy. Because single omics studies cannot accurately predict anticancer targets, we must use ML and computational biology investigation to effectively incorporate multiple omics data, address the complexity of cancer caused by interactions between genes and their products, and advance our understanding of carcinogenesis. How to integrate multiomics data and uncover new anticancer targets using AI biological analytical techniques will thus be a key focus of future research.

There is still much room for development before this technology becomes genuinely widespread. It takes time to adjust and develop methods that are not just trustworthy but also understandable and accessible for incorporation of this magnitude. The major problem with AI as well as DL is that they effectively rely on the vast volumes of data that are provided to them in order to learn and grow [67]. Issues arise because datasets are not readily available, which may limit their expansion [67]. The necessity for drawing relevant inferences from the massive amounts of information that are currently available may be addressed with the use of tools like data mining, but these techniques have limits since additional datasets result in more accurate and significant data [68].

Despite these difficulties, the adoption of AI in the treatment of cancer looks promising in the age of personalized medicine. It may be considered as an aid for endoscopic diagnostics to catch sickness early and determine how deep the invasion has gone. Digital pathology can also be used to categorize the many types of cancer and determine how each one responds to various pharmacological treatments. AI's application in detecting stomach cancer is expanding rapidly due to the quick the advancement of ML and digital pathology techniques. AI has been used in a variety of settings, such as endoscopic diagnosis, assessing the degree of membrane invasion, histopathologically diagnosis, and classification, analyzing gastric smears, molecular and genetic screening, and prognosis prediction.

Applications of AI technology in the diagnosis of gastrointestinal cancer have demonstrated rapidity and precision comparable to or even superior to that of conventional pathologists. However, pathologists' breadth and contextual knowledge will not be replaced by AI; rather, accuracy and effectiveness of pathologists in diagnosing stomach cancer can only be increased by their combination. The generalization of AI models [56], black boxes [54–56], as well as a scarcity of datasets of excellent quality are only a few of the issues that researchers have discovered with AI technology. Future work in this area of AI will probably concentrate on finding solutions to these issues. First, there is a lack of consensus regarding the inner workings of AI systems. One difficulty is deciphering and comprehending the decision-making processes of sophisticated AI models. One of the primary obstacles to the clinical use of algorithms that use DL is a situation known as the 'black box problem,' which is one of the key obstacles, and is the difficulty of reading and comprehending how sophisticated AI models arrive at judgments. The accuracy of DL may be impacted by flaws including spectral bias (class imbalance), over fitting, and selection bias. Graph neural networks (GNN) offer an edge over DL AI techniques like CNN models because they have demonstrated a lack of interpretability. GNNs are likely to be used increasingly in the diagnosis of stomach cancer in the future. The GNN's comprehensibility will make it possible as medical AI models acquire novel understandings beyond what is currently known to humans, researchers are able to use these new insights to better understand the biochemical mechanisms underlying disease.

Additionally, adopting AI frequently involves data problems. For instance, there aren't many high-quality datasets accessible for validation and training. To address the issue of insufficient data, we might take the Federated Learning (FL) method into consideration [57]. With the assumption of restricted data sharing, by transferring system parameters from the main database, FL is a multi-distributed joint learning approach that can learn across several databases and create a high-precision system. We show that FL allows us to efficiently build without the hassle of direct information exchange; weakly guided DL models are created from scattered data repositories and with differential privacy maintained via random noise creation.

The application of AI models and technologies for supporting medical decisions in general is the final crucial question. When presented with data from different sources, AI models using a single source of data could not work properly. Additionally, the ability to train AI models and validate them using datasets from many sources will increase generalization. The thorough examination of AI can also include multidisciplinary data from fields like gastroenterology, radiation therapy, pathological conditions, medical care, surgery, and radiation oncology for difficult situations. On the other hand, researchers may not always have access to the substantial computational power and massive data support that AI technology is relying on. Given these conditions, it is foreseeable that the specialization of AI technology for stomach cancer (a single illness or even a single subgroup) may be a practical solution. The entire surgical procedure will be supported by AI-assisted technologies. A harmonious coexistence of humans and technology is the best situation for achieving peak performance, thus AI will not entirely replace doctors.

The study of stomach cancer has advanced significantly thanks to improvements in AI approaches, particularly ML and DL. This chapter offers a thorough overview of the current state and potential developments in AI-assisted diagnosis and prognosis. In comparison to traditional statistical methods, many researchers have observed that AI produces outstanding outcomes. The diagnosis and prognosis of stomach cancer will be revolutionized by AI's effective computational power and learning capabilities, despite the technology's drawbacks and difficulties, for instance, the need for interpretable models and well-annotated data.

EGC detection is challenging and necessitates thorough endoscopic evaluation. According to studies, roughly 10% of instances of stomach cancer had previously negative endoscopies. This number can be lowered with better endoscopic assessment. Real-time systems that are capable of identifying and characterizing premalignant/malignant gastric lesions are being created thanks to the availability of more modern endoscopic imaging techniques and AI. Cross-sectional imaging techniques might not be able to detect these small malignant gastric lesions, hence adequate endoscopic evaluation of EGC is essential for choosing the best resection procedure. ESD provides a surgical resection substitute for a subset of EGC patients. It is also essential to plan endoscopic monitoring of high-risk individuals, premalignant lesions, and after EGC resection for the early detection and successful therapy of gastric cancer.

To summarize, current studies of AI in relation to GC primarily focus on diagnosis. While AI technology is impressive, it may not be widely applicable in clinical settings just yet. It is possible that few AI researchers have a background in clinical practice. However, the development of less invasive laparoscopic surgical techniques might be used for AI and other computer-assisted procedures. The majority of clinical problems may be replaced with AI-based queries in the near future. While global medical resource imbalances may hinder the usage of AI widely, locations with sufficient AI and medical resources may accelerate its development. Clinicians with AI backgrounds may be critical players in advancing AI technology. By utilizing AI-based tools to standardize clinical administration, they can lessen the detrimental effects of accidents in their working life.

References

[1] Ajani J A, Bentrem D J, Besh S *et al* 2013 National comprehensive cancer network. Gastric cancer, version 2.2013 *J. Natl. Compr. Canc. Netw.* **11** 531–46

[2] Isobe Y, Nashimoto A, Akazawa K *et al* 2011 Gastric cancer treatment in Japan: 2008 annual report of the JGCA nationwide registry *Gastric Cancer* **14** 301–16

[3] Veitch A M, Uedo N, Yao K *et al* 2015 Optimizing early upper gastrointestinal cancer detection at endoscopy *Nat. Rev. Gastroenterol. Hepatol.* **12** 660–7

[4] Pimentel-Nunes P, Dinis-Ribeiro M, Ponchon T *et al* 2015 Endoscopic submucosal dissection: European society of gastrointestinal endoscopy (ESGE) guideline *Endoscopy* **47** 829–54

[5] Wagner A D, Syn N L, Moehler M *et al* 2017 Chemotherapy for advanced gastric cancer *Cochrane Database Syst. Rev.* **8** CD004064

[6] Gravalos C and Jimeno A 2008 HER2 in gastric cancer: a new prognostic factor and a novel therapeutic target *Ann. Oncol.* **19** 1523–9

[7] Sauerbruch T, Schreiber M, Schussler P *et al* 1984 Endoscopy in the diagnosis of gastritis *Endoscopy* **16** 101–4

[8] Watanabe K, Nagata N, Shimbo T *et al* 2013 Accuracy of endoscopic diagnosis of *Helicobacter pylori* infection according to level of endoscopic experience and the effect of training *BMC Gastroenterol.* **13** 128

[9] Menon S and Trudgill N 2014 How commonly is upper gastrointestinal cancer missed at endoscopy? A meta-analysis *Endosc. Int. Open* **2** E46–50

[10] Gillies R J, Kinahan P E and Hricak H 2016 Radiomics: images are more than pictures, they are data *Radiology* **278** 563–77

[11] Andreu-Perez J, Poon C C, Merrifield R D, Wong S T and Yang G Z 2015 Big data for health *IEEE J. Biomed. Health Inform.* **19** 1193–208

[12] Colom R, Karama S, Jung R E and Haier R J 2010 Human intelligence and brain networks *Dialogues Clin. Neurosci.* **12** 489–501

[13] Li L *et al* 2020 Convolutional neural network for the diagnosis of early gastric cancer based on magnifying narrow band imaging *Gastric Cancer* **23** 126–32

[14] Hashimoto D A, Rosman G, Rus D and Meireles O R 2018 Artificial intelligence in surgery: promises and perils *Ann. Surg.* **268** 70–6

[15] Fard M J, Ameri S, Darin Ellis R, Chinnam R B, Pandya A K and Klein M D 2018 Automated robot-assisted surgical skill evaluation: predictive analytics approach *Int. J. Med. Robot.* **14** e1850

[16] Biglarian A, Hajizadeh E, Kazemnejad A and Zayeri F 2010 Determining of prognostic factors in gastric cancer patients using artificial neural networks *Asian Pac. J. Cancer Prev.* **11** 533–6

[17] Lee J *et al* 2018 deep learning-based survival analysis identified associations between molecular subtype and optimal adjuvant treatment of patients with gastric cancer *JCO Clin. Cancer Inform.* **2** 1–14

[18] Chien C W, Lee Y C, Ma T *et al* 2008 The application of artificial neural networks and decision tree model in predicting post-operative complication for gastric cancer patients *Hepato-Gastroenterology* **55** 1140–5

[19] Turing A M 1950 Computing machinery and intelligence *Mind* **59** 433–60

[20] Russell S and Norvig P 2009 Artificial intelligence: a modern approach, *Appl. Mech. Mater.* **263** 2829–33

[21] Rajpurkar P, Chen E, Banerjee O and Topol E J 2022 AI in health and medicine *Nat. Med.* **28** 31–8

[22] Jordan M I and Mitchell T M 2015 Machine learning: trends, perspectives, and prospects *Science* **349** 255–60

[23] Topol E J 2019 High-performance medicine: the convergence of human and artificial intelligence *Nat. Med.* **25** 44–56

[24] Lecun Y, Bengio Y and Hinton G 2015 Deep learning *Nature* **521** 436–44

[25] Deo R C 2015 Machine learning in medicine *Circulation* **132** 1920–30

[26] Yeung S, Downing N L, Fei-Fei L *et al* 2018 Bedside computer vision—moving artificial intelligence from driver assistance to patient safety *N. Engl. J. Med.* **378** 1271–3

[27] Gulshan V, Peng L, Coram M *et al* 2016 Development and validation of a deep learning algorithm for detection of diabetic retinopathy in retinal fundus photographs *JAMA* **316** 2402–10

[28] Esteva A, Kuprel B, Novoa R A *et al* 2017 Dermatologist-level classification of skincancer with deep neural networks *Nature* **542** 115–8

[29] Ehteshami Bejnordi B, Veta M, Johannes van Diest P *et al* 2017 Diagnostic assessment of deep learning algorithms for detection of lymph node metastases in women with breast cancer *JAMA* **318** 2199–210

[30] Yang Y J and Bang C S 2019 Application of artificial intelligence in gastroenterology *World J. Gastroenterol.* **25** 1666–83

[31] Le Berre C, Sandborn W J, Aridhi S *et al* 2020 Application of artificial intelligence to gastroenterology and hepatology *Gastroenterology* **158** 76–94, e2

[32] Karakitsos P, Stergiou E B, Pouliakis A *et al* 1996 Potential of the back propagation neural network in the discrimination of benign from malignant gastric cells *Anal. Quant. Cytol. Histol.* **18** 245–50

[33] Karakitsos P, Stergiou E B, Pouliakis A *et al* 1997 Comparative study of artificialneural networks in the discrimination between benign from malignant gastric cells *Anal. Quant. Cytol. Histol.* **19** 145–52

[34] Karakitsos P, Pouliakis A, Koutroumbas K *et al* 2000 Neural network application inthe discrimination of benign from malignant gastric cells *Anal. Quant. Cytol. Histol.* **22** 63–9

[35] Amin M B, Greene F L, Edge S B, Compton C C, Gershenwald J E, Brookland R K, Meyer L, Gress D M, Byrd D R and Winchester D P 2017 The eighth edition AJCC cancer staging manual: continuing to build a bridge from a population-based to a more 'personalized' approach to cancer staging *CA Cancer J. Clin.* **67** 93–9

[36] Sano T, Coit D G, Kim H H, Roviello F, Kassab P, Wittekind C, Yamamoto Y and Ohashi Y 2017 Proposal of a new stage grouping of gastric cancer for TNM classification: international gastric cancer association staging project *Gastric Cancer* **20** 217–25

[37] Liu D Y, Gan T, Rao N N, Xing Y W, Zheng J, Li S, Luo C S, Zhou Z J and Wan Y L 2016 Identification of lesion images from gastrointestinal endoscope based on feature extraction of combinational methods with and without learning process *Med. Image Anal.* **32** 281–94

[38] Ali H, Yasmin M, Sharif M and Rehmani M H 2018 Computer assisted gastric abnormalities detection using hybrid texture descriptors for chromo endoscopy images *Comput. Methods Programs Biomed.* **157** 39–47

[39] Luo H *et al* 2019 Real-time artificial intelligence for detection of upper gastrointestinal cancer by endoscopy: a multicentre, case-control, diagnostic study *Lancet Oncol.* **20** 1645–54

[40] Sakai Y, Takemoto S, Hori K, Nishimura M, Ikematsu H, Yano T and Yokota H 2018 Automatic detection of early gastric cancer in endoscopic images using a transferring convolutional neural network *Conf. Proc. IEEE Eng. Med. Biol. Soc.* pp 4138–41

[41] Bollschweiler E H, Mönig S P, Hensler K, Baldus S E, Maruyama K and Hölscher A H 2004 Artificial neural network for prediction of lymph node metastases in gastric cancer: a phase II diagnostic study *Ann. Surg. Oncol.* **11** 506–11

[42] Hensler K, Waschulzik T, Mönig S P, Maruyama K, Hölscher A H and Bollschweiler E 2005 Quality-assured efficient engineering of feedforward neural networks (QUEEN) - pretherapeutic estimation of lymph node status in patients with gastric carcinoma *Methods Inf. Med.* **44** 647–54

[43] Wang H, Ding S, Wu D S, Zhang Y T and Yang S L 2019 Smart connected electronic gastroscope system for gastric cancer screening using multi-column convolutional neural networks *Int. J. Prod. Res.* **57** 6795–806

[44] Bergholt M S, Zheng W, Lin K, Ho K Y, Teh M, Yeoh K G, Yan So J B and Huang Z 2011 *In vivo* diagnosis of gastric cancer using Raman endoscopy and ant colony optimization techniques *Int. J. Cancer* **128** 2673–80

[45] Duraipandian S, Sylvest Bergholt M, Zheng W, Yu Ho K, Teh M, Guan Yeoh K, Bok Yan So J, Shabbir A and Huang Z 2018 Real-time Raman spectroscopy for *in vivo*, online gastric cancer diagnosis during clinical *Proceedings of the 15th IEEE Int. Symposium on Biomedical Imaging* (Washington, DC: IEEE) pp 182–5

[46] Sharma H, Zerbe N, Klempert I, Hellwich O and Hufnagl P 2017 Deep convolutional neural networks for automatic classification of gastric carcinoma using whole slide images in digital histopathology *Comput. Med. Imaging Graph.* **61** 2–13

[47] Leon F, Gelvez M, Jaimes Z, Gelvez T and Arguello H 2019 Supervised classification of histopathological images using convolutional neuronal networks for gastric cancer detection *STSIVA 2019: Proceedings of the 22nd Symposium on Image, Signal Processing and Artificial Vision (Bucaramanga, Colombia, 2019 April 24–26)* (New York: IEEE)

[48] Iizuka O, Kanavati F, Kato K, Rambeau M, Arihiro K and Tsuneki M 2020 Deep learning models for histopathological classification of gastric and colonic epithelial tumours *Sci. Rep.* **10** 1504

[49] Yoshida H, Shimazu T, Kiyuna T, Marugame A, Yamashita Y, Cosatto E, Taniguchi H, Sekine S and Ochiai A 2018 Automated histological classification of whole-slide images of gastric biopsy specimens *Gastric Cancer* **21** 249–57

[50] Garcia E, Hermoza R, Castanon C B, Cano L, Castillo M and Castaneda C 2017 Automatic lymphocyte detection on gastric cancer IHC images using deep learning *CBMS 2017: Proc. 30th IEEE Int. Symp. on Computer-Based Medical Systems(2017 June 22–24) (Thessaloniki, Greece)* (New York: IEEE) pp 200–4

[51] Liang Q, Nan Y, Coppola G, Zou K, Sun W, Zhang D, Wang Y and Yu G 2019 Weakly supervised biomedical image segmentation by reiterative learning *IEEE J. Biomed. Health Inform.* **23** 1205–14

[52] Qu J, Hiruta N, Terai K, Nosato H, Murakawa M and Sakanashi H 2018 Gastric pathology image classification using stepwise fine-tuning for deep neural networks *J. Healthc. Eng.* **2018** 8961781

[53] Huang Z, Liu D, Chen X, Yu P, Wu J, Song B, Hu J and Wu B 2020 Retrospective imaging studies of gastric cancer: study protocol clinical trial (SPIRIT Compliant) *Medicine (Baltimore)* **99** e19157

[54] Gao Y *et al* 2019 Deep neural network-assisted computed tomography diagnosis of metastatic lymph nodes from gastric cancer *Chin. Med. J. (Engl.)* **132** 2804–11

[55] Li C, Shi C, Zhang H, Chen Y and Zhang S 2015 Multiple instance learning for computer aided detection and diagnosis of gastric cancer with dual-energy CT imaging *J. Biomed. Inform.* **57** 358–68

[56] Li C, Zhang S, Zhang H, Pang L, Lam K, Hui C and Zhang S 2012 Using the K-nearest neighbor algorithm for the classification of lymph node metastasis in gastric cancer *Comput. Math. Methods Med.* **2012** 876545

[57] Horiuchi Y *et al* 2020 Performance of a computer-aided diagnosis system in diagnosing early gastric cancer using magnifying endoscopy videos with narrow-band imaging (with videos) *Gastro. Intest. Endosc.* **92** P856–65

[58] Luo H Y *et al* 2019 Real-time artificial intelligence for detection of upper gastrointestinal cancer by endoscopy: a multicentre, case control, diagnostic study *Lancet Oncol.* **20** 1645–54

[59] Horiuchi Y *et al* 2020 Convolutional neural network for differentiating gastric cancer from gastritis using magnified endoscopy with narrow band imaging *Dig. Dis. Sci.* **65** 1355–63

[60] Ikenoyama Y *et al* 2020 Detecting early gastric cancer: comparison between the diagnostic ability of convolutional neural networks and endoscopists *Dig. Endosc* **33** 141–50

[61] Wu L *et al* 2019 A deep neural network improves endoscopic detection of early gastric cancer without blind spots *Endoscopy* **51** 522–31

[62] Correa P 1988 A human model of gastric carcinogenesis *Cancer Res.* **48** 3554–60

[63] De Vries A C, van Grieken N C, Looman C W *et al* 2008 Gastric cancer risk in patients with premalignant gastric lesions: a nationwide cohort study in the Netherlands *Gastroenterology* **134** 945–52

[64] Van Cutsem E, Sagaert X, Topal B *et al* 2016 Gastric cancer *Lancet Dig. Health* **388** 2654–64

[65] Amin A, Gilmour H, Graham L *et al* 2002 Gastric adenocarcinoma missed at endoscopy *J. R. Coll. Surg. Edinb.* **47** 681–4

[66] Yalamarthi S, Witherspoon P, McCole D *et al* 2004 Missed diagnoses in patients with upper gastrointestinal cancers *Endoscopy* **36** 874–9

[67] Voutilainen M E and Juhola M T 2005 Evaluation of the diagnostic accuracy of gastroscopy to detect gastric tumours: clinicopathological features and prognosis of patients with gastric cancer missed on endoscopy *Eur. J. Gastroenterol. Hepatol* **17** 1345–9

[68] Hosokawa O, Hattori M, Douden K *et al* 2007 Difference in accuracy between gastroscopy and colonoscopy for detection of cancer *Hepatogastroenterology* **54** 442–4

[69] Diao W, Huang X, Shen L *et al* 2018 Diagnostic ability of blue laser imaging combined with magnifying endoscopy for early esophageal cancer *Dig. Liver Dis.* **50** 1035–40

[70] Robbins S L and Cotran R S 1979 *Pathologic Basis of Disease* 2nd edn (Philadelphia, PA: Saunders)

[71] Huang C-R, Sheu B-S, Chung P-C *et al* 2004 Computerized diagnosis of *Helicobacter pylori* infection and associated gastric inflammation from endoscopic images by refined feature selection using a neural network *Endoscopy* **36** 601–8

[72] Shichijo S, Nomura S, Aoyama K *et al* 2017 Application of convolutional neural networks in the diagnosis of *Helicobacter pylori* infection based on endoscopic images *EBio Med.* **25** 106–11

[73] Nakashima H, Kawahira H, Kawachi H *et al* 2018 Artificial intelligence diagnosis of *Helicobacter pylori* infection using blue laser imaging-bright and linked colour imaging: a single centre prospective study *Ann. Gastroenterol.* **31** 462–8

[74] Shichijo S, Endo Y, Aoyama K *et al* 2019 Application of convolutional neural networks for evaluating *Helicobacter pylori* infection status on the basis of endoscopic images *Scand. J. Gastroenterol.* **54** 158–63

[75] Yasuda T, Hiroyasu T, Hiwa S *et al* 2020 Potential of automatic diagnosis system with linked colour imaging for diagnosis of *Helicobacter pylori* infection. *Dig. Endosc.* **32** 373–81

[76] Guimaraes P, Keller A, Fehlmann T *et al* 2020 Deep-learning based detection of gastric precancerous conditions *Gut* **69** 4–6

[77] Zhang Y, Li F, Yuan F *et al* 2020 Diagnosing chronic atrophic gastritis by gastroscopy using artificial intelligence *Dig. Liver Dis.* **52** 566–72

[78] Yan T, Wong P K, Choi I C *et al* 2020 Intelligent diagnosis of gastric intestinal metaplasia based on convolutional neural network and limited number of endoscopic images *Comput. Biol. Med.* **126** 104026

[79] Zhang X, Hu W, Chen F *et al* 2017 Gastric precancerous diseases classification using CNN with a concise model *PLoS One* **12** e0185508

[80] Cho B-J, Bang C S, Park S W *et al* 2019 Automated classification of gastric neoplasms in endoscopic images using a convolutional neural network *Endoscopy* **51** 1121–9

[81] Lee J H, Kim Y J, Kim Y W *et al* 2019 spotting malignancies from gastric endoscopic images using deep learning *Surg. Endosc.* **33** 3790–7

[82] Miyaki R, Yoshida S, Tanaka S *et al* 2013 Quantitative identification of mucosal gastric cancer under magnifying endoscopy with flexible spectral imaging colour enhancement. *J. Gastroenterol. Hepatol.* **28** 841–7

[83] Miyaki R, Yoshida S, Tanaka S *et al* 2015 A computer system to be used with laser-based endoscopy for quantitative diagnosis of early gastric cancer *J. Clin. Gastroenterol.* **49** 108–15

[84] Hirasawa T, Aoyama K, Tanimoto T *et al* 2018 Application of artificial intelligence using a convolutional neural network for detecting gastric cancer in endoscopic images *Gastric Cancer* **21** 653–60

[85] Liu X, Wang C, Hu Y *et al* 2018 Transfer learning with convolutional neural network for early gastric cancer classification on magnifying narrow-band imaging images *25th IEEE Int. Conf. on Image Processing (ICIP)* (Piscataway, NJ: IEEE) pp 1388–92

[86] Luo H, Xu G, Li C *et al* 2019 Real-time artificial intelligence for detection of upper gastrointestinal cancer by endoscopy: a multicentre, case-control, diagnostic study *Lancet Oncol.* **20** 1645–54

[87] Hsu C-C, Ma H-T and Lee J-Y 2019 SSSNet: small-scale-aware siamese network for gastric cancer detection *2019 16th IEEE Int. Conf. on Advanced Video and Signal Based Surveillance (AVSS)* (Piscataway, NJ: IEEE) pp 1–5

[88] Yoon H J, Kim S, Kim J-H *et al* 2019 A lesion-based convolutional neural network improves endoscopic detection and depth prediction of early gastric cancer *JCM* **8** 1310

[89] Ikenoyama Y, Hirasawa T, Ishioka M *et al* 2021 Detecting early gastric cancer: comparison between the diagnostic ability of convolutional neural networks and endoscopists *Dig. Endosc.* **33** 141–50

[90] Mori H and Miwa H 2019 A histopathologic feature of the behavior of gastric signet-ring cell carcinoma; an image analysis study with deep learning *Pathol. Int.* **69** 437–9

[91] Qu J, Hiruta N, Terai K, Nosato H, Murakawa M and Sakanashi H 2018 Gastric pathology image classification using stepwise fine-tuning for deep neural networks *J. Healthc. Eng.* **2018** 896–1781

[92] Sun M Y, Zhang G H, Dang H, Qi X Q, Zhou X G and Chang Q 2019 Accurate gastric cancer segmentation in digital pathology images using deformable convolution and multi-scale embedding networks *IEEE Access* **7** 75530–41

[93] Cao G T, Song W L and Zhao Z W 2019 Gastric cancer diagnosis with mask R-CNN *IHMSC: Proc. 11th Int. Conf. on Intelligent Human-Machine Systems and Cybernetics (2019 August 24–25) (Hangzhou, China)* (New York: IEEE) pp 60–3

[94] Vollmer S *et al* 2020 Machine learning and artificial intelligence research for patient benefit: 20 critical questions on transparency, replicability, ethics, and effectiveness *BMJ* **368** 6927

[95] Joo M *et al* 2019 A Deep learning model for cell growth inhibition IC50 prediction and its application for gastric cancer patients *Int. J. Mol. Sci.* **20** 6276

[96] Namikawa K *et al* 2020 Utilizing artificial intelligence in endoscopy: a clinician's guide *Expert Rev. Gastroenterol. Hepatol.* **14** 689–706

[97] Lee H L, Eun C S, Lee O Y *et al* 2010 When do we miss synchronous gastric neoplasms with endoscopy? *Gastrointest. Endosc.* **71** 1159–65

[98] Gotoda T 2007 Endoscopic resection of early gastric cancer *Gastric Cancer* **10** 1–11

[99] Probst A, Schneider A, Schaller T *et al* 2017 Endoscopic submucosal dissection for early gastric cancer: are expanded resection criteria safe for Western patients? *Endoscopy* **49** 855–65

[100] Abe S, Oda I, Minagawa T *et al* 2018 Metachronous gastric cancer following curative endoscopic resection of early gastric cancer *Clin. Endosc.* **51** 253–9

[101] Zhu Y, Wang Q C, Xu M D *et al* 2019 Application of convolutional neural network in the diagnosis of the invasion depth of gastric cancer based on conventional endoscopy *Gastrointest. Endosc.* **89** 806–815.e1

[102] Odagiri H and Yasunaga H 2017 Complications following endoscopic sub mucosal dissection for gastric, esophageal, and colorectal cancer: a review of studies based on nationwide large-scale databases *Ann. Transl. Med.* **5** 189

[103] Andras I *et al* 2019 Artificial intelligence and robotics: a combination that is changing the operating room *World J. Urol.* **38** 2359–66

[104] Yang J, Gong Y, Lam V K *et al* 2020 Deep sequencing of circulating tumor DNA detects molecular residual disease and predicts recurrence in gastric cancer *Cell Death Dis.* **11** 346

[105] Li Z, Chen S, Feng W *et al* 2020 A pan-cancer analysis of HER2 index revealed transcriptional pattern for precise selection of HER2-targeted therapy *EBioMed.* **62** 103074

[106] Ishii H, Sasaki H, Aoyagi K *et al* 2013 Classification of gastric cancer subtypes using ICA, MLR and Bayesian network *Stud. Health Technol. Inf.* **192** 1014

[107] Yan Z, Xu W, Xiong Y *et al* 2013 Highly accurate two-gene signature for gastric cancer *Med. Oncol.* **30** 584

[108] Ghanat Bari M, Ung C Y, Zhang C, Zhu S and Li H 2017 Machine learning-assisted network inference approach to identify a new class of genes that coordinate the functionality of cancer networks *Sci. Rep.* **7** 6993

[109] Muzio G, O'Bray L and Borgwardt K 2021 Biological network analysis with deep learning *Brief. Bioinform.* **22** 1515–30

[110] Camacho D M, Collins K M, Powers R K, Costello J C and Collins J J 2018 Next-generation machine learning for biological networks *Cell* **173** 1581–92

[111] Johnson C H, Ivanisevic J and Siuzdak G 2016 Metabolomics: beyond biomarkers and towards mechanisms *Nat. Rev. Mol. Cell Biol.* **17** 451–9

[112] Hasin Y, Seldin M and Lusis A 2017 Multi-omics approaches to disease *Genome Biol.* **18** 1–15

[113] Kim H and Kim Y-M 2018 Pan-cancer analysis of somatic mutations and transcriptomes reveals common functional gene clusters shared by multiple cancer types *Sci. Rep.* **8** 6041

[114] Vinayagam A *et al* 2016 Controllability analysis of the directed human protein interaction network identifies disease genes and drug targets *Proc. Natl. Acad. Sci. USA* **113** 4976–81

[115] Do Valle Í F *et al* 2018 Network integration of multi-tumour omics data suggests novel targeting strategies *Nat. Commun.* **9** 1 10

[116] Yang K *et al* 2017 A comprehensive analysis of metabolomics and transcriptomics in cervical cancer *Sci. Rep.* **7** 43353

[117] Medi K, Kazim Y A and Craig M 2018 Potential biomarkers and therapeutic targets in cervical cancer: insights from the meta-analysis of transcriptomics data within network biomedicine perspective *PLoS One* **13** e0200717

[118] Cantini L, Medico E, Fortunato S and Casella M 2015 Detection of gene communities in multi-networks reveals cancer drivers *Sci. Rep.* **5** 17386

[119] Ong S-E and Mann M 2005 Mass spectrometry–based proteomics turns quantitative *Nat. Chem. Biol.* **1** 252–62

[120] Li Z *et al* 2017 The OncoPPi network of cancer-focused protein–protein interactions to inform biological insights and therapeutic strategies *Nat. Commun.* **8** 14356

[121] Kalman R E 1963 Mathematical description of linear dynamical systems *J. Soc. Ind. Appl. Math. Ser. A Control* **1** 152–92

[122] Johnson C H, Ivanisevic J, Siuzdak and Metabolomics G 2016 beyond biomarkers and towards mechanisms *Nat. Rev. Mol. Cell Biol.* **17** 451–9

[123] Basler G, Nikoloski Z, Larhlimi A, Barabási A-L and Liu Y-Y 2016 Control of fluxes in metabolic networks *Genome Res.* **26** 956–68

[124] Chakraborty S, Hosen M, Ahmed M and Shekhar H U 2018 Onco-Multi-OMICS approach: a new frontier in cancer research *BioMed. Res. Int.* **2018** 9836256

[125] Zhang C *et al* 2017 The identification of key genes and pathways in hepatocellular carcinoma by bioinformatics analysis of high-throughput data *Med. Oncol.* **34** 101

[126] Gov E, Kori M and Arga K Y 2017 Multiomics analysis of tumor microenvironment reveals Gata2 and miRNA-124-3p as potential novel biomarkers in ovarian cancer *OMICS* **21** 603–15

[127] Biglarian A, Hajizadeh E, Kazemnejad A and Zali M 2011 Application of artificial neural network in predicting the survival rate of gastric cancer patients *Iran J. Public Health* **40** 80–6

[128] Amiri Z, Mohammad K, Mahmoudi M, Parsaeian M and Zeraati H 2013 Assessing the effect of quantitative and qualitative predictors on gastric cancer individuals survival using hierarchical artificial neural network models *Iran. Red Crescent Med. J.* **15** 42–8

[129] Nilsaz-Dezfouli H, Abu-Bakar M R, Aras an J, Adam M B and Pourhoseingholi M A 2017 Improving gastric cancer outcome prediction using single time-point artificial neural network models *Cancer* **16**

[130] Korhani Kangi A and Bahrampour A 2018 Predicting the survival of gastric cancer patients using artificial and Bayesian neural networks *Asian Pac. J. Cancer Prevent.* **19** 487–90

[131] Jiang Y *et al* 2018 Immunomarker support vector machine classifier for prediction of gastric cancer survival and adjuvant chemotherapeutic benefit *Clin. Cancer Res.* **24** 5574–84

[132] Lu F, Chen Z K, Yuan X, Li Q, Du Z D, Luo L and Zhang F Y 2017 MMHG: Multi-modal hypergraph learning for overall survival after D2 gastrectomy for gastric cancer *DASC/PiCom/DataCom/CyberSciTech 2017: Proc. of the 15th Int. Conf. on Dependable, Autonomic and Secure Computing, 15th Int. Conf. on Pervasive Intelligence and Computing, 3rd Int. Conf. on Big Data Intelligence and Computing and Cyber Science and Technology Congress; 2017 (Nov. 6-10; Orlando, FL)* 164–9

[133] Zhang W *et al* 2020 Development and validation of a CT-based radiomic nomogram for preoperative prediction of early recurrence in advanced gastric cancer *Radiother. Oncol.* **145** 13–20

[134] Liu B, Tan J, Wang X and Liu X 2018 Identification of recurrent risk-related genes and establishment of support vector machine prediction model for gastric cancer *Neoplasm* **65** 360–6

[135] Bollschweiler E H, Mönig S P, Hensler K, Baldus S E, Maruyama K and Hölscher A H 2004 Artificial neural network for prediction of lymph node metastases in gastric cancer: a phase II diagnostic study *Ann. Surg. Oncol.* **11** 506–11

[136] Jagric E *et al* 2014 Nanostring- based multigene assay to predict recurrence for gastric cancer patients after surgery *PLoS One* **9** e90133

[137] Su F *et al* 2020 Development and validation of a deep learning system for ascites cytopathology interpretation *Gastric Cancer*

[138] Lai K C, Chiang H C, Chen W C, Tsai F J and Jeng L B 2008 Artificial neural network-based study can predict gastric cancer staging *Hepatogastroenterology* **55** 1859–63

[139] An P, Yang D, Wang J *et al* 2020 A deep learning method for delineating early gastric cancer resection margin under chromo endoscopy and white light endoscopy *Gastric Cancer* **23** 884–92

[140] Wang X *et al* 2021 Predicting gastric cancer outcome from resected lymph node histopathology images using deep learning *Nat. Commun.* **12** 1–13

[141] Jiang Y *et al* 2021 Development and validation of a deep learning CT signature to predict survival and chemotherapy benefit in gastric cancer: a multicenter, retrospective study *Ann. Surg.* **274** e1153–61

[142] Ling T, Wu L, Fu Y *et al* 2021 A deep learning-based system for identifying differentiation status and delineating margins of early gastric cancer in magnifying narrow-band imaging endoscopy *Endoscopy* **53** 469–77

[142] Meier A *et al* 2020 Hypothesis-free deep survival learning applied to the tumor micro-environment in gastric cancer *J. Pathol. Clin. Res.* **6** 273–82

[143] Zhang L *et al* 2020 A deep learning risk prediction model for overall survival in patients with gastric cancer: a multicenter study *Radiother. Oncol.* **150** 73–80

[144] Hyung W J *et al* 2017 Superior prognosis prediction performance of deep learning for gastric cancer compared to Yonsei prognosis prediction model using Cox regression *J. Clin. Oncol.* **35** 164

[146] Tan J-W, Wang L, Chen Y *et al* 2020 Predicting chemotherapeutic response for far-advanced gastric cancer by radiomics with deep learning semi-automatic segmentation *J. Cancer* **11** 7224–36

[147] Joshi S S and Badgwell B D 2021 Current treatment and recent progress in gastric cancer *CA A Cancer J. Clin.* **71** 264–79

IOP Publishing

Nanobiotechnology and Artificial Intelligence in Gastrointestinal Diseases

Vivek K Chaturvedi, Anurag Kumar Singh, Jay Singh and Dawesh P Yadav

Chapter 11

Nanomedicines in liver fibrosis

Saras Tiwari, Bhaskar Sharma, Jugasmita Deka, Prabhakar Singh and Vivek K Chatruvedi

Chronic infection of liver cells causes scarring on liver tissue, resulting in Liver Fibrosis (LF), which is now a major global health concern. Hepatitis C, Hepatitis B, and alcohol abuse are the leading causes of liver damage, which results in the deposition of Extracellular cell matrix (ECM) and liver fibrosis. Ultrasonography and magnetic resonance imaging are commonly used as non-invasive diagnostic methods for hepatic fibrosis. The conventional therapy used to treat liver diseases is ineffective because it does not deliver a sufficient amount of drug concentration in the liver and is imprecise. Several clinical and preclinical Study has shown that the utilisation of nanotechnology to deliver therapeutic agents including drug molecules, and nucleic acids, in adequate amount and to target specifically the HSC (hepatic stellate cells) could be the future treatment to cure Liver diseases caused by LF. According to research, nanomedicines can reverse premature hepatic fibrosis. Many nanoparticulate systems (NPs) such as Liposomes, Inorganic NPs, and Nano-micelles have been studied because of their diverse properties for drug delivery and in addition to some therapeutic moieties. Out of these, Liposomal NPs have shown very promising results in clinical trials and are being considered as an extremity for the treatment of hepatic fibrosis. This book chapter discusses the causes, pathogenesis, diagnosis, and nanoparticulate systems used in the treatment of chronic liver diseases.

11.1 Introduction

The liver plays a vital role in filtering blood continuously. Its healthy hue, a deep reddish-brown, reflects its saturation with blood [3]. Remarkably, the liver holds about a pint of blood at any given time, accounting for approximately 13% of the body's total blood volume. Every minute, it filters over a liter of blood, equivalent to around 22 gallons per hour and surpassing 250 gallons within a 24 h period.

doi:10.1088/978-0-7503-6134-7ch11

This immense filtering capacity is sustained by two primary blood sources: the hepatic artery, delivering oxygen-rich blood to the liver, and the hepatic portal vein, through which blood from the digestive system enters, carrying nutrients, medications, or toxins [1]. Liver fibrosis, characterized by the abnormal accumulation of collagen and other extracellular matrix proteins, is a common occurrence in various chronic liver diseases. Chronic Hepatitis C Virus infection, alcohol abuse, and non-alcoholic steatohepatitis (NASH) are the primary factors contributing to liver fibrosis in industrialized countries [1]. The excessive buildup of extracellular matrix (ECM) proteins leads to the formation of fibrous scars, distorting the normal structure of the liver. As the condition progresses, cirrhosis develops, characterized by the emergence of regenerating hepatocyte nodules. Cirrhosis, in turn, causes hepatocellular dysfunction and elevates resistance to blood flow within the liver, resulting in hepatic insufficiency and portal hypertension [2]. In recent years, significant advancements have been made in understanding the mechanisms underlying liver fibrosis, along with the exploration of clinical interventions. It has been discovered that addressing the root causes of liver fibrosis, such as eliminating viral infections or eradicating pathogens, holds promise for reversing the condition. However, despite promising results in animal models with several anti-fibrotic candidates, obtaining effective anti-fibrotic effects in clinical trials remains a challenge [2].

11.2 Stages of liver fibrosis

Liver fibrosis staging encompasses various scales used by doctors to assess the extent of liver damage. This evaluation is conducted through diverse approaches, including blood tests, imaging techniques, and the analysis of tissue biopsies under a microscope. Before staging and treating fibrosis, it is important for doctors to first diagnose liver diseases such as fatty liver or liver cirrhosis so that the root cause of inflammation can be identified. [3].

The process of assessing the extent of fibrosis is referred to as staging. It involves categorizing fibrosis into five distinct stages.

Stage 0: No Fibrosis (F0): In this stage, there is no evidence of fibrosis in the liver tissue. Liver cells are healthy, and there is minimal to no scarring present. The liver functions normally, and individuals with stage 0 fibrosis may not exhibit any symptoms of liver disease [4].

Stage 1: Portal Fibrosis without Septa (F1): At this stage, fibrosis begins to develop around the portal areas of the liver, where blood vessels and bile ducts are located [1]. Fibrous tissue accumulates in these areas but does not extend to form septa (bridges of scar tissue between portal areas). Liver function may remain relatively unaffected, and individuals may not experience noticeable symptoms [3].

Stage 2: Portal Fibrosis with Few Septa (F2): In stage 2 fibrosis, there is further progression of scarring, with the formation of a few septa extending from portal areas into the liver parenchyma. While fibrosis is more pronounced than in stage 1, liver function may still be relatively preserved, and symptoms may not be evident in all cases [4].

Stage 3: Numerous Septa without Cirrhosis (F3): This stage is characterized by the presence of numerous septa extending into the liver parenchyma, resulting in significant distortion of the liver architecture. Fibrosis is advanced, but cirrhosis has not yet developed [1]. Liver function may start to decline, and individuals may begin to experience symptoms such as fatigue, abdominal discomfort, or jaundice [3].

Stage 4: Cirrhosis (F4): Cirrhosis represents the most advanced stage of liver fibrosis, where extensive scarring and nodular regeneration disrupt the normal structure of the liver. The liver becomes hardened and nodular, impairing its function significantly. Symptoms of cirrhosis can be severe and may include jaundice, ascites, peripheral edema, easy bruising or bleeding, confusion, and other signs of liver failure [4].

Distinct cut-off values can help differentiate between these stages of fibrosis, although determining the optimal cut-off values for individuals with alcoholic liver disease remains an ongoing challenge [4].

11.3 Etiology of liver fibrosis

Liver fibrosis arises from diverse forms of chronic hepatic diseases and involves a complex process characterized by an overabundance of hepatocellular death. It primarily stems from different underlying causes, including schistosome and chronic viral hepatitis infections, non-alcoholic fatty liver disease (NAFLD), alcoholic liver disease (ALD), as well as cholestatic and autoimmune liver diseases [5].

11.3.1 Chronic viral hepatitis

Hepatitis B Virus (HBV) Infection: Chronic infection with HBV can lead to persistent liver inflammation, causing progressive liver fibrosis over time [4]. Hepatitis C Virus (HCV) Infection: HCV is a major cause of chronic liver disease worldwide. Chronic HCV infection can result in ongoing liver inflammation and fibrosis, leading to cirrhosis if left untreated [5].

11.3.2 Alcohol-related liver disease (ALD)

Chronic Alcohol Abuse: Excessive and prolonged alcohol consumption can cause liver inflammation (alcoholic hepatitis) and promote the accumulation of fat in the liver (alcoholic fatty liver disease), both of which can contribute to liver fibrosis and eventually cirrhosis [2].

11.3.3 Non-alcoholic fatty liver disease (NAFLD) and non-alcoholic steatohepatitis (NASH)

NAFLD encompasses a spectrum of liver conditions characterized by the accumulation of fat in the liver in individuals who do not consume excessive alcohol. In some cases, NAFLD can progress to NASH, characterized by inflammation and liver cell damage, ultimately leading to fibrosis and cirrhosis [3].

Autoimmune Hepatitis: Autoimmune hepatitis is a chronic autoimmune disorder in which the body's immune system mistakenly attacks the liver, leading to inflammation and damage [5]. Persistent inflammation can result in liver fibrosis and, in severe cases, cirrhosis [1].

Chronic Bile Duct Diseases: Primary Biliary Cholangitis (PBC): PBC is a chronic autoimmune liver disease characterized by inflammation and destruction of the small bile ducts within the liver [3]. Progressive bile duct damage and inflammation can lead to liver fibrosis and cirrhosis over time [5].

Primary Sclerosing Cholangitis (PSC): PSC is a chronic inflammatory condition characterized by inflammation and scarring (fibrosis) of the bile ducts both within and outside the liver. Liver fibrosis and cirrhosis are common complications of PSC [5].

Hemochromatosis: Hemochromatosis is a genetic disorder characterized by excessive iron absorption and accumulation in various organs, including the liver. Iron overload in the liver can lead to chronic liver injury, inflammation, and fibrosis [5].

Viral Hepatitis Coinfection: Coinfection with multiple hepatitis viruses, such as HBV and HCV, or human immunodeficiency virus (HIV) can accelerate liver disease progression, leading to more severe liver fibrosis and cirrhosis [3, 5].

Toxic Liver Injury: Exposure to certain toxins, chemicals, medications, or environmental pollutants can cause liver damage and inflammation, leading to fibrosis. Examples include long-term exposure to certain medications (e.g., methotrexate, amiodarone) or industrial chemicals [1].

Metabolic Disorders: Metabolic disorders such as glycogen storage diseases, alpha-1 antitrypsin deficiency, and hereditary fructose intolerance can cause liver damage and inflammation, potentially leading to fibrosis and cirrhosis [5].

Liver fibrosis can stem from various underlying factors, including autoimmune disorders, obstructions in the bile ducts, specific medications, conditions that reduce blood flow to the liver, and hereditary metabolic disorders. Additionally, there is a congenital form of liver fibrosis that manifests from birth [3].

11.4 Pathogenesis

Chronic inflammation from infections, autoimmune diseases, metabolic diseases, chemicals and specific diseases are some of the factors that can cause liver fibrosis. The balance of pro-fibrotic and anti-fibrotic systems reduces the severity of hepatic fibrosis. Damage to the hepatocytes causes them to release Damage-Associated Molecular Patterns (DAMPs) that directly stimulate the activation of quiescent Hepatic stellate cells (HSCs). The stimulated HSCs produce an extracellular matrix composed of type 1 and type 3 collagen and fibronectin. In healthy conditions, the balance of Matrix metalloproteinases (MMPs) and Tissue inhibitors of metalloproteinases (TIMPs) regulates the formation and mortification of the Extracellular Matrix (ECM). There is a disturbed balance in the body, The amount of MMPs responsible for ECM inhibition decreases, whereas TIMPs that block the MMPs increase. There is a lack of regulation of ECM and scar formation in the spaces of Disse due to an imbalance between MMPs and TIMPs [7, 8]. Liver fibrosis occurs due to the imbalance between pro-fibrosis and anti-fibrosis activities, leading to substantial effects on the structure of liver tissue and its overall function. The activation of hepatic stellate cells (HSCs) increases contractility, elevates expression of α-Smooth Muscle Actin, and the production of various cytokines, including Transforming Growth Factor-1 (TGF-1) and Connective Tissue Growth Factor (CTGF). These activated HSCs are regulated by autocrine signalling pathways. Activated HSCs maintain their activation through autocrine signalling, while chemokines released by other cells attract them to the site of liver injury, where they aggregate in the inflammatory compartment and contribute to further inflammatory damage. Moreover, the release of damage-associated molecular patterns (DAMPs) by damaged liver cells triggers the activation of Kupffer cells and other components of the immune system. These activated immune cells further support HSC activation and survival by secreting proinflammatory and profibrotic factors, including platelet-derived growth factor (PDGF), tumour necrosis factor-alpha (TNF-α), and interleukin-1-beta (IL-1β). Various signalling pathways, such as the TGF-β1/Smad pathway and the mitogen-activated protein kinase (MAPK) pathways, are involved in these processes [9–11]. Furthermore, Kupffer cells play a vital role in recruiting monocytes to the site of inflammation and injury by releasing chemokines like chemokine (C-C motif) ligand 2 (CCL2) and CCL5. These recruited monocytes contribute to hepatocyte damage by synthesizing and releasing substances like apoptosis signal-regulated kinase 1 (ASK1), Pan-caspase, and Galectin-3 which have both anti-inflammatory and pro-fibrotic properties. Their presence enhances the activation of HSCs, leading to intensified inflammation and fibrosis within the liver [12]. Moreover, the liver microenvironment contains TGF-β1, which promotes the differentiation of monocytes into macrophages. These macrophages are crucial in the inflammatory response, as they secrete inflammatory molecules like interleukin 1 (IL-1) and interleukin 6 (IL-6). The presence of these inflammatory mediators further amplifies the inflammatory response, thereby sustaining the activation and survival of HSCs. Paracrine signalling between Kupffer cells, macrophages and HSCs further influences the development of liver fibrosis by helping to regulate HSC activation and function [3, 6] (figure 11.1).

11.5 Symptoms

Although liver fibrosis may not exhibit noticeable symptoms, its impact on the liver's functionality can be significant. The scarring resulting from fibrosis can hinder the liver's efficient operation. It's worth noting that individuals can have liver fibrosis without being aware of it, since mild to moderate stages are often challenging for doctors to diagnose [6]. Symptoms typically emerge when a considerable portion of the liver is damaged due to fibrosis. Research suggests that approximately 6%–7% of the global population is affected by liver fibrosis without experiencing noticeable symptoms, which makes it difficult for individuals to be aware of their condition. The absence of symptoms often leads to a lack of awareness regarding the presence of liver fibrosis among this portion of the population [3, 6].

Fatigue and Weakness: It is one of the early signs of liver fibrosis. It is a persistent feeling of tiredness and weakness. This fatigue can be exhausting and may interfere with daily activities, making individuals feel lethargic even after adequate rest.

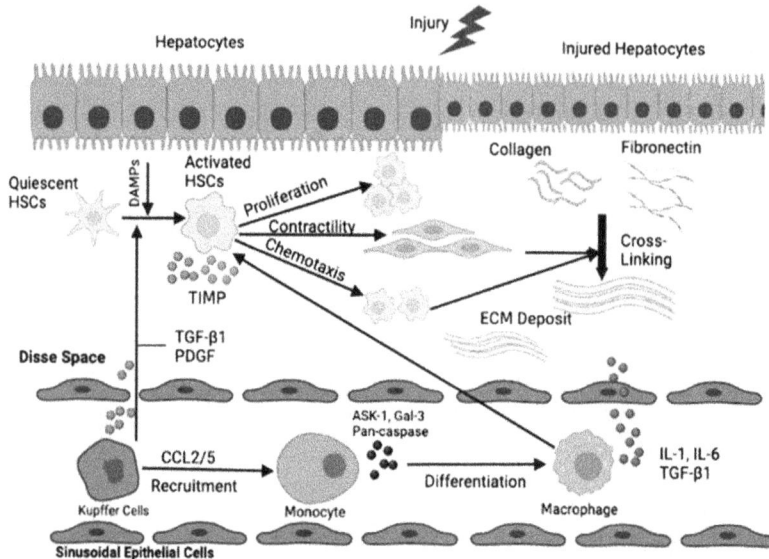

Figure 11.1. Pathogenesis of liver fibrosis. The activation of hepatic stellate cells (HSCs) plays a crucial role in the pathogenesis of liver fibrosis, contributing to its formation and progression. Initially quiescent, HSCs are activated upon exposure to damage-associated molecular patterns (DAMPs) released by injured hepatocytes, leading to the development of a fibrotic phenotype. Activated HSCs perpetuate their activation through both paracrine and autocrine processes. They secrete increased amounts of fibrotic cytokines and generate excessive extracellular matrix (ECM), which disrupts the balance between pro-fibrotic and anti-fibrotic mechanisms. These pro-fibrotic mechanisms contribute to the abnormal formation of scar tissue, ultimately leading to the development of liver fibrosis [2].

Abdominal Discomfort: People also experience vague discomfort or pain in the abdomen. This discomfort can range from a dull ache to a more severe, stabbing pain. It may be located in the upper right part of the abdomen, where the liver is situated.

Jaundice: Advanced liver fibrosis can impair the liver's ability to process bilirubin, a yellow pigment produced by the breakdown of red blood cells. This can result in jaundice, a condition characterized by yellowing of the skin, eyes, and mucous membranes. Jaundice can also cause dark urine and pale stools (figure 11.2).

Ascites: In later stages of liver fibrosis, fluid may accumulate in the abdominal cavity, leading to a condition called ascites. Ascites can cause abdominal swelling, discomfort, and a feeling of fullness. It may also contribute to weight gain and difficulty breathing.

Peripheral Edema: Liver fibrosis can impair the liver's ability to produce proteins involved in regulating fluid balance, leading to fluid retention in the body. This can cause swelling, particularly in the legs, ankles, and feet, a condition known as peripheral edema.

Portal Hypertension: As fibrosis progresses, it can lead to increased pressure in the portal vein, a major blood vessel that carries blood from the digestive organs to the liver. This condition, known as portal hypertension, can cause a variety of symptoms, including:

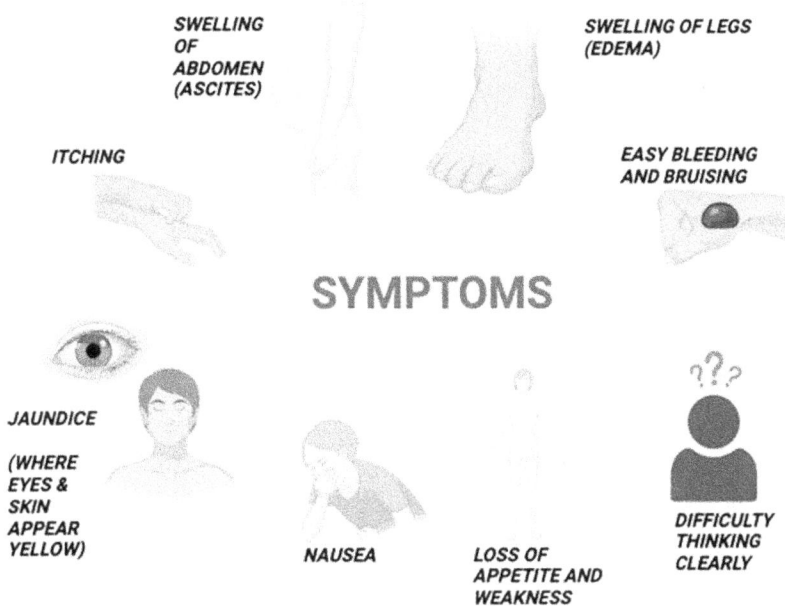

Figure 11.2. Symptoms of liver fibrosis. Symptoms like abdomen swelling, swelling of legs, easy bleeding and bruising, difficulty in clear thinking, loss of appetite and weakness, nausea, jaundice, itching are seen in liver fibrosis.

Gastrointestinal Bleeding: Portal hypertension can cause the development of enlarged veins, called varices, in the esophagus and stomach. These varices are prone to bleeding, which can result in vomiting of blood (hematemesis) or passing of black, tarry stools (melena).

Encephalopathy: Portal hypertension can impair the liver's ability to remove toxins from the blood, leading to a buildup of ammonia and other harmful substances in the brain. This can cause cognitive impairment, confusion, and even coma, a condition known as hepatic encephalopathy.

Easy Bruising and Bleeding: Liver fibrosis can impair the production of proteins involved in blood clotting, leading to a tendency to bruise easily and prolonged bleeding from minor cuts or injuries.

Loss of Appetite and Weight Loss: Liver fibrosis can cause a loss of appetite and unintentional weight loss due to factors such as nausea, abdominal discomfort, and metabolic disturbances associated with liver dysfunction.

11.6 Diagnosis

To initiate the diagnostic process, your doctor will inquire about your medical history and symptoms. A physical examination will also be conducted. To aid in the diagnosis of liver fibrosis, the doctor may recommend blood tests to assess liver function. These tests will specifically evaluate the levels of liver enzymes such as ALT and AST. Elevated levels of these enzymes can indicate the presence of fatty liver conditions [6].

11.7 Invasive approach

11.7.1 Liver biopsy

In the past, liver biopsy was commonly regarded as the definitive method for testing liver fibrosis. Medical practices are continually evolving, and there may be alternative methods or advancements in diagnostic techniques available. It is always recommended to consult with a healthcare provider for the most up-to-date information and options regarding liver fibrosis testing [3]. When it comes to invasive approaches, liver biopsy allows for a histopathological evaluation of liver tissue. The biopsy can be performed through different methods, including percutaneous, transvenous (trans jugular or transfemoral), or surgical (open or laparoscopic) procedures. A liver biopsy is indicated for diagnostic, prognostic, and treatment planning purposes. It allows for a comprehensive evaluation of liver tissue to aid in the diagnosis and management of liver fibrosis [13].

11.7.2 Limitations of liver biopsy

The utilization of liver biopsy as a routine clinical tool is hindered by various issues, such as the limited availability of manpower to perform biopsies for all patients in need, associated costs, and the potential risk of patient injury. However, it is crucial to highlight three specific limitations that directly impact the use of serum marker models.

11.7.2.1 Fibrosis staging system

Although histological staging of fibrosis is widely used, it is a bilateral misconception. First, it is inappropriate to use categorical values (e.g., fibrosis level) and second, the staging system assumes that the progression of fibrosis is severe in stage, which is incorrect. It is known that fibrosis does not increase linearly. Alternatively, blood samples are assigned a score based on an algorithm which provides a fixed variable that may represent a better method for assessing fibrosis [14].

11.7.2.2 Sampling error

Biopsies are prone to errors. A small sample of 10–15 mg is taken from a small part of the body which weighs about 1500 grams. Even in diseases that equally affect the liver, such as Hepatitis C, fibrosis can vary from lobe to lobe, although not more than once. In a study involving simultaneous laparoscopic biopsies of the left and right liver lobes in 124 patients with hepatitis C, at least some degree of lobular differentiation was observed in 33% of patients. This difference cannot be attributed to the small inter-observer differences. Only two patients differed between the two stages of fibrosis. Sampling is especially noticeable when dealing with small biopsies [14, 15].

11.7.2.3 Inter-observation variations

A third limitation concerns up to 20% difference in the classification of fibrosis grade by physicians. Differences between various observers indicate the fibrosis assessment study, making it difficult to compare results from different studies using different scores, such as Ishak and METAVIR. The lack of standardized measures makes it difficult to interpret and compare findings on the severity of fibrosis in research and clinical settings [16].

11.8 Non-invasive approach

11.8.1 Ultrasonographic based

11.8.1.1 Transient elastography

Transient elastography is a non-invasive diagnostic technique used to assess liver fibrosis by measuring the stiffness of the liver [17]. It has gained popularity as a reliable and convenient alternative to liver biopsy, which is invasive and carries risks of complications.

Principle: Transient elastography works on the principle of ultrasound-based elastography, where mechanical waves, generated using a specialized ultrasound probe are used to measure their propagation speed through liver tissue. The speed of these waves is directly correlated with tissue stiffness, allowing for the estimation of severity of liver fibrosis [55].

Procedure: During transient elastography procedure, the patient lies on their back with their right arm raised above their head. A small probe, connected to an ultrasound machine, is placed on the skin over the right lobe of the liver, typically at the level of the right lower rib cage [55]. The probe emits a low-frequency vibration, generating shear waves that propagate through the liver. The ultrasound machine measures the speed of these shear waves, which is directly related to liver stiffness. The results are displayed on the machine as a numerical value in kilopascals (kPa), representing the degree of liver fibrosis. The higher the stiffness measurement, the more severe the fibrosis [56].

Accuracy and Validity: Transient elastography has been extensively studied and validated for assessing liver fibrosis in various chronic liver diseases, including hepatitis B and C, nonalcoholic fatty liver disease (NAFLD), and alcoholic liver disease [55]. Studies have shown that transient elastography has good accuracy for detecting significant fibrosis (F2–F4) and cirrhosis (F4), with sensitivity and specificity rates ranging from 75% to 90% or higher, depending on the underlying liver disease and fibrosis stage [55, 56].

11.8.1.2 Advantages

Non-invasive: Transient elastography does not require an incision or tissue sampling, making it more tolerable for patients compared to liver biopsy [55, 56].

Rapid: The procedure is quick, usually taking only a few minutes to perform, and provides immediate results [55].

Repeatable: Transient elastography can be easily repeated over time to monitor disease progression or response to treatment [55].

Risk-free: Unlike liver biopsy, transient elastography carries minimal risk of complications such as bleeding or infection [57].

Limitations:
1. **Obesity:** In individuals with a high body mass index (BMI) or significant abdominal fat, transient elastography may be less accurate due to the attenuation of ultrasound waves by adipose tissue [57].

2. **Ascites:** The presence of ascites (fluid accumulation in the abdominal cavity) can interfere with transient elastography measurements, leading to unreliable results.

3. **Operator dependence:** Proper technique and operator experience are essential for obtaining accurate and reproducible transient elastography measurements [55].

11.8.1.3 Magnetic resonance elastography (MRE)

Magnetic Resonance Elastography (MRE) utilizes mechanical shear waves (with a frequency range of 20–200 Hz) to investigate and analyze the mechanical characteristics of different tissues. This non-invasive imaging technique provides valuable information about the tissue's elasticity and can aid in the diagnosis and monitoring of various medical conditions [17]. MRE can be integrated into conventional MR systems by adding custom hardware and software for data collection and processing to create non-invasive systems. In a commercial MRE setup, the device usually has an acoustic driver located outside the MRI machine. This driver is connected to a disc-shaped non-metallic passive driver located on the right side of the chest wall just above the heart. Elastic bands are used to improve their performance. While measuring pressure, a passive driver is used to send a continuous sound, usually 60 Hz, to the abdomen. Importantly, these vibrations are beneficial and the person undergoing the MRE method should not be disturbed. [18] (figure 11.3).

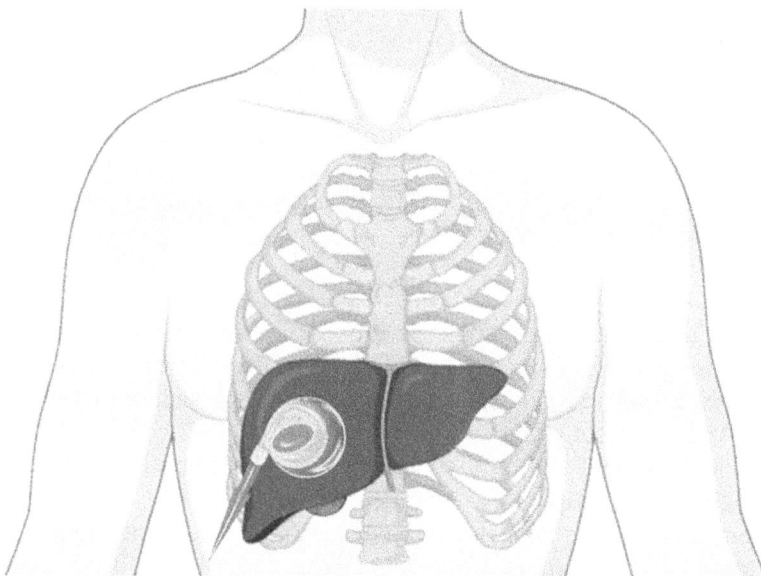

Figure 11.3. Performing MRE of liver. This image shows the position of the driver of the right lobe of the liver with its position near the level of the xiphisternum. This particular location has been carefully chosen to visualize the liver during end-trial breath hold. This zonal strategy ensures adequate print is focused and improves the quality of the MRE images obtained during the examination.

11.9 Non-surgical tests

Although symptoms may not be present during the early stages, healthcare professionals have implemented alternative non-surgical methods to evaluate the likelihood of liver fibrosis in different individuals. These methods encompass assessments of serum hyaluronate, matrix metalloproteinase-1 (MMP), tissue inhibitor of matrix metalloproteinase-1 (TIMP-1) levels, as well as calculations such as the aminotransferase-to-platelet ratio (APRI) or a comprehensive blood test called FibroSURE. The latter specifically measures six distinct indicators of liver function and employs an algorithm to generate a score [13]. However, it is important to note that these tests typically do not allow doctors to determine the specific stage of liver fibrosis. Ideally, doctors aim to diagnose liver fibrosis at an early stage when treatment options are more effective. Unfortunately, due to the typically asymptomatic nature of the condition in its initial stages, early diagnosis is uncommon [2, 3].

11.9.1 Serum biomarkers

Fibrosis-4 Index (FIB-4): FIB-4 is a simple calculation based on routine laboratory tests, including age, aspartate aminotransferase (AST), alanine aminotransferase (ALT), and platelet count. It provides a non-invasive estimation of liver fibrosis stage and has been validated in various liver diseases, including hepatitis B and C.

Enhanced Liver Fibrosis (ELF) Test: The ELF test measures serum levels of three fibrosis-related biomarkers: hyaluronic acid, tissue inhibitor of metalloproteinase 1 (TIMP-1), and procollagen III N-terminal peptide (PIIINP). The combination of these biomarkers provides a quantitative assessment of liver fibrosis severity and has been validated in chronic liver diseases.

AST to Platelet Ratio Index (APRI): APRI is another simple calculation based on routine laboratory tests, including AST and platelet count. It provides a non-invasive estimation of liver fibrosis severity, particularly in patients with chronic hepatitis C infection.

11.10 Treatment

The treatment of liver fibrosis depends on the underlying cause of the condition. To minimize the effects of liver disease, medical professionals primarily focus on treating the root cause whenever possible. For individuals who excessively consume alcohol, healthcare providers may recommend a treatment program to aid in alcohol cessation. In the case of non-alcoholic fatty liver disease (NAFLD), dietary changes for weight loss and medications to improve blood sugar control may be suggested. Engaging in regular exercise and losing weight can also help in slowing down the progression of the disease.

Treatment approaches for liver fibrosis include:

- **Chronic liver disease:** ACE inhibitors like benazepril, lisinopril, and ramipril may be prescribed.
- **Hepatitis C virus:** Direct-acting antiviral medications such as Epclusa, Harvoni, and Mayvret are commonly used.

- **Nonalcoholic steatohepatitis:** PPAR-alpha agonists are often recommended.
- **Autoimmune hepatitis:** Immunosuppressive therapy is the standard treatment.
- **Alcohol-related liver disease:** The key approach is complete abstinence from alcohol. [3, 5]

Additionally, doctors may suggest antifibrotic drugs that could potentially reduce the risk of permanent liver scarring (cirrhosis). Antifibrotics are classified based on their mechanisms of action:
- **Anti-inflammatories:** Examples include belapectin, cenicriviroc, and liraglutide.
- **Hepatocyte apoptosis inhibitors:** These include emricasan, pentoxifylline, and selonsertib.
- **Oxidative stress inhibitors:** Possibilities include methyl ferulic acid and losartan.
- **Hepatic stellate cell (HSC) inhibitors:** These drugs target various cytokines that can activate HSCs and contribute to fibrosis [4].

Note that although some are used for other purposes, such as hypertension and vascular disease, not all of these drugs are approved for the treatment of liver fibrosis. While animal studies are promising, the availability of human clinical trials is limited. When liver fibrosis progresses to a serious stage and the liver stops functioning normally, the most obvious treatment option is a liver transplant. However, the scarcity of organ donors and strict criteria for surgical eligibility lead to long waiting lists for transplants and not everyone is a suitable candidate [1, 3, 6].

11.11 Limitations of antifibrotic therapy

Various critical aspects related to the treatment of hepatic fibrosis have been addressed. Currently, there is a lack of a single therapeutic drug for hepatic fibrosis, but researchers are exploring combination therapies to alleviate symptoms and potentially reverse fibrosis. Although certain antifibrotic agents, like simtuzumab, have shown promise in experimental models, they have not successfully translated into clinical use. This is because these drugs are often tested against HSCs *in vitro*, whereas *in vivo* this issue is difficult with different cell types in the liver during the development of fibrosis. Consequently, targeted antifibrotics have not effectively addressed the multifaceted functions of myofibroblasts (MFBs), which include activation, proliferation, secretion of profibrogenic cytokines, and extracellular matrix synthesis. Instead, they have focused on specific modes of action, such as inhibiting PDGF or TGF-β or activating PPARγ [19, 20]. Although herbal-derived compounds have demonstrated beneficial effects in experimental liver fibrosis, challenges remain in terms of their solubility, bioavailability, and targeted delivery. While some new synthetic drugs are being developed, they are not specific to MFB in fibrotic liver and the possibility of further inflammation cannot be excluded. Nanomedicines offer an innovative approach by allowing the delivery of poorly soluble and bioavailable antifibrotic compounds, and they can also serve as theranostic agents. Nanoparticle-based anti-fibrotic therapy has emerged as a strategy to deliver retinol-modified anti-fibrotic compounds to activate HSCs, inhibit HSC activation and address liver fibrosis. Using nanotechnology and targeting MFB in the fibrotic liver, this approach shows promise for reversing liver fibrosis [21–23].

11.12 Role of nanomedicines in the treatment of hepatic fibrosis

Due to the complex nature of cancer, nanotechnology has been evolved and utilized in the field of medicine as a delivery system of therapeutic agents. Nanomedicines have wide use in the health sector such as: diagnostics, monitoring, therapy etc. Studies have shown the use of nanomedicines in the treatment of Liver Fibrosis. Numerous natural compounds derived from plants exhibit low solubility in water, leading to limited bioavailability. As a solution to overcome this challenge, researchers have developed nano-formulations. These novel formulations involve the use of liposomes, liposomes, nanoparticles (NPs), micelles, nanosuspensions, nano-capsules, nano-emulsions, and other herbal particle formulations. By employing these techniques, the efficiency of drug delivery systems (DDSs) can be enhanced, specifically targeting receptors found on hepatic stellate cells (HSCs), hepatocytes, macrophages, and other cell types. In experimental studies, both synthetic and plant-derived compounds, when formulated as nano-systems, have shown successful results against liver fibrosis. [20, 24]. kind of delivery system. For RNA therapeutic agents like siRNA, miRNA, mRNA, and other non-coding RNA, several nanoparticle system like Lipid Nanoparticles (LNPs), Polymeric nano-particles and Lipid–Polymer hybrid nanoparticles have eased their delivery with promising safety and efficiency.

11.13 Type of nanoparticles currently in use for LF

11.13.1 Phytochemical compound for LF

Biologically, the utilization of plant-derived compounds such as silymarin, quercetin, and berberine as reducing agents has been employed in the synthesis of nanoparticles (NPs). In an experiment, the administration of silymarin-assisted gold nanoparticles (AuNPs) via intragastric route demonstrated notable efficacy in preventing the activation of hepatic stellate cells (HSCs) and inducing the degradation of extracellular matrix (ECM) in rats with CCl4-induced hepatic fibrosis. In a recent study, quercetin was incorporated into nanocages made from hepatitis B core (HBc) protein for imaging. Integrin-targeted multifunctional nano-particles can selectively deliver quercetin to activate HSCs in the injured liver, showing promise as an anti-fibrotic theragnostic strategy [25]. In addition, berberine was combined with glucose and bovine Serum Albumin (BSA) to form a drug carrier nanoparticle. This complex containing glucose-berberine-BSA effectively inhibited the growth of HSCs *in vitro* and attenuated CCl4-induced liver fibrosis in mice.

Curcumin has many anti-inflammatory properties, but its bioavailability is difficult due to poor intestinal absorption and rapid metabolism. To solve this problem, nano-formulations have been developed to improve the bioavailability of curcumin. Micronized powder and liquid curcumin micelles have been shown to have improved solubility, stability and reduced initial metabolism. In the carbon tetrachloride (CCl4)-induced fibrosis model, polymeric curcumin nanoformulations (NanoCurc™) stably deliver curcumin to hepatocytes and HSCs, showing good solubility and bioavailability. Curcumin-encapsulated polylactide hyaluronic acid nanoparticles (CEHPNPs) reduced hepatotoxicity makers and hepatic collagen levels in a mouse model of thioacetamide (TAA)-induced liver fibrosis. *In vitro*, nano-formulations induce significant apoptosis in active HSCs while sparing dormant HSCs and parenchymal cells. However, it is worth noting that the curative effect of CEHPNPs in the *in vitro* test was approximately 1/30 of the group treated with free drugs. A phosphatidylserine-modified curcumin nanoparticle system examined in a CCl4-induced liver fibrosis model showed that proinflammatory cytokines, collagen, α-SMA reduction, collagenase activity improved by 204.6 ± 1.97 nm, encapsulation efficiency was 89.06% ± 0.47% [26–28].

Salvianolic acid B (SAB), derived from the herbal plant *Salvia miltiorrhiza* (SM), exhibits anti-fibrotic effects. However, its efficacy in treating hepatic fibrosis is limited due to poor water solubility and bioavailability. To overcome this challenge, previous studies have explored nano-based drug delivery systems (DDS). One such system is SAB@MSNs-RhB, where rhodamine B (RhB) is covalently grafted onto mesoporous silica nanoparticles (MSNs) with a size of 400 nm. This nano-formulation enhances cellular uptake, bioaccessibility and anti-fibrotic performance of SAB through the antioxidant mechanism. *In vitro* studies indicate that endocytosis in LX-2 cells mediates enhanced drug release. Nanoparticles that participate in globulins can be digested and biodegraded by the liver, facilitating their release in the liver, and thereby reducing fibrosis scores and development [29].

11.13.2 Synthetic antifibrotic nano formulations

Sorafenib, a widely used drug approved for the treatment of liver cancer, acts as a tyrosine kinase inhibitor with inhibitory effects on the vascular endothelial growth factor receptor (VEGF) and PDGF. However, its long-term prophylactic use as a fibrotic therapy has two main problems. First, sorafenib paradoxically activated the mitogen-activated protein kinase (MAPK) pathway in malignant and normal stromal cells, including during liver fibrosis, where MAPK contributes to HSC activation. Second, the elimination of sorafenib from normal tissues can cause side effects such as pain in the hand, diarrhea and high blood pressure [30]. To address these issues, CXCRA-targeted nanoparticles (NPs) loaded with sorafenib/MEK inhibitors at 140 nm size were developed. Interestingly, this combination inhibited MAPK-induced HSC activation *in vitro* and attenuated liver fibrosis in a CCl4-induced rat model. In addition, sorafenib-loaded poly lactic-glycolic acid (PLGA) nanoparticles with sizes of 100 to 300 nm and encapsulation efficiency (EE) greater than 82% reduced α-SMA and collagen in fibrotic liver tissue rats treated with CCl4. More importantly, increasing the PLGA content in the PEG-PLGA/PLGA mixture resulted in a smaller size and higher EE for sorafenib in nanoparticles while reducing drug release [31, 32].

Taxol® (paclitaxel) is an anti-cancer drug that acts against cancer by targeting the TGF-β pathway. However, its clinical application in the treatment of liver fibrosis is limited due to its side effects such as neutropenia. To overcome this limitation, a recent study introduced carboxymethylcellulose-docetaxel conjugated nanoparticles (Cellax) as albumin-dependent drug delivery. These Cellax nanoparticles are 120 nm in size and target selectively activated hepatocytes (aHSCs). Importantly, Cellax nanoparticles reduced the *in vitro* pro-fibrotic capacity of HSCs and attenuated CCl4-induced liver fibrosis in mice [33–36]. Hyaluronic acid (HA), an important component of the ECM, is biocompatible, biodegradable and non-toxic. CD44, an HA-related receptor whose expression is increased during liver fibrosis, plays a vital role in the activation and migration of HSCs. Thus, CD44 has become a target for the development of HA-based micelles as a drug delivery system (DDS). Specifically, micelles with an HA polymer backbone are designed to deliver losartan-loaded HA micelles that are selectively retained in the liver and exhibit significant anti-fibrotic effects. These micelles significantly reduced α-SMA expression in *in vitro* and *in vivo* models of TAA- and ethanol-induced fibrosis, demonstrating their potential as a promising anti-fibrotic therapy [37–40].

11.13.3 siRNA derived NPs

Liver fibrosis/cirrhosis is lead due to the addition of many ECM proteins in the damaged liver due to which silencing of ECM-associated gene expression using siRNA is a successful therapeutic approach to decrease accumulation. However, efficient and stable production of siRNA to activate HSCs in the injured liver remains a challenge. The delivery of siRNA faces many challenges *in vivo*. Therefore, the use of nanoparticles (NPs) to provide siRNAs has emerged to treat liver fibrosis [41–43]. Cationic polymers and lipid nanoparticles were used for liver-specific siRNA delivery. Since siRNA is highly degradable in nature, it needs protection for delivery. To overcome this problem lipid nanoparticles are mostly studied agents to deliver siRNA inside the cells and release the cargo into the cytosol. Two different kinds Catanionic and Ionisable lipids are used to provide a barrier for safe delivery of the siRNA as therapeutic agents. siRNA carries highly negative charge and these lipid particles with positive charge form complexes and self-assemble around it to form safe cores to provide protection. Lipid agents compose three major components such as hydrophilic head, hydrophobic tail, and this both groups joined with the linker group. This formulation starts their assembly with electrostatic interaction and grows with hydrophobic and van der Waals interaction. Lipoplexes comprising cationic lipids (CLs) are commonly used for delivering nucleic acids, but as CLs have been replaced by pH-sensitive ionizable lipids (ILs) due to concerns about toxicity and *in vivo* efficacy. When formulated into LNPs, these lipids are designed to be electrically neutral at physiological pH but become positively charged inside acidic endosomes. This pH-dependent ionizability makes ILs suitable for nucleic acid delivery, leading to improved efficacy and reduced toxicity. ILs typically constitute 30%–50% of the total lipids in a formulation, and significant research has been dedicated to refining IL properties to further improve efficiency, especially in hard-to-reach tissues.

One crucial component of LNPs that influences their duration in the body and their uptake by cells is the presence of PEG-anchored lipids. When LNPs are assembled, the PEG chain is positioned on the outer surface of the nanoparticle due to its hydrophilic nature and bulkiness. Similar to other nanocarriers, PEG serves to provide LNPs with an external polymeric layer that inhibits the absorption of serum proteins and the mononuclear phagocyte system, thereby extending their circulation time *in vivo*. PEG also prevents the aggregation of nanoparticles during storage and in the bloodstream. Furthermore, the quantity of PEG-lipids may impact the size of the particles. Another potential function of PEG-lipids is to customize the surface of LNPs. Functionalized PEG-lipids allow for the bioconjugation of LNPs with ligands or biomacromolecules. Polymer-based carriers are commonly utilized and studied as promising options for gene delivery due to their easy production and adaptable properties. The ability to easily modify the chemical and physical characteristics of polymer-based carriers provides advantages over lipid-based carriers, including effective protection of unstable siRNA from degradation, improved skin penetration through the skin barrier, and controlled release and targeting abilities. Several polymers such as Polyethyleneimine (PEI), PLGA chitosan are developed for safe gene delivery.

PEI is a positively charged polymer with a high concentration of amino groups that can be protonated. Among various polymers, PEI was the first to be made commercially available and is the most effective non-viral polymeric gene carrier both in laboratory settings and in living organisms. This is due to its polycations being highly effective in binding to DNA and its high transfection ability at physiological pH, thanks to its pH buffering capacity. The pH buffering capacity of PEI helps gene carriers to escape the endosomal barrier to avoid lysosomal degradation, which is crucial for achieving high gene transfection.

Chitosan is a naturally occurring linear polycationic polysaccharide made up of β-(1–4)-linked D-glucosamine and N-acetyl-D-glucosamine. Specifically, chitosan has been the subject of research as a carrier for different methods of gene delivery due to its positive charge, which allows it to form electrostatic complexes or multilayer structures with negatively charged oligonucleotides such as miRNAs and siRNAs.

FDA approved copolymer PLGA made of poly (lactic acid) (PLA) and poly (glycolic acid) (PGA) which is highly biodegradable in nature and shows biocompatibility is also one of the most common polymers for the delivery of genes. Since this polymer has low retention in blood and rapidly cleared, modification is essential to overcome this problem. PEGylated PLGA has reduced this problem and due to hydrophilic nature PEG prevents the opsonization of PLGA from immune cells.

Specifically, NPs targeting G-protein-linked C–X–C chemokine receptor 4 (CXCR4) were designed to potentiate anti-angiogenesis by delivering siRNA against vascular endothelial growth factor (VEGF) to the fibrotic liver [44, 45]. CXCR4-targeted nanoparticles loaded with VEGF siRNA reduce VEGF expression and ameliorate CCl4-induced liver fibrosis in mice. Similarly, tissue growth factor (CTGF) siRNA was delivered to HSCs using polyethyleneimine functionalized magnetic iron oxide nanoparticles. It causes decreased CTGF expression and collagen production Tenascin-C, another ECM component synthesized by HSCs during liver fibrosis, was effectively activated in HSCs using mesoporous silica NPs, resulting in decreased Tenascin-C mRNA and protein levels [46–49].

11.13.4 Mesenchymal stem cells coated nanoparticles in hepatic fibrosis

Nanoparticles (NPs) have been used to enable targeted delivery of mesenchymal stem cells (MSCs) to the injured liver. After MSCs are injected into the bloodstream, they will be filtered through the lungs before reaching the heart. In addition, resident liver macrophages known as Kupffer cells (KCs) can act on MSCs, further influencing their distribution to specific areas in the damaged liver. But the researchers developed a solution that uses MSC-conditioned medium-loaded poly lactic-glycolic acid (PLGA) nanoparticles, called MSC/RBC-inspired nanoparticles, These nanoparticles are less absorbed by macrophages when given intravenously [50, 51].

Therefore, they reduce proinflammatory cytokines, promote apoptosis, improve liver regeneration and increase survival in mice with CCl4-induced liver failure. The long-term therapeutic effect of MSCs/RBSs-NPs is due to red blood cell mechanisms. MSCs secrete an anti-fibrotic cytokine calcium loaded with MSC-phosphate. These nanoparticles were shown to be liver-specific in a mouse model of CCl4-induced liver fibrosis, reduced fibrosis and inflammatory markers. Thus, the use of NPs in the treatment of MSC plays an important role in increasing the lifespan of MSCs, inhibiting the activity of Kupffer cells, enabling the *in vivo* recording of MSCs and directing them to a specific location in the injured heart [29, 52, 53] (table 11.1).

11.14 HSC targeted nanoparticle delivery

The concept of targeted nanoparticle delivery to hematopoietic stem cells (HSCs) is a promising area of research in the field of gene therapy and regenerative medicine. This approach aims to improve the efficiency and specificity of gene delivery, addressing some of the challenges associated with traditional gene therapy methods [58].

One of the key strategies in targeted nanoparticle delivery involves the use of polymer nanoparticles to mediate the delivery of gene editing reagents into HSCs [59]. This method has been demonstrated to be efficient, allowing for the precise targeting and modification of HSCs *in vivo*. The use of nanoparticles for gene delivery of gene editing reagents into human hematopoietic stem and progenitor cells demonstrated the potential of this technology for the treatment of hematological diseases [59, 60].

Another approach to targeted nanoparticle delivery to HSCs involves the use of targeted lipid nanoparticles. These nanoparticles are designed to bind specifically to HSCs, enabling the delivery of RNA or other therapeutic agents directly to these cells [58]. This targeted delivery method has been studied by researchers at the Massachusetts Institute of Technology, who developed a targeted lipid nanoparticle system for the *in vivo* delivery of RNA to HSCs. This system leverages the specificity of lipid nanoparticles to bind to HSCs, ensuring that the RNA is delivered only to the target cells. This research highlights the potential of lipid nanoparticles as a powerful tool for targeted gene therapy of hematological diseases [60].

Table 11.1. Treatment for liver fibrosis (cell type, cellular target, targeting ligand, carrier, name of drug, references.)

Sl. No.	Cell type	Cellular target	Targeting ligand	Carrier	Drug	References
1.	Hepatocytes	Asialoglycoprotein (ASGP) receptor	Galactose, galactosylated lipid (lactobionic acid)	Liposomes Solid lipid nanoparticles	Quercetin, Cucurbitacin B, TLR4 siRNA	[64–66]
2.	Kupffer cells (macrophages)	Mannose receptor Scavenger Receptor	Mannose	Liposomes, nanoparticles Liposomes	Dexamethasone, TNFα-siRNA Dexamethasone	[67, 68] [69]
3.	Hepatic Stellate Cells	Mannose-6-Phosphate receptor	Mannose-6-phosphate	HSA, Liposomes	Doxorubicin, pentoxifylline, rosiglitazone, 15dPGJ2, Gliotoxin, Losartan, Y27632, rho-kinase inhibitor, ALK5 inhibitor LY-3694	[70–75]
		Retinol Binding Protein (RBP)	Vitamin A	Liposomes, RcP nanoparticles	HSP47 siRNA, antisense oligonucleotides (ASO)	[76, 82]
		Platelet-derived growth factor receptor	Cyclic peptide and bicyclic peptide	HSA, peptide, liposomes	Interferon gamma (IFNγ) and mimetic IFNγ	[77, 78, 81]
		Integrins	RGD peptide	Liposomes, polymerosomes	Inteferon alpha 1 beta (IFN-α −1b), hepatocyte growth factor, oxymatrine	[79, 80]
4.	Liver Sinusoidal Endothelial Cells (LSECs)	Endoglin (CD105) receptor	Endoglin (CD105)	Lentiviral particles	Erythropoietin gene	[83]
		Hyaluronic acid (HA) receptor	Hyaluronic acid	Micelles	—	[84]

Targeted nanoparticle delivery to HSCs represents a promising avenue for the treatment of hematological diseases [59]. Through the use of polymer and lipid nanoparticles, researchers have developed methods to efficiently deliver gene editing reagents and RNA directly to HSCs, bypassing many of the limitations associated with traditional gene therapy approaches. These advancements hold great promise for the future of regenerative medicine and gene therapy [58, 60].

11.15 Advantage of nanomedicine for LF

Nanomedicine offers various advantages for the treatment of liver fibrosis. These advantages stem from the unique properties of nanoparticles as therapeutic agents and drug carriers, which can be tailored to target specific cells or pathways involved in fibrosis.

11.15.1 Specific targeting and minimized side effects

Nanoparticles can be designed to target specific cells or pathways involved in liver fibrosis. The use of nanoparticles with targeting ligands, such as those conjugated with vitamin A, has shown promising results in treating liver fibrosis. These nanoparticles can be designed to target HSCs, which are crucial for the progression of liver fibrosis, Studies have demonstrated that vitamin A-coupled liposomes can deliver drugs to the liver with a significantly higher accumulation compared to non-targeted treatments, leading to reduced expression of profibrotic mediators and improved therapeutic outcomes. For example: lipid-based nanoparticles have been used to deliver RNA oligonucleotides that can upregulate CEBPA, a transcription factor that helps reduce fibrosis and reverse liver dysfunction. This targeted delivery minimizes the systemic effects of the treatment, reducing side effects and ensuring that the therapeutic effect is localized to the liver [63].

11.15.2 Enhanced drug delivery

Nanoparticles can serve as drug carriers, improving the delivery and bioavailability of antibiotic drugs. For example: cationic lipid nanoparticles loaded with small interfering RNA targeting the procollagen $\alpha 1(I)$ gene have been shown to accumulate in the liver and specifically block procollagen expression, thereby inhibiting liver fibrosis progression. This method enhances the therapeutic effect of the drug by ensuring that it is delivered directly to the site of fibrosis [62, 63].

11.15.3 Modulation of inflammatory and oxidative stress pathways

Nanoparticles can modulate the activity of inflammatory and oxidative stress pathways, which are key factors in the development of liver fibrosis [63]. Studies have shown that gold nanoparticles can reduce liver fibrosis by inhibiting the activity of Kupffer cells and HSCs, thereby reducing pro-inflammatory cytokine secretion and oxidative stress. Similarly, vitamin E-modified selenium NPs have been shown to attenuate liver fibrosis by reducing oxidative stress [61].

11.15.4 Reduced adverse effects

Targeting drug delivery systems can reduce the adverse associated with traditional anti-fibrotic drugs. By focusing the drug delivery on specific cells or pathways involved in fibrosis, the overall toxicity and side effects can be minimized, making nanomedicine a more effective and safer treatment option for liver fibrosis [61].

11.15.5 Improved pharmacokinetic properties

Nanoparticles system helps to improve the pharmacokinetic properties like absorption, distribution, metabolism and excretion. For example the molecules which are highly degradable in nature like: siRNA can be safely delivered by using nanoparticle systems and the other parameters like distribution in specific tissue, renal clearance can also be improved [61, 63].

Nanomedicine offers a promising approach for the treatment of liver fibrosis with the ability to target specific cells or pathways, and reduce adverse effects. These advantages make nanomedicine a valuable tool in the fight against liver fibrosis, potentially offering more effective and safer treatments than traditional methods.

11.16 Challenges of nm for LF

Targeting the liver with nanoparticles (NPs) poses a significant challenge due to the liver's unique anatomical location and the presence of Kupffer cells (macrophages) and other immune cells that possess efficient immune clearance abilities. Depleting macrophages in the liver has been shown to increase the internalization of NPs into hepatocytes. The surface charge of NPs plays a crucial role in their internalization, as only positively charged NPs can enter hepatocytes. The formation of a protein corona on NPs, depending on the type of NPs, can modify their biological properties. However, this can be mitigated by coating the NPs with polyethylene glycol (PEG), which imparts hydrophilicity to the NPs' surface and prevents opsonization. There are several challenges that need to be addressed before clinical translation, despite promising advancements in nanotechnology-based experimental therapeutics for chronic liver diseases (CLD) [54].

Before using inorganic nanoparticles (NPs) as a drug delivery system (DDS), it is important to consider the potential toxicity associated with these nanomaterials. In experimental animal models, silica nanoparticles were used as a model to induce liver fibrosis, emphasizing the importance of assessing the toxicity risk of inorganic nanoparticles, On the other hand, organic nanoparticles made from natural or biocompatible polymers such as PEG are considered less toxic. In the case of liver fibrosis, most nanoparticles are given intravenously due to poor absorption from the intestinal tract. However, it should be noted that intravenously administered nanoparticles will be removed by macrophages (such as Kupffer cells) in the liver, Nanoparticles can interact with other liver cells, including hepatocytes, via sinusoidal fenestrations. Therefore, according to Almedia *et al* larger nanoparticles are more likely to be absorbed by the liver than smaller nanoparticles [52].

11.17 Future of nm in the treatment of LF

In the past, evaluation of anti-fibrotic drugs did not generally focus on the cell types that cause liver fibrosis. However, the focus has shifted as most current studies focus on the activation and regulation of hepatic stellate cells (HSCs) in the fibrotic liver. Notably, liver fibrosis has multiple cell types, including resident hepatocytes, HSCs, Kupffer cells, liver sinusoidal endothelial cells, and portal fibroblasts. For cells involved in other cell types involved in liver fibrosis, more research is true, although there are some studies using nanomaterials modified with HSC-specific markers such as retinol to target active HSCs or myofibroblasts (MFBs). Promising results have been demonstrated for different targets in different cell types [50].

In addition, Giannitrapani *et al* propose the development of nano-vigilance or regulatory responsibility as a scientific research goal to enable monitoring of the field. In the past, evaluation of anti-fibrotic drugs did not generally focus on the cell types that cause liver fibrosis However. The focus has shifted as most current studies focus on the activation and regulation of hepatic stellate cells (HSCs) in the fibrotic liver [53]. More research is needed on cells involved in other cell types involved in liver fibrosis, although there are some studies using nanomaterials modified with HSC-specific markers such as retinol to target active HSCs or myofibroblasts (MFBs). Promising results have been demonstrated for targeted drug delivery using such devices, indicating the need for future studies with different targets in different cell types. In addition, Giannitrapani *et al* recommended the establishment of a nano-vigilance or management role as a research objective to enable monitoring of the region [51].

References

[1] Bataller R and Brenner D A 2005 Liver fibrosis *J. Clin. Invest.* **115** 209–18
[2] Tan Z, Xue T, Gan C, Liu H, Xie Y, Yao Y and Ye T 2021 Liver fibrosis: therapeutic targets and advances in drug therapy *Front. Cell Dev. Biol* 18
[3] Nall R and Cherney K 2023 *Healthline* www.healthline.com/health.liver-fibrosis#outlook.
[4] Pavlov C S, Casazza G, Nikolova D, Tsochatzis E, Burroughs A K, Ivashkin V T and Gluud C 2017 Transient elastography for diagnosis of stages of hepatic fibrosis and cirrhosis in people with alcoholic liver disease *Ultrasound Med. Biol.* **43** S150
[5] Zhang C Y, Yuan W G, He P, Lei J H and Wang C X 2016 Liver fibrosis and hepatic stellate cells: etiology, pathological hallmarks and therapeutic targets *World J. Gastroenterol* **22** 10512
[6] Lewis S 2022 *Healthgrades* https://healthgrades.com/right-care/liver-conditions/liver-fibrosis.
[7] Brenner D A 2009 Molecular pathogenesis of liver fibrosis *Trans. Am. Clin. Climatol. Assoc* **120** 361
[8] Pinzani M and Macias-Barragan J 2010 Update on the pathophysiology of liver fibrosis *Expert Rev. Gastroenterol. Hepatol* **4** 459–72
[9] de Alwis N M W and Day C P 2008 Non-alcoholic fatty liver disease: the mist gradually clears *J. Hepatol* **48** S104–12

[10] Zhu Y K, Wang B E, Shen F J, Wang A M, Jia J D and Ma H 2004 Dynamic evolution of MMP-13, TIMP-1, type I and III collagen and their interaction in experimental liver fibrosis *Zhonghua Gan Zang Bing Za Zhi* **12** 612–5

[11] Tacke F and Weiskirchen R 2021 Non-alcoholic fatty liver disease (NAFLD)/non-alcoholic steatohepatitis (NASH)-related liver fibrosis: mechanisms, treatment and prevention *Ann. Transl. Med* **9**

[12] Aydın M M and Akçalı K C 2018 Liver fibrosis *Turk. J. Gastroenterol* **29** 14

[13] Cheng J Y K and Wong G L H 2017 Advances in the diagnosis and treatment of liver fibrosis *Hepatoma Res.* **3** 156–69

[14] Rossi E, Adams L A, Bulsara M and Jeffrey G P 2007 Assessing liver fibrosis with serum marker models *Clin. Biochem. Rev.* **28** 3–10

[15] Rosenberg W M, Voelker M, Thiel R, Becka M, Burt A, Schuppan D, Hubscher S, Roskams T, Pinzani M and Arthur M JEuropean Liver Fibrosis Group 2004 Serum markers detect the presence of liver fibrosis: a cohort study *Gastroenterology* **127** 1704–13

[16] Regev A, Berho M, Jeffers L J, Milikowski C, Molina E G, Pyrsopoulos N T, Feng Z Z, Reddy K R and Schiff E R 2002 Sampling error and intraobserver variation in liver biopsy in patients with chronic HCV infection *Am. J. Gastroenterol* **97** 2614–8

[17] Sudhakar K, Venkatesh MD M Y P and Richard L 2013 Ehman MD, Magnetic resonance elastography of liver: technique, analysis, and clinical application *J. Magn. Reson. Imaging* **37** 544–55

[18] Yin M, Talwalkar J A, Glaser K J, Manduca A, Grimm R C, Rossman P J, Fidler J L and Ehman R L 2007 Oct Assessment of hepatic fibrosis with magnetic resonance elastography *Clin. Gastroenterol. Hepatol* **5** 1207–1213.e2

[19] Ezhilarasan D *et al* 2016 Silibinin inhibits proliferation and migration of human hepatic stellate LX-2 cells **6** 167–74

[20] Ezhilarasan D *et al* 2014 Plant derived antioxidants and antifibrotic drugs: past, present and future **2** 738–45

[21] Singh R P *et al* 2015 Population pharmacokinetics modeling and analysis of foretinib in adult patients with advanced solid tumors **55** 1184–92

[22] Friedman S L J D D 2015 Hepatic fibrosis: emerging therapies **33** 504–7

[23] Friedman S L J T 2008 Hepatic fibrosis—overview **254** 120–9

[24] Cengiz M *et al* 2015 A comparative study on the therapeutic effects of silymarin and silymarin-loaded solid lipid nanoparticles on D-GaIN/TNF-α-induced liver damage in Balb/c mice **77** 93–100

[25] Kabir N *et al* 2014 Silymarin coated gold nanoparticles ameliorates CCl_4-induced hepatic injury and cirrhosis through down regulation of hepatic stellate cells and attenuation of Kupffer cells

[26] Zhang Q *et al* 2019 Theranostic quercetin nanoparticle for treatment of hepatic fibrosis **30** 2939–46

[27] Lam P-L *et al* 2015 Evaluation of berberine/bovine serum albumin nanoparticles for liver fibrosis therapy **17** 1640–6

[28] Schiborr C *et al* 2014 The oral bioavailability of curcumin from micronized powder and liquid micelles is significantly increased in healthy humans and differs between sexes **58** 516–27

[29] Ezhilarasan D J E J O P 2021 Advantages and challenges in nanomedicines for chronic liver diseases: a hepatologist's perspectives **893** 173832

[30] Jamwal R J J o I M 2019 Corrigendum: bioavailable curcumin formulations: a review of pharmacokinetic studies in healthy volunteers **17** 310 310

[31] Sung Y-C *et al* 2018 Combined delivery of sorafenib and a MEK inhibitor using CXCR4-targeted nanoparticles reduces hepatic fibrosis and prevents tumor development **8** 894

[32] Lin T-T *et al* 2016 Development and characterization of sorafenib-loaded PLGA nanoparticles for the systemic treatment of liver fibrosis **221** 62–70

[33] Chang C-C *et al* 2018 Docetaxel-carboxymethylcellulose nanoparticles ameliorate CCl4-induced hepatic fibrosis in mice **26** 516–24

[34] Wang C *et al* 2013 Low-dose paclitaxel ameliorates pulmonary fibrosis by suppressing TGF-β1/Smad3 pathway via miR-140 upregulation **8** e70725

[35] Zhou J *et al* 2010 Paclitaxel ameliorates fibrosis in hepatic stellate cells via inhibition of TGF-β/Smad activity **16** 3330

[36] Cella D *et al* 2003 Measuring the side effects of taxane therapy in oncology: the functional assessment of cancer therapy–taxane (FACT-taxane) **98** 822–31

[37] Chen Y-N *et al* 2017 Ameliorative effect of curcumin-encapsulated hyaluronic acid–PLA nanoparticles on thioacetamide-induced murine hepatic fibrosis **14** 11

[38] Kikuchi S *et al* 2005 Role of CD44 in epithelial wound repair: migration of rat hepatic stellate cells utilizes hyaluronic acid and CD44v6 **280** 15398–404

[39] Sudha P N, Rose and M H J A i f 2014 Beneficial effects of hyaluronic acid **72** 137–76

[40] Thomas R G *et al* 2015 Effectiveness of losartan-loaded hyaluronic acid (HA) micelles for the reduction of advanced hepatic fibrosis in C3H/HeN mice model **10** e0145512

[41] Schuppan D *et al* 2018 Liver fibrosis: direct antifibrotic agents and targeted therapies **68** 435–51

[42] Zhao Y *et al* 2017 Heat shock protein 47 effects on hepatic stellate cell-associated receptors in hepatic fibrosis of *Schistosoma japonicum*-infected mice **398** 1357–66

[43] Mussi S V and VPJJoMCB 2013 Torchilin, recent trends in the use of lipidic nanoparticles as pharmaceutical carriers for cancer therapy and diagnostics **1** 5201–9

[44] Kong W H *et al* 2013 Cationic solid lipid nanoparticles derived from apolipoprotein-free LDLs for target specific systemic treatment of liver fibrosis **34** 542–51

[45] Jia Z *et al* 2018 pPB peptide-mediated siRNA-loaded stable nucleic acid lipid nanoparticles on targeting therapy of hepatic fibrosis **15** 53–62

[46] Bisht S *et al* 2011 A polymeric nanoparticle formulation of curcumin (NanoCurc™) ameliorates CCl4-induced hepatic injury and fibrosis through reduction of pro-inflammatory cytokines and stellate cell activation **91** 1383–95

[47] Jiménez Calvente C *et al* 2015 Specific hepatic delivery of procollagen α1 (I) small interfering RNA in lipid-like nanoparticles resolves liver fibrosis **62** 1285–97

[48] Kaps L *et al* 2015 Nanomedicine: *in vivo* gene-silencing in fibrotic liver by siRNA-loaded cationic nanohydrogel particles (*Adv. Healthcare Mater.* 18/2015) **4** 2737

[49] Liu C H *et al* 2016 Dual-functional nanoparticles targeting CXCR4 and delivering antiangiogenic siRNA ameliorate liver fibrosis **13** 2253–62

[50] Bai X, Su G and Zhai S J 2020 Recent advances in nanomedicine for the diagnosis and therapy of liver fibrosis **10** 1945

[51] Peng W *et al* 2021 Advances in the research of nanodrug delivery systems for targeted treatment of liver fibrosis. **137** 111342

[52] Almeida J P M *et al* 2011 *In vivo* biodistribution of nanoparticles **6** 815–35

[53] Giannitrapani L *et al* 2014 Nanotechnology applications for the therapy of liver fibrosis **20** 7242

[54] Yu Y *et al* 2017 Silica nanoparticles induce liver fibrosis via TGF-β1/Smad3 pathway in ICR mice 6045–57

[55] Lédinghen de V *et al* 2008 Transient elastogrphy (Fibroscan) **32** 18973847

[56] Castera L *et al* 2008 Non-invasive evaluation of liver fibrosis using transient elastography **48** 18334275

[57] Rockey C 2008 Noninvasive assessment of liver fibrosis and portal hypertension with transient elastography **134** 18166342

[58] Shi D *et al* 2023 *In vivo* RNA delivery to hematopoietic stem and progenitor cells via targeted lipid nanoparticles **23** 2938–44

[59] Han X *et al* 2023 Ligand-tethered lipid nanoparticles for targeted RNA delivery to treat liver fibrosis **14** 36650129

[60] Breda L *et al* 2023 *In vivo* hematopoietic stem cell modification by mRNA delivery **381** 436–43

[61] Ezhilarasan D 2021 Advantages and challenges in nanomedicines for chronic liver diseases: a hepatologist's perspectives **893** 173–832

[62] Gu L *et al* 2022 Nanotechnology in drug delivery for liver fibrosis **8** 804–396

[63] Bai X *et al* 2020 Recent advances in nanomedicine for the diagnosis and therapy of liver fibrosis **10** 33003520

[64] Autio A *et al* 2013 Preclinical evaluation of a radioiodinated fully human antibody for *in vivo* imaging of vascular adhesion protein-1-positive vasculature in inflammation **54** 1315–9

[65] Ali A H *et al* 2015 Current research on the treatment of primary sclerosing cholangitis **4** 25674381

[66] Wang W *et al* 2010 Galactosylated solid lipid nanoparticles with cucurbitacin B improves the liver targetability **17** 114–22

[67] He C *et al* 2013 Multifunctional polymeric nanoparticles for oral delivery of TNF-α siRNA to macrophages **34** 2843–54

[68] Melgert B N *et al* 2001 Targeting dexamethasone to Kupffer cell: effects on liver inflammation and fibrosis in rats **1** 719–28

[69] Bartneck M *et al* 2015 Fluorescent cell-traceable dexamethasone-loaded liposomes for the treatment of inflammatory liver diseases **37** 367–82

[70] Greupink R *et al* 2006 The antiproliferative drug doxorubicin inhibits liver fibrosis in bile duct-ligated rats and can be selectively delivered to hepatic stellate cells *in vivo* **317** 514–21

[71] Gonzalo T *et al* 2006 Selective targeting of pentoxifylline to hepatic stellate cells using a novel platinum-based linker technology **111** 193–203

[72] Hagens W I *et al* 2007 Targeting 15d-prostaglandin J2 to hepatic stellate cells: two options evaluated **24** 566–74

[73] Beige M M *et al* 2011 Increased liver uptake and reduced hepatic stellate cell activation with a cell-specific conjugate of the Rho-kinase inhibitor Y27632 **28** 2045–54

[74] Klein S *et al* 2012 HSC-specific inhibition of Rho-kinase reduces portal pressure in cirrhotic rats without major systemic effects **57** 1220–7

[75] Zhang Z *et al* 2015 Corona-directed nucleic acid delivery into hepatic stellate cells for liver fibrosis therapy **9** 2405–19

[76] Bansal R *et al* 2011 Peptide-modified albumin carrier explored as a novel strategy for a cell-specific delivery of interferon gamma to treat liver fibrosis **8** 1899–909

[77] Li F *et al* 2012 Effects of interferon-gamma liposomes targeted to platelet-derived growth factor receptor-beta on hepatic fibrosis in rats **159** 261–70

[78] Yang J *et al* 2014 Targeted delivery of the RGD-labeled biodegradable polymersomes loaded with the hydrophilic drug oxymatrine on cultured hepatic stellate cells and liver fibrosis in rats **52** 180–90

[79] Li F *et al* 2008 Effect of hepatocyte growth factor encapsulated in targeted liposomes on liver cirrhosis **131** 77–82

[80] Kim W H *et al* 2005 Growth inhibition and apoptosis in liver myofibroblasts promoted by hepatocyte growth factor leads to resolution from liver cirrhosis **166** 1017–2005

[81] Bansal R 2011 Novel engineered targeted interferon-gamma blocks hepatic fibrogenesis in mice **54** 586–96

[82] Sato Y *et al* 2008 Resolution of liver cirrhosis using vitamin A—coupled liposomes to deliver siRNA against a collagen-specific chaperone **26** 431–42

[83] Abel T *et al* 2013 Specific gene delivery to liver sinusoidal and artery endothelial cells **122** 2030–8

[84] Ohya Y *et al* 2011 Evaluation of polyanion-coated biodegradable polymeric micelles as drug delivery vehicles **155** 104–10

IOP Publishing

Nanobiotechnology and Artificial Intelligence in
Gastrointestinal Diseases

Vivek K Chaturvedi, Anurag Kumar Singh, Jay Singh and Dawesh P Yadav

Chapter 12

Artificial intelligence (AI) based colonoscopy

Akbar Hamid, Rajesh Kumar, Vivek K Chaturvedi, Sunil Dutt, Gira Sulabh,
Vinod Kumar and D P Yadav

With the increase in the world's population and development, a number of health-related issues are also increasing in gastroenterology. One of the major causes is poor food habits. To deal with this, constant advancement is required in the field of the medical sector, which will not only help in easy and earlier diagnosis of the underlying health issue but also in accurate diagnosis. In this chapter advancement and collaboration of artificial intelligence with the medical sector are discussed below. How one technique helps is the accurate detection of colorectal cancer (CRC) as well as other diseases such as IBD or any other abnormalities in the colon. A different version of colonoscopy has been developed along with artificial intelligence, discussed in this chapter with future prospects and advancement.

12.1 Introduction

Colonoscopy is a very important modern medicine procedure that is crucial for diagnosis, treatment and prevention of various gastrointestinal diseases, especially CRC screening. It helps in identifying CRC, inflammatory bowel disease (IBD) like Crohn's disease or ulcerative colitis, diverticular disease, and other conditions through detection of gastrointestinal diseases [1]. At its core, a colonoscopy entails the careful insertion of a flexible and slender tube known as a colonoscope into the rectum, which is then advanced through the colon. With its own source of light and camera, the colonoscope allows medical practitioners to get a good view of the lining inside the intestines (colon), thus making it easy to identify any abnormalities on it that may qualify as possible growths such as polyps, tumors or inflammation among other things [2].

The process of preparing for a colonoscopy is critical because it has a profound impact on the efficacy and precision of the procedure. In order to have an optimal

doi:10.1088/978-0-7503-6134-7ch12

view of the colon while inspecting it, patients are generally recommended to follow some dietary restrictions and go through bowel cleansing. While others may find this preparation regimen tiresome, its significance cannot be undermined as it helps eliminate any fecal matter or debris that might obstruct the view by the colonoscope and potentially hide lesions or anomalies [3].

During the actual procedure itself, sedation is frequently given to patients so that they feel no pain and can relax. The physician gently guides the colonoscope along all parts of the organ after positioning the patient comfortably. The colonoscope offers real-time visualization allowing healthcare providers to immediately evaluate the condition of their colons and identify any abnormalities which require further investigation or intervention [4]. If there are any abnormalities such as polyps during the examination, they can be removed or biopsied for further examination. This part of colonoscopy is very important in early identification and prevention of CRC since removing precancerous polyps decreases the risk of further developing CRC. Polyps refer to small growths that can develop on the inner lining of the colon and are believed to be an antecedent of cancer. By detecting and eliminating these polyps at the time of colonoscopy, medical professionals can actually prevent progression of CRC, thereby improving outcomes for patients. In addition, colonoscopy has a vital role in surveillance and management of people at high risk or with previous gastrointestinal diseases [5]. These individuals should have regular colonoscopies done so as to check on new growths that may occur within their colons over time, allowing for early detection and appropriate interference when required.

One of the key advantages of colonoscopy is its ability to provide real-time visualization of the colon, allowing for immediate assessment and intervention if necessary. This can be particularly beneficial in cases where other diagnostic modalities may not provide sufficient information or where a rapid response is required. Furthermore, colonoscopy is considered a safe and well-tolerated procedure for the majority of patients, with minimal risks of complications when performed by experienced healthcare professionals in a controlled clinical setting. There are some risks associated with it, including bleeding, perforation of the colon, and adverse reactions to sedation. However, these risks are relatively rare and are typically outweighed by the benefits of early detection and intervention in preventing CRC and other gastrointestinal disorders [6].

It is essential to recognize that colonoscopy may not be suitable for everyone and alternative screening methods such as fecal occult blood testing (FOBT) or sigmoidoscopy may be recommended based on individual circumstances and preferences. However, for the vast majority of individuals, colonoscopy remains the gold standard for CRC screening and surveillance due to its exceptional sensitivity and specificity in detecting abnormalities within the colon [7].

Colonoscopy is considered to be a vital tool in the field of gastroenterology, offering unparalleled insights into the health and function of the colon and rectum. From its role in early cancer detection to its capacity for monitoring and managing gastrointestinal conditions, colonoscopy plays a pivotal role in improving patient outcomes and reducing the global burden of colorectal disease. As technology continues to advance and techniques evolve, the future of colonoscopy holds promise for further enhancing its diagnostic capabilities and expanding its utility in the prevention and treatment of gastrointestinal disorders.

12.2 Medical requirement for colonoscopy

Colonoscopy is considered a significant instrument of preventive healthcare whereby the entire large intestines are explored thoroughly for any abnormalities ranging from polyps to tumors or inflammation. Patients therefore must comply with certain medical requirements before it can be done, hence ensuring its effectiveness and safety. One of such preparations involves restrictive dietary measures [8]. Generally, patients are advised to take low-fiber foods in the days leading to their colonoscopies. This is because these foods help to evacuate an individual's bowel system making it easier for a physician to see inside the gut during the process. For instance, there is limitation or complete avoidance of foods rich in fiber contents, such as fruit, vegetables, whole grains and nuts, so as not to allow residues capable of obstructing the view during colonoscopy. Instead of this, people may drink transparent fluids including water, broth and juice without pulp as well as gelatin and ice lollies [9]. Henceforth red or purple-colored liquids should be avoided alongside alcoholic drinks or beverages containing caffeine since they can either interfere with results from the colonoscopy or lead to complications after that procedure has been completed. Apart from that, modification of dieting thus prescribed involves having bowels prepared, which entails emptying them entirely of excrement and other waste materials contained therein. This is often achieved through the use of laxatives or oral solutions that induce diarrhea. Adequate bowel preparation is crucial for the success of the colonoscopy as residual stool can obscure the physician's view and compromise the accuracy of the examination. Patients must carefully follow the instructions provided by their healthcare provider regarding the timing and dosage of bowel preparation medications to ensure thorough cleansing of the colon [10].

Moreover, there may be a need to adjust some medications or temporarily stop them for a short time before colonoscopy can be done. Procedures such as non-steroidal anti-inflammatory drugs (NSAIDs), blood thinners, and iron supplements are among the medications that can hinder this process or promote bleeding during colonoscopy. Patients should usually be told to provide information regarding all kinds of medication used such as prescription medication, over the counter medicine and even nutritional supplement so that necessary changes can be effected in case any is required. Sometimes alternative drugs may be given, or doses may be changed to minimize risks associated with this type of colonoscopy [11].

Furthermore, patients who are undergoing a colonoscopy might have to undergo certain medical evaluations to assess their general health and fitness for the procedure. This might involve blood tests which checks clotting factors and looks out for conditions like anaemia which could put at risk the safety or outcome of the colonoscopy. Before having any procedure done on them, individuals suffering from some medical problems like heart disease, diabetes or kidney problem must take extra care with regard to how they are treated by their physician [12]. Close coordination between the patient's primary care physician and the gastroenterologist performing the colonoscopy is essential to ensure a comprehensive pre-procedural evaluation and optimization of medical management.

Moreover, the patient is also adequately informed about the risks and benefits associated with colonoscopy, as well as any alternative screening options available to them. While colonoscopy is considered the gold standard for detecting CRC and precancerous lesions, it carries certain risks, including perforation of the colon, bleeding, and adverse reactions to sedation medications. Patients should have the opportunity to discuss these risks with their healthcare provider and address any concerns or questions they may have before undergoing the procedure. In some cases, individuals may opt for alternative screening modalities such as fecal occult blood testing (FOBT), fecal immunochemical testing (FIT), or sigmoidoscopy, which may be more suitable based on their medical history, preferences, or risk factors [13].

Therfore, adherence to specific medical requirements is crucial to ensuring the safety and efficacy of colonoscopy as a screening and diagnostic tool for CRC and other gastrointestinal conditions. From dietary modifications and bowel preparation to medication adjustments and medical evaluations, comprehensive pre-procedural planning is essential to optimize patient outcomes and minimize risks associated with the procedure. Effective communication between patients and healthcare providers is paramount to ensure that individuals are well-informed and actively engaged in the decision-making process regarding their CRC screening options.

12.3 Limitation of colonoscopy

In the field of gastrointestinal health, colonoscopy is regarded as a key procedure which is useful in diagnosing and preventing CRC among other bowel diseases. However, there are some limitations that need to be taken into consideration when dealing with this kind of medical examination. Its major limitation is its inability to cover entire areas of the colon. Although there has been introduction of advanced solutions intending to improve colonoscopy experiences, including high-definition cameras and flexible scopes, portions within the colon still pose visualization problems at times [14]. This may be as a result of various factors including intricate nature like complex curvature and tortuosity which might prevent the endoscopist's effective navigation through the scope, thereby leading to missed lesions or incomplete examinations. In addition, poor bowel cleansing poses one more significant challenge in successful completion of colonoscopy. Incompletely cleansed bowels with residual stool matter or fecal debri may reduce visibility for the endoscopist and compromise detection of abnormalities, hence reducing accuracy during such procedures. Suboptimal bowel cleaning has remained a common problem in practice despite attempts towards optimizing protocols on patient literacy and the use of split-dose regimens [15].

The colonoscopy, besides being extremely effective in the detection of large polyps and early-stage CRC, may not be so sensitive in smaller lesions or flat or serrated polyps, especially within the proximal colon. In fact these types of polyps are very difficult to detect during a colonoscopy, hence false-negative results may be obtained and thus delay the diagnosis of colorectal neoplasia. To overcome this shortcoming, chromoendoscopy, narrow-band imaging as well as virtual chromoendoscopy have been invented to improve lesion detection rate and diagnostic yield of colonoscopy, particularly among high risk groups [16].

Furthermore, colonoscopy carries an inherent procedural risk even though it is relatively low when compared to other invasive procedures. Colon perforation and post-polypectomy bleeding are rare but serious complications associated with the procedure. Complications related factors such as age advancement, concurrent sicknesses or specific diseases put patients at a higher chance of experiencing problems, hence a pre-procedural evaluation is necessary. Despite this, since the advantages of doing a colonoscopy for prevention against CRC generally outweigh its demerits, there must be awareness among patients about possible complications and surveillance strategies in advance before doing one [17].

In addition, there are practical challenges like the cost of performing a colonoscopy. Moreover, patient acceptance poses challenges, and accessibility to colonoscopy-based screening programs presents problems towards its widespread adoption among patients. Although colonoscopy is effective, it is both time consuming and expensive as it requires expensive equipment that needs skilled hands to operate it as well as for sedation services unlike non-invasive forms of CRC screening. Some geographical areas still do not have sufficient access to colonoscopy services, making poor people in these regions lag behind in terms of CRC screening and detection disparities [18]. Additionally, some individuals may experience anxiety disorder prior to or during the process of being screened through a colonoscope due to the fear of pain or humiliation from this type of examination, which tends toward violation particularly when addressing these issues in public places, making it necessary for patients to be educated on such matters, undergo counseling about them and make decisions based on how they feel.

Challenges such as incomplete examination, suboptimal bowel preparation, missed lesions, procedural complications, and practical barriers underscore the need for ongoing research and innovation in gastrointestinal endoscopy. Continued efforts to improve colonoscopy technology, enhance bowel preparation protocols, refine lesion detection techniques, and address accessibility and patient acceptance issues are essential to maximize the effectiveness and accessibility of CRC screening and surveillance programs.

12.4 Advancement of colonoscopy

The goal of continuous improvement in colonoscopic technology has been to enhance the efficiency, security, and comfort of patients undergoing colonoscopy operations. With the advent of high-definition and ultra-high-definition imaging equipment, abnormalities like polyps and lesions may now be more easily seen during colonoscopies. Endoscopists can see further with certain colonoscopes because they have panoramic views or wide-angle lenses [19]. This makes it easier to navigate the colon and improves lesion identification, especially in hard-to-reach places.

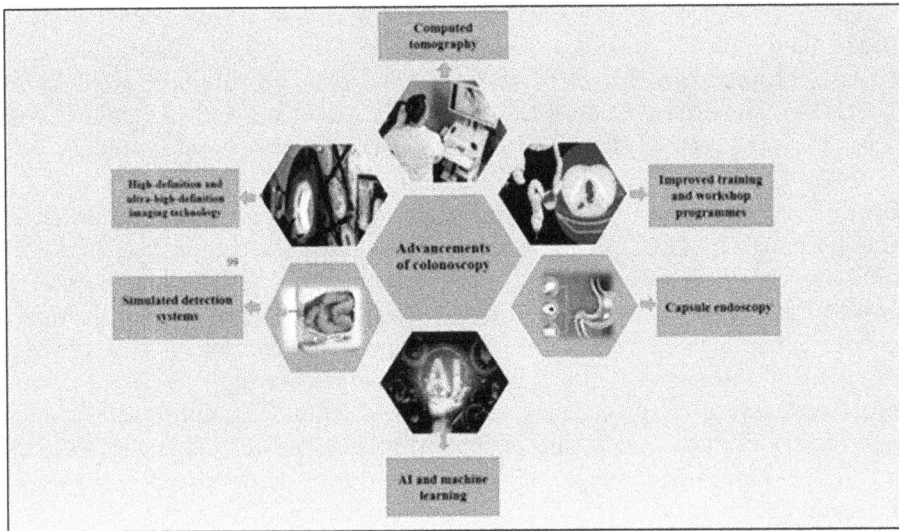

Figure 12.1. Advancement of colonoscopy. Reprinted from [19], Copyright (2000), with permission from Elsevier.

New technologies that offer real-time high-magnification and microscopic images of the mucosa include magnifying narrow-band imaging (M-NBI) and confocal laser endomicroscopy (CLE). By helping to characterise worrisome lesions *in vivo*, these approaches may help avoid the need for biopsy. These developments enhance the efficacy of colonoscopy in CRC screening and monitoring by facilitating the more precise identification and characterisation of colorectal lesions (figure 12.1) [20].

12.5 High-definition and ultra-high-definition imaging technology

With better visualisation and diagnostic capabilities, high-definition (HD) and ultra-high definition (UHD) imaging technologies have revolutionised the area of colonoscopy. A number of characteristics of colonoscopy operations, including as detection rates, diagnostic precision, patient comfort, and overall procedural efficiency, have been greatly influenced by these technologies [21]. When it comes to sharpness and clarity, HD and UHD imaging surpasses conventional standard-definition imaging. Better visualisation of the colon mucosa makes it possible for physicians to identify subtle lesions, polyps, and anomalies more successfully. HD and UHD colonoscopes are able to identify and describe lesions that standard-definition imaging may miss or fail to notice, such as flat lesions, tiny polyps, and early-stage malignancies. This is because they have superior picture quality [22].

Better patient outcomes and increased adenoma detection rates (ADRs) may result from this. With the use of HD and UHD imaging, lesions may be thoroughly characterised, giving physicians more accurate information about the shape, size, and surface features of polyps and other anomalies. This data is essential for choosing the right treatment tactics, including changing up the frequency of surveillance or removing problematic lesions right away. Advanced endoscopic methods that improve mucosal visualisation and lesion identification, such as electronic chromoendoscopy, NBI and chromoendoscopy, are supported by HD and UHD colonoscopes. These methods enhance contrast and highlight mucosal patterns by using certain filters and light wavelengths, which helps identify subtle lesions and dysplastic alterations [23].

Optical enhancement technologies, such Pentax i-scan, Fujinon Intelligent Chromo Endoscopy (FICE), and i-scan, are included in certain HD and UHD colonoscopes. These technologies offer further image enhancing choices for improved tissue characterisation and lesion diagnosis. These technologies improve diagnostic capabilities by providing a range of image enhancement modes suited to diverse clinical settings. HD and UHD colonoscopes are made with the patient's comfort and safety in mind, even with their increased resolution and imaging powers. In addition to minimising patient pain, slimmer and more flexible scopes lower the possibility of damage or perforation during insertion and colonoscopy manoeuvres [24].

By enabling students and working physicians to see and study detailed, high-quality endoscopic pictures, HD and UHD imaging technologies also contribute to the training and education of endoscopists. This promotes the growth of abilities, mastery of lesion identification, and ongoing quality enhancement in colonoscopy procedures. By enhancing visualisation, detection rates, and diagnostic accuracy, HD and UHD imaging technologies have transformed colonoscopy and, in the process, improved patient outcomes and the prevention of CRC through early diagnosis and intervention [25].

12.6 Computed tomography

Computed tomography colonography (CTC) is a minimally invasive imaging technology used for colon and rectal examination and CRC screening. It is often referred to as virtual colonoscopy or CT colonoscopy. For people who are unable or reluctant to have a standard colonoscopy, CTC is a non-invasive substitute for visual colonoscopy. Patients often take it well and don't require sedation. Using CT technology, CTC creates three-dimensional, high-resolution pictures of the whole colon and rectum. Radiologists can see the interior architecture of the colon using these pictures and can identify anomalies including polyps, tumours, and inflammatory diseases. The patient lays on a table that passes through a CT scanner during CTC [26].

Multiple x-ray pictures of the colon are captured by the scanner from various angles. After that, a computer processes these pictures to produce an intricate 3D model of the colon. With the use of specialised software, radiologists may move through the virtual colon, mimicking the sensation of navigating through the colon during an optical colonoscopy. This makes it possible to thoroughly assess the colon as a whole and identify any anomalies [27]. Characterising and identifying polyps—growths that may eventually turn into CRC—is a task that CTC excels at. Radiologists can determine whether a discovered polyp is precancerous by evaluating its size, shape, and other characteristics. Similar to optical colonoscopy, CTC necessitates bowel preparation in order to guarantee unobstructed colon visualisation [28].

Furthermore, individuals with specific medical illnesses or anatomical defects that might compromise picture quality or interpretation may not be appropriate candidates for CTC. In the event that CTC reveals abnormalities or polyps, patients would need a further visual colonoscopy for assessment and possible lesion removal.

12.7 Artificial intelligence and machine learning

To increase lesion identification, characterization, and overall quality improvement, artificial intelligence and machine learning are being included in colonoscopy practices more and more. Real-time analysis of colonoscopy images by artificial intelligence algorithms may identify and classify worrisome lesions, including tumours and polyps. Based on the form, texture, and colour features of aberrant structures, these systems recognise those using deep learning techniques and pattern recognition. Colonoscopy recordings may be analysed by artificial intelligence algorithms to evaluate a range of quality measures, including cecal intubation rate, mucosal visibility, and withdrawal time. Artificial intelligence can assist pinpoint opportunities for development and enhance colonoscopy practice by automatically assessing procedure quality [29].

Based on endoscopic appearance, machine learning models trained on histological data can forecast the histology of polyps. These models aid in the guidance of management decisions about surveillance intervals and the necessity of biopsy or excision by providing a high degree of accuracy in differentiating between adenomatous and hyperplastic polyps. Artificial intelligence systems can assist endoscopists in real time during a colonoscopy by making suggestions for biopsy or polyp excision depending on the features of the lesion and the patient's medical history. Artificial intelligence can enhance patient outcomes and diagnostic accuracy by supporting decision-making [30].

Large-scale analysis of colonoscopy data, including pictures, videos, and clinical results, is made possible by artificial intelligence algorithms. Researchers can find trends, patterns, and predictive characteristics associated with colorectal neoplasia by utilising big data analytics, which can lead to improvements in screening protocols and therapeutic modalities. Artificial intelligence-driven features like automatic lesion detection and characterisation software are available on some endoscopic systems. During colonoscopy operations, these integrated technologies boost workflow efficiency and endoscopists' skills [31].

12.8 Advancement in patient experience

In recent years, innovation has focused on improving the patient experience during colonoscopy treatments. Enhancing patient comfort, safety, and happiness is essential to guaranteeing colonoscopy programme success and promoting adherence to CRC screening recommendations [32]. In an effort to reduce anxiety and guarantee that patients understand the colonoscopy process, healthcare practitioners are placing a greater emphasis on patient education and preparation. Educational resources, such as leaflets and films, describe the process of bowel preparation, the significance of screening, and the actual procedure. Patients prepare more efficiently when given clear instructions and nutritional restrictions, which increases their comfort and confidence [33].

Bowel preparation regimen innovations strive to maximise colon hygiene while reducing patient burden. To enhance tolerance and compliance, split-dose regimens, low-volume preparations, and acceptable formulations are used. Pre-packaged kits that make preparation easier and come with options for flavouring further improve the patient experience. Technological developments in sedation and anaesthesia enable customised methods based on the medical requirements and preferences of each patient. Options include heavy sedation or general anaesthesia provided by an anesthesiologist, as well as conscious sedation using drugs like benzodiazepines and opioids. Patients with patient-controlled sedation devices feel more in control and have less anxiety since they may gradually increase the amount of sedative they take [34].

Modern colonoscopy technology aims to reduce pain and enhance manoeuvrability through the use of tools with variable stiffness, thin scope designs, and high-definition images. Methods like cap-assisted colonoscopy and water immersion colonoscopy improve mucosal visualisation even more and lessen the need for excessive insufflation, which improves patient comfort. Streamlining the colonoscopy technique and cutting down on time spent on it enhances the overall patient experience [35]. The inspection of the colon may now be completed more quickly and effectively because of advancements in endoscopic technology, including high-speed processors and effective irrigation and suction systems. Lesion identification algorithms and scope positioning systems are two examples of automated elements that can streamline procedure flow and reduce patient pain. Throughout the colonoscopy process, patient safety is guaranteed by constant monitoring of vital indicators, such as blood pressure and oxygen saturation [36]. Real-time identification of adverse occurrences is made possible by innovations like automatic warnings and remote monitoring systems, which enable healthcare practitioners to promptly intervene to reduce risks and guarantee patient well-being. Encouraging patients to recuperate with clear instructions and extensive post-procedure care improves their overall experience [37].

Patients are further involved in their treatment and are able to make well-informed decisions about recommended screening and monitoring in the future when they have follow-up meetings with the endoscopist to examine biopsy results, discuss findings, and address any concerns. Healthcare professionals may enhance patient satisfaction, increase compliance with CRC screening recommendations, and ultimately improve health outcomes for those who are at risk of colorectal illness by implementing these developments into colonoscopy procedures [38].

12.9 Capsule endoscopy

Using a tiny wireless capsule camera, capsule endoscopy is a minimally invasive imaging method that allows for the visualisation of the gastrointestinal system, including the small intestine. Nonetheless, colonoscopy is not usually performed using capsule endoscopy exclusively. Rather, its main application is in the evaluation of the small intestine, where conventional endoscopic methods like colonoscopy might not be as effective in visualising things. The patient eats a tiny capsule that contains a tiny camera, light source, battery, and transmitter during capsule endoscopy [39]. The capsule takes excellent pictures of the intestinal mucosa as it passes through the digestive system. The examination of unclear gastrointestinal bleeding, suspected small bowel pathology (such as Crohn's disease), and other disorders affecting the small intestine are the main indications for capsule endoscopy [40].

It is especially helpful in cases when other imaging modalities, such as conventional endoscopy and radiographic tests, have not been able to reach the small intestine or have produced conflicting results. Several benefits of capsule endoscopy include its non-invasiveness, the fact that it doesn't require anaesthesia, and its capacity to view parts of the small intestine that conventional endoscopy can't reach. It can identify lesions such ulcers, tumours, and vascular anomalies and offers thorough visualisation of the mucosa [41].

Due to a number of drawbacks, capsule endoscopy is not commonly utilised for colonoscopy, even if it is useful for examining the small intestine. Furthermore, real-time visualisation and biopsy of lesions—two crucial aspects of colonoscopy for the diagnosis and treatment of colorectal diseases—are not possible with capsule endoscopy. Because traditional optical colonoscopy can give real-time visualisation, biopsy, and therapeutic procedures such polyp removal, it continues to be the gold standard for examining the colon and rectum. Depending on the clinical situation and the patient's wishes, additional modalities including flexible sigmoidoscopy and virtual colonoscopy (CT colonography) may also be utilised for colon examination and CRC screening [42].

12.10 Simulated detection systems

In colonoscopy, computer-based simulation platforms known as 'simulated detection systems' are used to teach endoscopists lesion identification and characterisation techniques. These technologies offer training settings that are immersive and replicate the experience of performing a colonoscopy operation via the use of realistic endoscopic simulators and virtual reality (VR) technology. VR technology is used by simulated detection systems to provide virtual colonoscopy settings that faithfully mimic the anatomy and disease experienced during actual procedures. In order to move through the virtual colon and recognise simulated lesions, endoscopists use VR headsets and virtual endoscopic tools, such as scopes and accessories [43].

Anatomically precise colon models with authentic mucosal textures, landmarks, and diseases are available in endoscopic simulators. These models add to the realism of the simulation experience by offering tactile input and resistance akin to what is experienced during real colonoscopy operations. Endoscopists are given a variety of lesion detection duties via simulated detection systems, including locating tumours, polyps, and other anomalies concealed in the virtual colon. Endoscopists are required to do a thorough examination of the mucosal surface, precisely detect and characterise simulated lesions, and manoeuvre the endoscope to see various colon segments. Real-time performance feedback and objective evaluation metrics are provided by simulated detection systems to measure the competency and talents of endoscopists in lesion identification [44]. Metrics might be mucosal examination, withdrawal time, accuracy, time to detection, and adherence to quality indicators. Endoscopists can enhance their lesion detection abilities with the use of curriculum modules and organised training programmes offered by simulated detection systems. Trainees progress through several degrees of difficulty and complexity, beginning with simple assignments and progressively learning intricate methods and demanding situations. Simulated detection systems are useful resources for endoscopic education and training research and development. They make it easier to conduct research on the best training approaches, the applicability of skills to actual practice, and the effects of simulation-based training on patient outcomes and care quality [45].

12.11 Improved training and workshop programs

Enhancing colonoscopy training and workshop programs is crucial to guaranteeing endoscopists get and retain the skills required to carry out high-quality procedures efficiently and securely. These courses use a range of cutting-edge teaching strategies and learning modalities to improve student experience and encourage ongoing professional growth. Colonoscopy training programs must to adhere to a defined curriculum that includes procedural competence, technical abilities, and fundamental knowledge. The curriculum needs to be thorough, well-structured, and compliant with accepted norms and standards of conduct. Learning by doing is the key to becoming proficient with colonoscopy techniques [46].

Workshop programs should give participants plenty of chances to practise colonoscopy procedures under the supervision of knowledgeable faculty members utilising live tissue training models, virtual reality simulators, and simulation models.

Through the use of simulation-based learning, instructors may hone their colonoscopy techniques in a secure setting without endangering patients. High-fidelity endoscopic simulators and virtual reality platforms should be used in training programs for simulation sessions that mimic real-world procedural circumstances and improve procedural competency. Through lectures, case-based discussions, in-person demonstrations, and practical practice sessions, interactive workshops encourage active learning among participants [47].

To encourage participation and information retention, interactive workshop components including case-based quizzes, audience response systems, and group discussions should be included. Training programs must include knowledgeable teachers and mentors with a wealth of colonoscopy experience [48].

Expert endoscopists may help trainees enhance their skills and make therapeutic decisions by offering insightful advice, constructive criticism, and support. Training programs should encourage interdisciplinary cooperation and teamwork amongst technologists, endoscopy nurses, gastroenterologists, and other medical professionals who provide care for colonoscopies. When performing colonoscopy procedures, collaboration improves communication, coordination, and efficiency in providing high-quality patient care [49].

Training programs must incorporate the latest technical innovations and break-throughs in colonoscopy, such as artificial intelligence, high-definition imaging, and sophisticated endoscopic methods. To be on the cutting edge of the profession, participants should be exposed to the newest tools and methods through interactive workshops, live case presentations, and hands-on demonstrations [50].

12.12 Future of colonoscopy

Significant advances in technology, procedures, and patient care are anticipated in the field of colonoscopy in the future. The goals of these advancements are to improve CRC screening and diagnosis in terms of efficacy, safety, and accessibility. More resolution and in-depth colon visualisation might result from advances in imaging technologies. To increase lesion detection rates, this may include the use of sophisticated optics, such as ultra-high resolution and high-definition scopes. More individualised methods of CRC screening may be made possible by developments in molecular diagnostics and biomarker identification. Biomarker testing may be used to stratify people according to their risk profile, enabling customised screening plans and the early identification of high-risk lesions (figure 12.2) [51].

12.13 Multi-spectral imaging

A sophisticated imaging technology used in colonoscopy is called multi-spectral imaging (MSI), which uses several light wavelengths to offer comprehensive information about the tissue being inspected. The colon lining is normally visible with traditional colonoscopes using white light; however, multi-spectral imaging

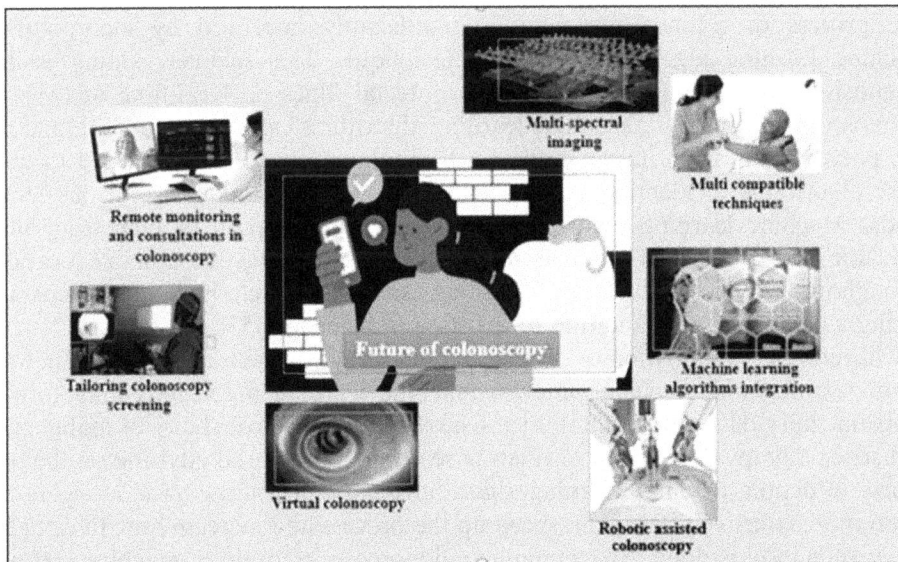

Figure 12.2. Future of colonoscopy. Reprinted from [19], Copyright (2000), with permission from Elsevier.

improves this procedure by obtaining pictures at various wavelengths, such as visible and near-infrared light. The way that different colon tissues absorb and reflect light varies based on their makeup and overall health [52].

Through the use of targeted light wavelengths, MSI can draw attention to certain characteristics or anomalies that might not be immediately apparent when illuminated by white light. As the colonoscope is inserted and moved into the colon, its multi-spectral imaging capabilities take pictures of the colon lining [53].

The doctor is then presented with the images in real time once they have been processed. By presenting more information beyond what is apparent under conventional white light, multi-spectral imaging improves visualisation. It can draw attention to minute variations in tissue architecture, colour, and vascularity that could point to anomalies such as polyps, inflammation, or early-stage malignancies. MSI can help doctors identify and characterise problems more accurately by giving more specific information about the colon tissue. This may result in early diagnosis of colorectal disorders and better diagnostic results [36].

MSI during a colonoscopy may provide several advantages, such as higher polyp and early-stage cancer detection rates, lower miss rates, and better patient surveillance for high-risk individuals. Additionally, it could aid in differentiating between benign and malignant tumours, assisting in the selection of the best course of action. Although MSI has the potential to improve colonoscopy results, there are several obstacles to overcome, including the requirement for specialised training and equipment and the interpretation of multi-dimensional data produced by the imaging system [54].

12.14 Machine learning algorithms integration

The process of colonoscopy may be significantly improved by incorporating machine learning algorithms into the technique. This includes aiding in the diagnosis, treatment, and detection of colorectal illnesses. Real-time analysis of colonoscopy images using machine learning algorithms can help identify anomalies like polyps and lesions. Large datasets of annotated photos may be used to train these algorithms to identify patterns and characteristics linked to various lesion kinds. Machine learning algorithms can assist endoscopists in increasing their detection rates and decreasing their miss rates by highlighting questionable locations throughout the operation. Machine learning can help characterise lesions discovered during a colonoscopy in addition to assisting in detection [55].

Through the examination of diverse characteristics of the lesions, including their form, texture, and vascular patterns, machine learning algorithms may furnish supplementary data that facilitates the assessment of the probability of malignancy and steers therapy choices. By evaluating real-time photos and advising on the best course of action, machine learning algorithms can help endoscopists navigate the colon more effectively. This can speed up the process and increase how thoroughly the examination is done. By examining colonoscopy recordings, machine learning may be applied to quality assurance to evaluate the sufficiency and comprehensiveness of the examination [56].

Segments of the colon that may not have been sufficiently visualised can be flagged by algorithms, enabling endoscopists to return to those areas if needed. Utilising patient data from imaging results, medical history, and demographics, machine learning algorithms may create prediction models for a range of outcomes, including prognosis, response to therapy, and chance of getting CRC. Clinical decision-making can benefit from the personalisation of patient care provided by these models [57].

To provide endoscopists with a realistic virtual environment in which to practise colonoscopy operations, machine learning algorithms can be implemented into training simulators. Furthermore, trainees can enhance their competence and abilities by receiving real-time feedback and coaching from machine learning-based instructional tools while they are doing actual processes. Machine learning algorithms can assist in simplifying the colonoscopy workflow and lessening the workload on endoscopists by automating tasks like picture processing and documentation. In endoscopic units, this may result in increased production and efficiency [58].

12.15 Robotic-assisted colonoscopy

A technical development in the field of endoscopy, robotic-assisted colonoscopy aims to increase the accuracy, manoeuvrability, and effectiveness of colonoscopic treatments. An endoscopist can control a robotic arm or endoscopic platform in robotic-assisted colonoscopy systems. Advanced imaging and navigation features are frequently included in these devices to improve visibility and mobility inside the colon. Compared to traditional colonoscopes, robotic devices are more flexible and dexterous, making it easier to navigate the intricate and winding architecture of the colon. In circumstances of difficult anatomy or prior abdominal operations, this can lead to less pain for the patient and higher procedural success rates [59].

Platforms for robotic-assisted colonoscopy may have features like image stabilisation technologies and stabilisation devices to reduce motion artefacts and keep a stable view of the colon. This can increase lesion detection rates and improve intestinal mucosa visualisation. Robotic technologies have the ability to enter the colon more deeply and access areas that conventional colonoscopes would find challenging to access. This might lessen the need for further diagnostic tests and enhance the identification of lesions in the proximal colon. With robotic-assisted colonoscopy, endoscopic tools, such as biopsy forceps and treatment devices, may be precisely controlled. This can enable more precise and safe targeted tissue sample, polyp removal, and other therapeutic procedures. By offering ergonomic control interfaces and eliminating the need for manual colonoscope manipulation, robotic platforms can lessen the physical strain on the endoscopist. Enhanced procedural efficiency and operator comfort during extended and intricate colonoscopic operations might result from this [60].

Robotic-assisted colonoscopy systems can be useful teaching and training aids because they let inexperienced endoscopists practise colonoscopic procedures in a safe, simulated setting. Additionally, these systems may offer learners immediate feedback and direction to help them advance their knowledge and abilities. Even though robotic-assisted colonoscopy has the potential to improve the effectiveness and quality of colonoscopic procedures, there are a number of drawbacks and difficulties to be aware of, such as the need for further clinical validation, training requirements, and expense. Further technological developments and clinical studies are required to establish the long-term clinical advantages of robotic-assisted colonoscopy devices and to optimise them [61].

12.16 Virtual colonoscopy

A non-invasive imaging method called virtual colonoscopy, sometimes referred to as CT colonography (CTC), is used to check for anomalies in the colon and rectum as well as CRC. With virtual colonoscopy, comprehensive pictures of the colon are created from outside the body using CT scanning, as opposed to standard colonoscopy, which entails inserting a flexible tube (colonoscope) into the rectum and colon. A table is brought into a CT scanner, and the patient rests there while the virtual colonoscopy is performed. The scanner creates comprehensive two- and three-dimensional pictures of the colon by taking a series of cross-sectional images (slices) of the abdomen and pelvis [20].

When examining the virtual colonoscopy pictures, radiologists look closely for anomalies including tumours, polyps, and other lesions. Concerning results could necessitate further assessment or a conventional colonoscopy as a follow-up to remove any lesions found or sample tissue. The non-invasive aspect of virtual colonoscopy is one of its main benefits. Virtual colonoscopy is less uncomfortable and less likely to result in problems like bleeding or perforation than traditional colonoscopy, which involves inserting a colonoscope into the colon. Virtual colonoscopy has drawbacks and limits despite its benefits, such as the requirement for intestinal preparation, exposure to ionising radiation from CT scanning, and the potential for false-positive or false-negative results. Furthermore, lesions seen during a virtual colonoscopy could still need to be confirmed or evaluated further via a regular colonoscopy. The choice to have a virtual colono-scopy, like any screening test, should be taken after discussing personal risk factors and preferences with a healthcare professional [62].

12.17 Tailoring colonoscopy screening

The process of tailoring colonoscopy screening entails adjusting screening protocols to each patient's unique risk factors, preferences, and medical background. Customised methods seek to reduce needless steps and related hazards while optimising the advantages of colonoscopy. Customising screening recommendations for CRC requires evaluating each person's unique risk factors. The timing and frequency of colonoscopy screening can be affected by a number of factors, including age, a family history of CRC or polyps, a personal history of colorectal neoplasia, the presence of inflammatory bowel disease, and certain genetic disorders. Adenomatous polyps and CRC run in families, thus screening for these conditions may need to happen sooner or more frequently [20].

Customising screening to take into account factors including age at onset, number of afflicted relatives, and degree of relatedness might assist identify high-risk people who would benefit from closer monitoring. When customising colonoscopy screening, considerations such as life expectancy, general health, and the existence of comorbidities should be made. Individualised screening regimens that weigh the advantages and risks are necessary for individuals with substantial comorbidities or short life expectancies. Screening programmes should take into account factors that affect patient adherence and follow-up, including logistical obstacles, cultural attitudes, socioeconomic position, and healthcare access.

Adherence-boosting tactics including patient education, reminder systems, and navigation services can boost the efficacy of customised screening methods. Consequently, in order to maximise the benefits and acceptability of CRC screening while reducing any possible risks, colonoscopy screening must be customised using a personalised strategy that takes into account each patient's unique risk factors, preferences, and circumstances. Creating customised screening programmes that are evidence-based, patient-centered, and in line with patients' values and preferences requires cooperation between patients and healthcare professionals [63].

12.18 Patient-compatible techniques

In the context of colonoscopy, patient-compatible procedures are methods designed to maximise the comfort, security, and happiness of the patient during the process. These methods are designed to make colonoscopy patients feel as comfortable as possible while also lowering their chance of problems and enhancing their overall experience [64]. Warm blankets, cushioned armrests, and comfortable placement are a few examples of comfort measures that may be used to reduce discomfort and encourage relaxation throughout the process. Providing a cosy atmosphere in the endoscopic room, with proper lighting and temperature regulation, can help enhance patient comfort [65].

Managing expectations, resolving concerns, and providing an explanation of the process all depend on having open lines of communication with patients before, during, and after the treatment. Trust is cultivated and fear is reduced by giving patients information regarding the surgery, sedative alternatives, possible dangers, and post-surgical instructions. By lessening the strain of colon cleaning and minimising adverse effects including nausea, bloating, and abdominal discomfort, physicians can improve patient experience by making bowel preparation regimens more tolerable and effective. Improved bowel preparation and patient compliance can be achieved by providing split-dose regimens, low-residue meals, and clear instructions. Pain can be minimised and the possibility of mucosal damage lowered during colonoscope insertion by employing gentle insertion methods and topical anaesthetics or lubricants. In order to make the insertion procedure go more smoothly and painlessly, gradual progress, patient relaxing methods, and consideration of patient anatomy are helpful [66].

During the process, minimising colonic distention and insufflation aids in easing patients' pain and bloating. The pain associated with gas distention can be lessened by varying insufflation rates, utilising carbon dioxide instead of room air, and applying intermittent suction. Providing patients with a seamless and comfortable recuperation process is crucial to their happiness. Accurate post-procedure monitoring, pain control, and well-defined discharge instructions facilitate patients' safe and comfortable recovery from colonoscopy. Healthcare professionals may improve patient comfort, safety, and happiness during colonoscopies by using patient-compatible procedures. This will eventually improve adherence to CRC screening standards and promote overall well-being [67].

12.19 Remote monitoring and consultations

Using telemedicine and digital technology, remote monitoring and consultations for colonoscopies enable the provision of healthcare services, such as pre-operation planning, procedure monitoring, and post-procedure follow-up, from a distance. Patients can virtually confer with medical professionals before a colonoscopy to go over the process, go over their medical history, and ask any questions or address any concerns. Telemedicine solutions facilitate remote communication between patients and gastroenterologists or other medical experts, therefore decreasing the need for in-person appointments and saving time. Remote monitoring technologies allow medical professionals to keep an eye on patients' vital signs, level of sedation, and progress of the colonoscopy process from a distance [27].

Gastroenterologists can watch and direct endoscopists in real-time using telepresence or real-time video streaming technologies, offering support or criticism as required. Endoscopic pictures and results can be safely sent to gastroenterologists or other qualified reviewers for interpretation and analysis following a colonoscopy. Platforms for telemedicine make it possible for professionals to obtain imaging data remotely, evaluate and analyse the results, and offer prompt comments or recommendations. After a colonoscopy, telemedicine allows for remote follow-up discussions with patients to go over procedure outcomes, go over pathology reports, and give post-procedure care recommendations [68].

Virtual consultations can provide patients with tailored advice on post-procedure food, activity limitations, and medication management, therefore eliminating the need for in-person appointments. Patients have better access to care with remote monitoring and consultations for colonoscopies, especially those who live in underserved or rural locations and have restricted access to gastrointestinal services. Telemedicine improves access to and convenience of healthcare by removing geographical boundaries and enabling patients to get expert consultation and specialised care remotely. Patients and healthcare systems can save money with remote monitoring and consultations for colonoscopies by eliminating the need for in-person visits and optimising the care delivery process [44].

12.20 Alternative bowel preparation methods

Compared to conventional stool preparation regimens, alternative colonoscopy bowel preparation techniques seek to increase patient tolerance, adherence, and effectiveness. These substitutes could consist of altered bowel preparation procedures, dietary adjustments, pharmaceuticals, and innovative cleaning solutions. When using split-dose bowel preparation, the stool cleansing solution is divided into two doses, to be given the night before the treatment and again the morning of the surgery. By eliminating the possibility of insufficient intestinal preparation and enhancing colonoscopy quality, this method outperforms single-dose regimens in terms of stool cleansing efficacy and patient tolerance. Lower amounts of bowel cleaning solution are used in low-volume bowel preparation regimens than in high-volume preparations [69].

These formulations usually contribute to better patient acceptability and adherence since they are more pleasant and simpler to take. Low-volume sulfate-free preparations and reduced-volume polyethylene glycol (PEG) solutions are two examples. Dietary changes that decrease faecal matter and residue in the colon can improve stool cleaning. To enable successful stool preparation in the days preceding the colonoscopy, clear liquid diets, low-residue diets, and particular dietary restrictions (e.g., avoiding high-fiber foods, seeds, and nuts) may be advised. To improve colon motility and shorten the time it takes for the colon to empty, pharmacological medicines such prokinetic agents and adjunctive laxatives can be used in addition to stool cleansing solutions. More laxatives, such as magnesium citrate, and stimulant laxatives, such as bisacodyl, may be recommended to enhance the benefits of bowel preparation regimens, especially for patients who are constipated or do not respond well to conventional preparations [70].

The development of innovative bowel cleansing agents aims to enhance the ease, effectiveness, and tolerance of preparing the gut for a colonoscopy. These medicines might be oral sulfate-free preparations, more recent versions of PEG-based solutions, or combination regimens with agents that improve intestinal cleaning or supplementary drugs. Traditional bowel cleaning treatments can be supplemented or replaced with magnesium citrate solutions or citrus-based preparations. These formulations possess osmotic qualities and could be more palatable for some patients; nevertheless, they might not offer sufficient cleaning for certain individuals, especially those with substantial faecal loading. To maximise preparation quality and guarantee a successful colonoscopy, healthcare professionals should talk with patients about the many alternatives for bowel preparation, address any concerns, and give clear instructions [43].

12.21 Preventive measures enhancement

Improving colonoscopy preventative measures include putting initiatives into place targeted at raising the procedure's efficacy, safety, and quality in order to lower the risk of CRC and the morbidity and death that go along with it. For a colonoscopy to successfully identify colorectal lesions, adequate intestinal preparation is necessary. Optimising visualisation of the colonic mucosa and increasing lesion detection rates can be achieved by putting high-quality bowel preparation procedures into practice, such as split-dose regimens, explicit patient instructions, and pre-procedure evaluations. The efficacy of CRC prevention is correlated with the (ADR, a critical quality indicator in colonoscopies [23].

Endoscopists can find performance variances and areas for improvement by routinely monitoring and measuring ADRs. Lesion identification can be improved, as well as the overall quality of treatment, by providing feedback and instructional interventions to endoscopists who have unsatisfactory ADRs. Promoting adherence and participation in screening programmes requires educating patients about the value of colonoscopy, the necessity of bowel preparation, and the relevance of CRC screening. Enhancing patient happiness and results may be achieved by including patients in talks about shared decision-making, attending to their concerns, and giving them comprehensive information about the operation [24].

Comprehensive CRC prevention and management requires cooperation between gastroenterologists, primary care physicians, colorectal surgeons, pathologists, oncologists, and other medical specialists. Coordinated care delivery, prompt follow-up on aberrant results, and integration of preventative interventions across the care continuum are made possible by multidisciplinary methods. Healthcare professionals may lessen the incidence of CRC, enhance patient outcomes, and maximise the efficacy of surveillance and screening for the disease by including these preventative practices into colonoscopy procedures [51].

12.22 Conclusion

In summary, a key technique in the management, diagnosis, and prevention of CRC and other gastrointestinal disorders is colonoscopy. It is not without limitations, though, and efforts are constantly made to solve these issues and enhance patient outcomes through technological and clinical practice developments. Patients may find colonoscopy intrusive and unpleasant, which might result in low adherence rates and unwillingness to be screened. Lesion identification and characterisation are improved by advanced imaging methods such as virtual chromoendoscopy, chromoendoscopy, and high-definition endoscopy. Access to treatment, patient involvement, and procedural quality are all enhanced via virtual platforms for colonoscopies, remote monitoring, and consultations.

Real-time evaluation of tissue morphology and histology during colonoscopy is now possible thanks to advancements in microscopic imaging methods, such as magnifying endoscopy and confocal laser endomicroscopy. Patient preferences, values, and experiences are given priority in patient-centered care, collaborative decision-making, and customised methods to screening and monitoring. In conclusion, even though colonoscopy is still a crucial tool for managing and preventing CRC, continued efforts to overcome its drawbacks, welcome its advancements, and mould its future are necessary to ensure that colonoscopy fulfils its promise of enhancing patient outcomes and lowering the global incidence of CRC.

References

[1] Gimeno-García A Z and Quintero E 2023 Role of colonoscopy in colorectal cancer screening: available evidence *Best Pract. Res. Clin. Gastroenterol.* **66** 101838
[2] Rastogi A and Wani S 2016 Colonoscopy *Gastrointest. Endosc.* **85** 59–66

[3] Saltzman J S, Cash B D, Faulx A L *et al* 2015 Bowel preparation before colonoscopy *Gastrointest. Endosc.* **81** 781–94

[4] Romera R V and Mahadeva S 2013 Factor influencing quality of bowel preparation for colonoscopy *World J. Gastrointest. Endosc.* **5** 39–46

[5] Latos W, Aebisher D, Latos M *et al* 2022 Colonoscopy: preparation and potential complications *Diagnostics* **12** 747

[6] Amri R, Bordeianou L G and Sylla P 2013 Impact of screening colonoscopy on outcomes in colon cancer surgery *JAMA* **148** 747–54

[7] Lanas A, Balaguer F *et al* 2023 Fecal occult blood and calprotection testing to prioritize primary care patients for colonoscopy referral: the advantage study *United Eur. Gastroenterol. J.* **11** 692–9

[8] Belesey J, Epstein O and Heresbach D 2007 Systematic review: oral bowel preparation for colonoscopy *Aliment. Pharmacol. Ther.* **25** 373–84

[9] Leszczynski A M, MacArthur K L, Nelson K P *et al* 2018 The association among diet, dietary fiber, and bowel preparation at colonoscopy *Gastrointest. Endosc.* **88** 685–94

[10] Nguyen D L, Jamal M M *et al* 2016 Low-residue versus clear liquid diet before colonoscopy: a meta-analysis of randomized, controlled trials *Gastrointest. Endosc.* **83** 499–507

[11] Church J 2013 Complications of colonoscopy *Gastroenterol. Clin. North Am.* **42** 639–57

[12] Kastenberg D, Bertiger G and Brogadir S 2018 Bowel preparation quality scales for colonoscopy *World J. Gastroenterol.* **24** 2833–43

[13] Mousavinezhad M, Majdzadeh R, Sari A A *et al* 2016 The effectiveness of FOBT vs. FIT: a meta-analysis on colorectal cancer screening test *Med. J. Islam. Repub. Iran* **30** 366

[14] Hafner M 2007 Conventional colonoscopy: technique, indications, limits *Eur. J. Radiol.* **61** 409–14

[15] Gangwani M K, Aziz A *et al* 2023 History of colonoscopy and technological advances: a narrative review *Transl. Gastroenterol. Hepatol.* **8** 18

[16] Shahsavari D, Waqar M and Chandrasekar V T 2023 Image enhanced colonoscopy: updates and prospects- a review *Transl. Gastroenterol. Hepatol.* **8** 26

[17] Adiwinata R, Tandarto K, Arifputra J *et al* 2023 The impact of artificial intelligence in improving polyp and adenoma detection rate during colonoscopy: systematic-review and meta-analysis *Asian Pac. J. Cancer Prev.* **24** 3655–63

[18] Fraiman J, Brownlee S *et al* 2022 An estimate of the US rate of overuse of screening colonoscopy: a systematic review *J. Gen. Intern. Med.* **37** 1754–62

[19] Fujimoto J G, Pitris C, Boppart S A and Brezinski M E 2000 Optical coherence tomography: an emerging technology for biomedical imaging and optical biopsy *Neoplasia* **2** 9–25

[20] Scalise P, Mantarro A, Pancrazi F and Neri E 2016 Computed tomography colonography for the practicing radiologist: a review of current recommendations on methodology and clinical indications *World J. Radiol.* **8** 472–83

[21] Taghiakbari M, Mori Y and von Renteln D 2021 Artificial intelligence-assisted colonoscopy: a review of current state of practice and research *World J. Gastroenterol.* **2** 8103–22

[22] Rosvall A, Gershater M A, Kumlien C, Toth E and Axelsson M 2022 Patient-reported experience measures for colonoscopy: a systematic review and meta-ethnography *Diagnostics* **12** 1–16

[23] Gibbons E, Kelly O B and Hall B 2023 Advances in colon capsule endoscopy: a review of current applications and challenges *Front. Gastroenterol.* **2** 1–7

[24] Wen T, Medveczky D, Wu J and Wu J 2018 Colonoscopy procedure simulation: virtual reality training based on a real time computational approach *Biomed. Eng. Online* **17** 15

[25] Siau K, Pelitari S, Green S *et al* 2023 JAG consensus statements for training and certification in colonoscopy *Front. Gastroenterol.* **14** 201–21

[26] Ning D, Geng H, Guan J *et al* 2023 A novel approach to improving colonoscopy learning efficiency through a colonoscope roaming system: randomized controlled trial *PeerJ Comput. Sci.* **9** 1–16

[27] Shahsavari D, Waqar M and Chandrasekar V T 2023 Image enhanced colonoscopy: updates and prospects-a review *Transl. Gastroenterol. Hepatol.* **8** 0–2

[28] Li J W, Mun Wang L and Leong Ang T 2022 Artificial intelligence-assisted colonoscopy: a narrative review of current data and clinical applications *Singapore Med. J.* **63** 118–24

[29] Chun J, Kim J-H, Youn Y H and Park H 2023 Noninvasive testing for colorectal cancer screening: where are we now? *J. Dig. Cancer Res.* **11** 85–92

[30] Breekveldt E C H, Toes-Zoutendij E *et al* 2023 Personalized colorectal cancer screening: study protocol of a mixed-methods study on the effectiveness of tailored intervals based on prior f-Hb concentration in a fit-based colorectal cancer screening program (PERFECT-FIT) *BMC Gastroenterol.* **23** 10

[31] Cipolletta L and Rotondano G 2013 Patient-friendly bowel preparation for colonoscopy—another brick in the wall? *Dig. Liver Dis.* **45** 16–7

[32] Aghedo B O, Svoboda S *et al* 2021 Telehealth adaptation for multidisciplinary colorectal cancer clinic during the COVID-19 pandemic *Cureus* **13** 3–10

[33] Gimeno-García A Z, Benítez-Zafra F, Nicolás-Pérez D and Hernández-Guerra M 2023 Colon bowel preparation in the era of artificial intelligence: is there potential for enhancing colon bowel cleansing? *Medicina* **59** 1834

[34] Misawa M *et al* 2021 Current status and future perspective on artificial intelligence for lower endoscopy *Dig. Endosc* **33** 273–84

[35] Mohammed N and Subramanian V 2013 Screening colonoscopy: should we focus more on technique and less on technology? *F1000Prime Rep.* **5** 1–6

[36] Niederreiter M, Niederreiter L, Schmiderer A, Tilg H and Djanani A 2019 Colorectal cancer screening and prevention—pros and cons *Memo—Mag. Eur. Med. Oncol.* **12** 239–43

[37] Hull M A, Rees C J, Sharp L and Koo S 2020 A risk-stratified approach to colorectal cancer prevention and diagnosis *Nat. Rev. Gastroenterol. Hepatol.* **17** 773–80

[38] Patton E A, Cunningham P, Noneman M *et al* 2023 Acute administration of ojeok-san ameliorates pain-like behaviors in pre-clinical models of inflammatory bowel diseases *Nutrients* **15** 1559

[39] Seitz U, Seewald S, Bohnacker S and Soehendra N 2023 Advances in interventional gastrointestinal endoscopy in colon and rectum *Int. J. Colorectal Dis.* **18** 12–8

[40] Kudo S-Ei, Mori Y, Misawa M, Takeda K, Kudo T, Itoh H, Oda M and Mori K 2019 Artificial intelligence and colonoscopy: current status and future perspectives *Dig. Endosc.* **31** 363–71

[41] Cheng W B *et al* 2012 Overview of upcoming advances in colonoscopy *Dig. Endosc* **24** 1–6

[42] Vitulo M, Gnodi E, Meneveri R and Barisani D 2022 Interactions between nanoparticles and intestine *Int. J. Mol. Sci.* **23** 4339

[43] Swain P 2005 Colonoscopy: new designs for the future *Gastrointest. Endosc. Clin. North Am.* **15** 839–63

[44] Lee S H, Park Y K, Lee D J and Kim K M 2014 Colonoscopy procedural skills and training for new beginners *World J. Gastroenterol.* **20** 16984–95

[45] Ahmed R, Santhirakumar K, Butt H and Yetisen A K 2019 Colonoscopy technologies for diagnostics and drug delivery *Med. Dev. Sens.* **2** 1–16

[46] Häfner M 2007 Conventional colonoscopy: technique, indications, limits *Eur. J. Radiol.* **61** 409–14

[47] Yeung C K, Cheung J L K and Sreedha B 2019 Emerging next-generation robotic colonoscopy systems towards painless colonoscopy *J. Dig. Dis* **20** 196–205

[48] Romero R V 2013 Factors influencing quality of bowel preparation for colonoscopy *World J. Gastrointest. Endosc* **5** 39–43

[49] Ciuti G, Skonieczna-żydecka K, Marlicz W *et al* 2020 Frontiers of robotic colonoscopy: a comprehensive review of robotic colonoscopes and technologies *J. Clin. Med.* **9** 1648

[50] Da Silva G M and Vernava A M 2001 History of colonoscopy *Clin. Colon Rectal Surg.* **14** 303–8

[51] Witte T N and Enns R 2007 The difficult colonoscopy *Cancer J. Gastroenterol.* **21** 487–90

[52] Appleyard M N, Mosse C A, Mills T N *et al* 2000 The measurement of forces exerted during colonoscopy *Gastrointest. Endosc.* **52** 237–40

[53] Khan I, Saeed K and Khan I 2019 Nanoparticles: properties, applications and toxicities *Arabian J. Chem.* **12** 908–31

[54] Malone J C and Thavamani A 2023 *Physiology, Gastrocolic Reflex* (StatPearls)

[55] Taye M M 2023 Understanding of Machine Learning with Deep Learning: Architectures, Workflow, Applications and Future Directions *Computers* **12** 91

[56] Shen Y T, Chen L, Yue W W and Xu H X 2021 Artificial intelligence in ultrasound *Eur. J. Radiol.* **139** 109717

[57] Pei Q, Luo Y, Chen Y, Li J, Xie D and Ye T 2022 Artificial intelligence in clinical applications for lung cancer: diagnosis, treatment and prognosis *Clin. Chem. Lab. Med.* **60** 1974–83

[58] Vélez-Guerrero M A, Callejas-Cuervo M and Mazzoleni S 2021 Design, development, and testing of an intelligent wearable robotic exoskeleton prototype for upper limb rehabilitation *Sensors* **21** 5411

[59] Smolsky J, Kaur S, Hayashi C, Batra S K and Krasnoslobodtsev A V 2017 Surface-enhanced Raman scattering-based immunoassay technologies for detection of disease biomarkers *Biosensors* **7** 7

[60] Poghossian A and Schöning M J 2021 Recent progress in silicon-based biologically sensitive field-effect devices *Curr. Opin. Electrochem.* **29** 100811

[61] Bayda S, Adeel M, Tuccinardi T, Cordani M, Rizzolio F and Baeza A 2020 The history of nanoscience and nanotechnology: from chemical-physical applications to nanomedicine *Molecules* **25** 112

[62] Sun B, Liu J, Li S, Lovell J F and Zhang Y 2023 Imaging of gastrointestinal tract ailments *J. Imaging* **9** 115

[63] Ravanshad R, Zadeh A K, Amani A M *et al* 2017 Application of nanoparticles in cancer detection by Raman scattering based techniques *Nano Rev. Exp.* **9** 1373551

[64] Kumar A, Nandi M K, Kumar B *et al* 2022 Toxicity (acute and subacute) assessment and in-vivo antiurolithiatic activity of ethanolic extract of *Caesalpinia bonducella* seed in albino Wistar rat *J. Appl. Pharm. Sci.* **12** 187–97

[65] Kumar A, Kumar B, Kumar R *et al* 2022 Acute and subacute toxicity study of ethanolic extract of *Calotropis procera* (Aiton) dryand flower in *Swiss albino* mice *Phytomed. Plus* **2** 100224

[66] Cojocaru M I, Cojocaru M, Silosi I and Doina Vrabie C 2011 Gastrointestinal manifestations in systemic autoimmune diseases *Maedica (Bucur.)* **6** 45–51

[67] Young P E and Womeldorph C M 2013 Colonoscopy for colorectal cancer screening *J. Cancer* **4** 217

[68] McAlindon M E, Ching H L, Yung D, Sidhu R and Koulaouzidis A 2016 Capsule endoscopy of the small bowel *Ann. Transl. Med.* **4** 369

[69] Willis B H, Beebee H and Lasserson D S 2013 Philosophy of science and the diagnostic process *Family Pract.* **30** 501–5

[70] Silva A C, Moreira J N, Manuel J *et al* 2023 Advances with lipid-based nanosystems for siRNA delivery to breast cancers *Pharmaceuticals* **16** 970

www.ingramcontent.com/pod-product-compliance
Lightning Source LLC
Chambersburg PA
CBHW082135210326
41599CB00031B/5985